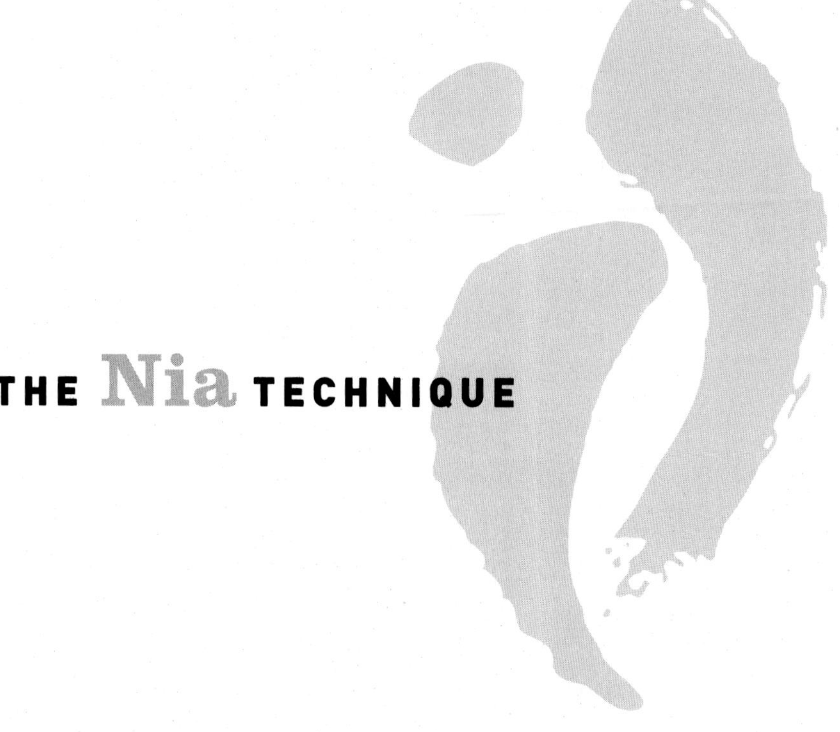

THE Nia TECHNIQUE

DEBBIE ROSAS & CARLOS ROSAS

Broadway Books
New York

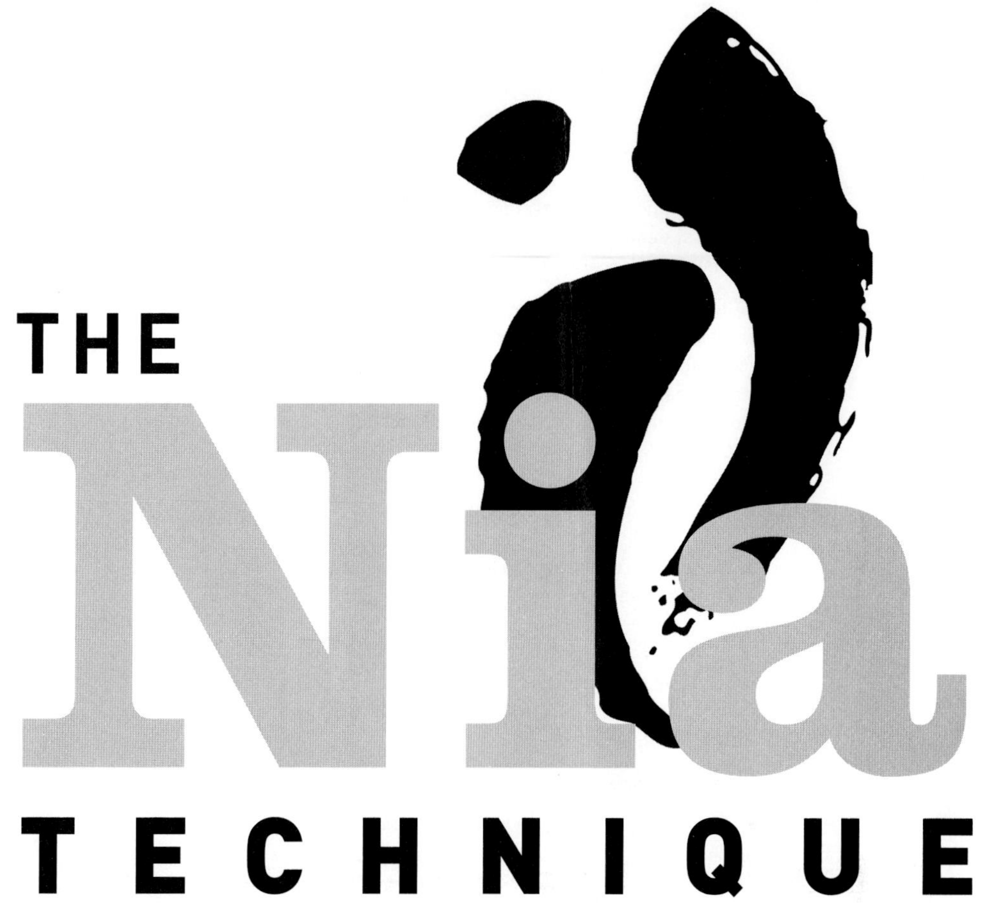

THE NIA TECHNIQUE

THE HIGH-POWERED ENERGIZING WORKOUT THAT GIVES YOU A NEW BODY AND A NEW LIFE

DISCLAIMER: The instructions and advice in this book are in no way intended as a substitute for medical counseling. We advise the reader to consult with his/her doctor before beginning this or any other exercise regimen. The author and the publisher disclaim any liability or loss, personal or otherwise, resulting from the exercises in this book.

PRINTED IN THE UNITED STATES OF AMERICA

Visit our Web site at www.broadwaybooks.com

First edition published 2004.

Library of Congress Cataloging-in-Publication Data

Rosas, Debbie, 1951–
The Nia technique: the high-powered energizing workout that gives you a new body and a new life / Debbie Rosas and Carlos Rosas.—1st. ed.
p. cm.
ISBN 0-7679-1730-8 (alk. paper)
1. Low impact aerobic exercises. 2. Physical fitness. 3. Exercise. 4. Health. I. Rosas, Carlos (Carlos Augustos) II. Title.

RA781.15.R658 2004
613'.1—dc22 2004053122

10 9 8 7 6 5 4

We dedicate

The Nia Technique

to the people in our lives whose support and encouragement made this book possible. To Jeff Stewart, for his love, clear sight, integrity, commitment, and enthusiasm, and for demanding that we step out, even when we felt like we weren't ready. To Jasmine Patten, for her unconditional love, playfulness, and unwavering support for the path we walk.

contents

introduction
Nia Is Like Chocolate

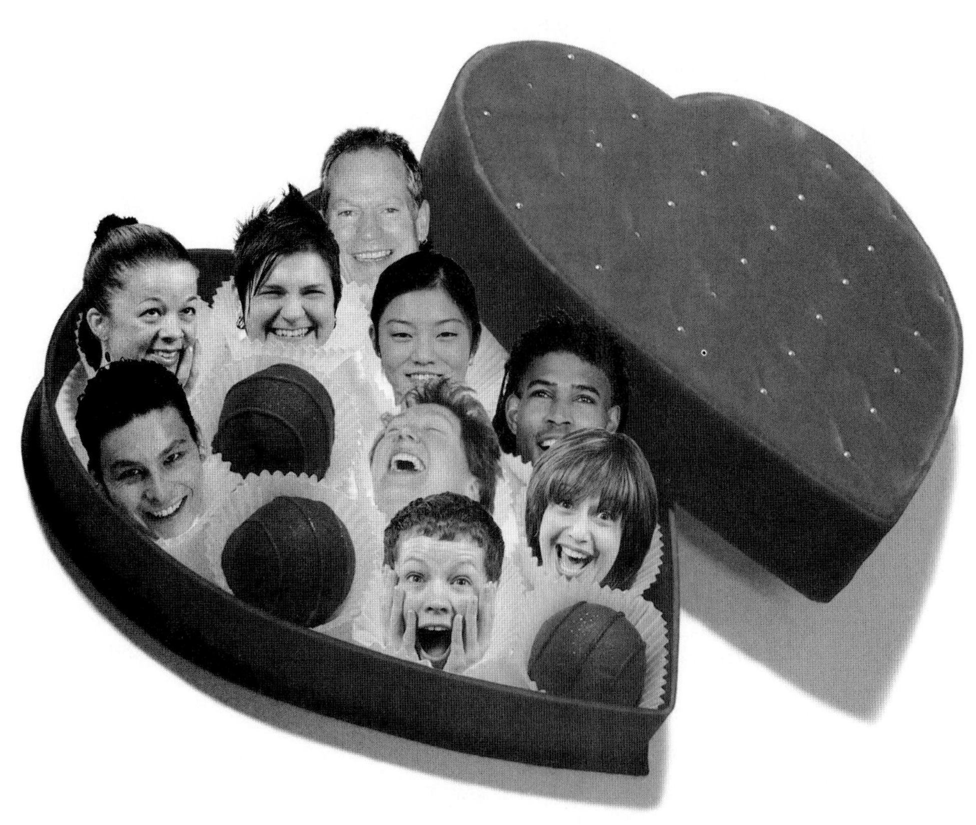

Nia is a revolutionary fitness technique that replaces the idea of punishment with pleasure.

Nia is a completely unique fitness program that tones and trims the body superbly—through pleasure, not pain. So kind to the joints, it is usually done barefoot.

Nia is a technique that starts with fitness and ends with comprehensive healing of the body, mind, spirit, and emotions.

Nia is to exercise what holistic medicine is to health care. It has many different components that help many different conditions such as asthma, depression, and pregnancy. Nia is movement as medicine.

Nia is the first and most advanced form of fusion fitness—the combining of classic movement forms. It encompasses the martial arts, the healing arts (including yoga), and dance. This combination creates a synergy that no isolated technique can match.

Nia is a cardiovascular program that uses whole-body, expressive, grounded movement, rather than repetitive jogging or lifting.

Nia is adaptable to every level of fitness, every age and type of body, even those with special limitations.

Nia is the first fitness program that advocates doing things the easy way instead of the hard way.

Nia is a worldwide fitness movement with more than twenty years of technical advancement.

Nia is a nonintimidating way of appreciating your body—indeed yourself—in class, or in the privacy of your own home, thanks to Nia's at-home video workouts.

Nia is effective and fun.

Nia is the Body's Way, a new way of being and living in your body.

When we first created Nia, back in 1983, we had no idea that it would change the entire fitness industry. But it has. Now mind–body fitness is in. So is fusion fitness, cross-training, yoga, martial arts for fitness, and dance exercise.

A great many major fitness programs are now patterned after Nia, and that is very gratifying to us.

Even so, most of the fitness industry still doesn't quite get Nia. People copy it, but don't really understand it.

It's easy for us to see why this is so. We're still learning new things about Nia. Nia is intricate. Ever changing. It's very special. It's in a class of its own.

Nia, in fact, is like chocolate. You can't describe it—you have to taste it.

Here is a taste of Nia.

one hour in the life of Nia

This *body!* This *body* of mine! How did it ever *get* like this?

Conny looks at all the beautiful, tightly muscled bodies around her and feels like fleeing. But she can't leave, because she's too desperate for help.

For eight years, Conny has been struggling to find a cure for the burning, biting torment of chronic pain and was recently told by her physical therapist in Hamburg, Germany, who's also here at this Nia class, that Nia may be her last viable option. Her therapist should know—she's an Olympic swimmer who's always on the cutting edge of fitness and healing. But Conny is dubious. It's been eight years since the accident that ripped apart her right shoulder, and for all that time, her body has been her worst enemy.

Almost every movement hurts, and her legs, torso, and arms are puffy, flabby, and flaccid. Before the accident, she'd been proud of how she looked. Not anymore. She's only in her mid-thirties, but when she looks in the mirror, she sees an old woman: a haggard face on a bloated and bent body, with eyes now empty of life.

Carlos enters the room and notices Conny right away. His first impression of her is: "She looks so *frightened.*" He catches her attention, holds her eyes with a smile, and says that he thinks she will enjoy the class.

Conny tries to smile back.

Carlos fiddles with the sound system and music seeps into the room. It's *nothing* like the usual hard-thump music of an aerobics class. It's soft and soothing and Conny relaxes a little as Carlos invites everyone to "step in"—to take a couple of paces toward the center of the group and to focus on how their bodies feel and what they hope to achieve in this class. It's a simple physical act, but Conny quickly sees it's also more than that. It's a live-action metaphor for leaving behind the past and filling the empty unknown that lies ahead with whatever you need most. Conny knows what she needs.

"Let's start by feeling the sensations in our fingertips," Carlos quietly urges, as he begins to flick out his fingers. "Are your fingers loose? Warm? Can you feel the energy in them? Now feel your wrists." Carlos twirls his wrists in languid circles and Conny is struck by his grace. He seems to be making every movement into a dance. "How do your elbows feel?" he asks. He moves his own luxuriously, as if the simple act provides great pleasure.

"This is a *workout*?" Conny thinks.

"Now feel your shoulders."

Carlos sees Conny tighten. Her arms go rigid.

"Now let's all pretend we're sinking into a pool of warm, flowing water," Carlos says, his melodic voice merging with the music. "Slowly now, very slowly, let's do the backstroke."

Conny hears him say her name. "Do it *your* way, Conny," he says. "Don't do it like anyone else. *Your* way is the best way for your body."

Carlos can see a deep breath leave Conny's chest as she relaxes into the movement. It doesn't hurt . . . *yet!*

"Listen to *all* of the music, not just the beat," Carlos says softly, as he begins to lead them in gentle yoga-like movements. Some of the exercises, Conny realizes, are not strictly yoga, but are drawn from the Alexander Technique and the Feldenkrais Method, which her therapist had used. This fusion of techniques feels natural—and powerful—and becomes a smooth waltz of motion.

"Feel the melody," Carlos says. "Doesn't it feel nice?"

Conny forgets herself for a moment and is submerged in the sounds of the violins, rich and dark, that wash over her in a tactile, visceral way, just like the imaginary water that's rushing past her shoulders and neck.

It's been so *long* since she's forgotten herself! Ever since she hurt her shoulder, she's learned to watch herself relentlessly, always guarding against those spontaneous, relaxed movements that stab her with pain.

She's lived this way ever since multiple surgeries failed to repair her shoulder's broken bones and shredded tendons. After the surgeries, she tried heavy painkillers, years of acupuncture, Reiki, bodywork, osteopathy, chiropractic, massage, and physical therapy. Nothing helped. Things just got worse. The pain and immobility of her frozen shoulder disrupted her muscular and skeletal systems so severely that now she suffers bursts of screaming-hot pain not in just her shoulder and neck, but also in her lower back, both knees, and her right ankle. She never sleeps through the night without awakening to pain, and simple tasks like housework are out of the question. Feelings of depression and helplessness shroud each of her days, and make the pain feel even more powerful.

The music changes. It's jazzier now. It's girls-night-out music—fun, with lots of attitude. Outside, the streets are gray and icy, but in here the lights are like sun and the jazzy music is adding heat to the room.

Carlos continues to lead them in unique, pleasant movements and somehow seems to know exactly what Conny's body will tolerate. Conny begins to feel her body grow warm and loose, energized by oxygen, and she's starting to experience something in her movements that has been gone for years. It's . . . she can't place it. Fearlessness? No. Grace? No. Energy? More than that.

It's . . . *joy.*

"My God!" Conny thinks. "I'm actually working *out,* and it *feels* good!"

Cut to a small gym in a small town in western Pennsylvania. It's the same day, the same time—although a different time zone—and approximately the same stage of the workout. In the back row, trying to remain unnoticed, we see Meghan, who's also at her first Nia class.

Meghan hates her body, too, but for a different reason. She doesn't have any appreciable aches or pains, but suffers from something she thinks is even worse than pain: obesity. She's just plain *fat,* is the way she sees it.

Meghan's gained about forty pounds in the past year and has nothing to blame for the weight but the fact that, in her own self-negating opinion, she eats like a *pig* and is too *lazy* to work it off. It wasn't always this way. Only thirteen months earlier, she had starved, purged, and exercised her way to just over a hundred pounds—a size four. Even then, however, she'd felt like she could pinch blobs of blubber all around her waist and thighs. All that fat had driven her crazy, because everyone had been telling her she was dangerously thin for a thirty-year-old woman, and should check into a hospital. They'd been trying to *control* her, she thought, just as they'd tried to control her years before, when she'd had a drinking problem. So she'd given up and had started stuffing her face, and *now* look at her: a *blimp.* Served everybody right.

Meghan is hoping she can drop a pound or two in this class, and as the music starts to rock that seems like a realistic possibility, because she's really starting to sweat, even though she isn't doing any conventional aerobics. In here, there's no pounding up and down, while some Fitness Bunny yells, "Feel the burn!" and "Smile!" The yoga that they'd been doing earlier had imperceptibly segued into slow, flowing dance movements, and has now shifted into faster, jazz-style dance steps that can be done with varying levels of intensity. Meghan's doing all of them at their highest level of intensity, of course, dropping almost all the way to the floor while others in the class are dipping only a few inches. Truth be told, Meghan thinks a lot of the other people are slackers—cheating *themselves!*—and that she's better than them.

Trouble is, even though she's pushing herself hard, the effort she's making isn't filling that hole that always seems to sit in the pit of her stomach. And that hole, she knows in her heart of hearts, is her *real* problem. It isn't the fat. She can trim off pounds and tame physical problems as well as anyone. What really hurts, now and always, is the feeling that no matter how well she does, she'll never live up to her own lofty standards and will always have that empty, anxious feeling inside. That anxiety is the emotional curse she lives with, and no antidepressant or tranquilizer has ever been able to touch it.

Even so, Meghan has hope. The friend who told her about this class said a study published in the journal *Women's Health Issues* had shown that Nia not only is effective against anxiety but is—because of its mind–body emphasis—notably more effective than regular aerobics. "Nia," her friend had said, "is about more than just thinner thighs."

Just the day before, while doing some Internet research of her own, Meghan had learned that Nia is recognized as a form of somatic psychotherapy, the branch of psychology that's based on the belief that certain physical actions, when channeled with thought, can help unlock emotional blocks.

So Meghan isn't just working out, but is, as some Nia students put it, "working in"—going inside herself physically as well as emotionally to see what's there and what she can do about it. And if this doesn't help emotionally, well, what's wrong with just thinner thighs? Meghan sighs, and some of that sick feeling in the pit of her stomach seems to whoosh out of her.

"Mustang Sally" starts to blast out of the speakers and the vibration seems to crawl right up Meghan's spine—What caused *that?*—as she focuses on her body, at the urging of her instructor, and starts to feel sensations that she hasn't felt in years, feelings that are part physical and part emotional, all wrapped together.

Now we cut to Portland, Oregon, on the same day, at about the same time, in an earlier still time zone, at approximately the same stage of the workout.

Debbie is leading the massive Portland class, shouting, "Kick! Block! Kick!" They're in the cardiovascular stage of the workout, which includes lots of martial arts. Almost everyone is smiling, though no one is telling them to.

For Debbie, one face—that of another first-time student—stands out, because the student's expression has just changed dramatically. "Wow!" Debbie's thinking, "she just *got* it!" Meaning, the new student just put her mind and body together, in perfect synchronization and harmony, for the first time that day, and maybe for the first time in a week or a month.

And the student's thinking, "This feels *great!*" as she does the martial arts kicks and blocks that she'd *felt* like doing all day long at work. She's Zan, a forty-year-old lawyer, and her day so far has consisted of one tense confrontation after another—all conducted quite civilly, of course—as her stress has mounted.

Worse yet, her work isn't even her biggest worry today. It's the divorce. From her husband of eighteen years. The father of her children. Her "soul mate." It's making her such a mental wreck that she can't even concentrate on her cases. Just this morning, she forgot something that would have been disastrous, if her assistant hadn't caught it. Lately she feels as if her head doesn't even belong on her own body anymore. It's in another world. There are just too many issues in her life to work through, so that's what she's doing here, not just working out, or even "working in," but hoping to work *through* the jumble of thoughts her divorce is causing. She's looking for mental clarity.

The magazine article she'd read about Nia said it helped people sort out their thoughts, and function better cognitively. But it didn't mention anything about the amazing thing she's experiencing right now, which is *not thinking*—just feeling and being. It feels like being ten years old! She feels clear, sharp—ready to tackle her work again.

This is Debbie's downtown class, set among the high-rises of inner-city Portland, and it's full of hard-charging urban professionals who make their livings with their minds. As Debbie looks at them, though—many of them wooden and mechanical, divorced from their own bodies—she can see the price people pay for living in their heads.

Zan's movements, Debbie notices, are already starting to change a little. They're softer. Looser. Zan's in relatively good physical condition, but early in the workout, she'd been much more stiff—almost masculine, which is common in exercise classes, since they were founded within the macho environment of weightlifting gyms and fitness clubs: Harder! Faster! Gimme ten more! Love the pain!

Debbie knows all about that environment, because she came from it. She once owned the most successful aerobics company in northern California. She learned, though, that there's a big problem with the pain-is-good approach: *It doesn't work.*

Already, Zan is learning to do her movements the Nia way: the *easy* way, instead of the hard way.

A hot salsa tune rockets around the room, and Debbie tells the group to pretend they're shoveling snow. Zan likes all this imagery—it makes the movements easy to follow. "Go easy," Debbie says. "Take the path of least resistance. Don't run up the hill—walk up the *mountain*!"

Debbie is breathing hard and looks happy, totally in her element. "*Taste* the movement!" Debbie shouts. "Nia's like chocolate! You can't describe it. You have to taste it!"

The next stop is San Diego, California, at a tony health spa. It's the same time zone as Portland, and the Nia class here is in approximately the same stage of the sixty-minute workout, which is just starting to wind down.

The diversity of the crowded class is astonishing: There's an eighty-two-year-old woman working out beside a buff-beyond-belief triathlete. In the front row is a man who's here on doctor's orders, recovering from a triple-bypass surgery, and in the rear is a twelve-year-old girl who's tired of being the heaviest kid in her class. Next to her, same age, is a budding ballerina. There's a woman who has lost over one hundred pounds, doing only Nia. She feels reborn and acts it. Over there, by the speakers, is a young woman, now a successful realtor but once a drug addict, who actually learned Nia in a correctional facility. Behind the realtor is a Black Belt Nia practitioner who does the workout so vigorously that she can match its intensity only by running hills. And, as usual, there are at least two dozen average people who just want to be fit and healthy without having to kill themselves in a gym.

There's also another first-timer who doesn't know what to expect. She's Claudine, thirty-one, a project coordinator for an immunology research lab—and she feels about half dead. Whatever spark of life she once had is gone. It's been gone so long she can't even remember why she keeps trying to find it.

Long ago, as a very young child, Claudine made a concerted effort to escape from her body—This *body* of mine!—because her body had betrayed her. She was born with severe asthma, and the asthma wouldn't tolerate the intrusion of *life.* Whenever Claudine became excited, or even really happy, the asthma smothered her. Any kind of fear or nervousness took her breath away. Exercise? Play with the other kids? Forget about it. So she built walls around herself and within herself and shut out life. Then she discovered that when you shut out life, life shuts you out, too, and your spirit (if you can still feel it) starts to die. So Claudine is now stuck in a spiritual desert—weak, overweight, overmedicated, wondering why she was singled out by God to suffer.

The music shifts from fast, high-tech sounds to slow, ambient music, soothing and peaceful, and the class's movements are mellowing back into sensuous yoga postures. Claudine notices the change and thinks, "Whoa! We're *done*—and I haven't had an attack!" She made it through an entire class, and breath and life are still flowing in and out of her.

She can't quite believe it, as her spark—her spirit—begins once again to glow.

In Hamburg, Germany. The music swells to completion and Carlos's voice fills the vacuum of silence. "Let's close today with three breaths," he says. "One breath is for the past, one breath is for the present, and on the third we take two steps forward and walk into the future."

Conny takes her third breath and steps forward. Her shoulder does not hurt. *Nothing* hurts. She has absolutely no idea why not. But she has a sneaking feeling, though she won't yet say it out loud, that her body has begun to heal.

At other times, she might have felt like crying at such an auspicious moment. Or laughing. Not now. Now Conny feels like going home and making love with her husband.

In western Pennsylvania. Meghan walks down the hallway of the little gym with a new feeling in the pit of her stomach. She doesn't feel the butterflies that tell her to go eat. She doesn't feel stuffed and ugly. Her stomach just feels like . . . a stomach.

Abruptly, she ducks into a restroom and cloisters herself in an empty stall. Tears—*Why?*—start to plop onto her cheeks.

She starts to think, but doesn't want to jinx it, that her emotions, after so long, have maybe, just maybe, begun to transform.

In Portland, Oregon. Zan leaves the downtown class and strides back to her law office.

She's clear and calm. She's not thinking about the divorce. That can wait. Right now, she just wants to get behind her desk, hit the phones, and kick a little butt on behalf of her clients.

For the first time in a long time, her head feels like it belongs on her body.

In San Diego. Claudine wraps a towel around her neck and stops at the watercooler with some other students. She doesn't know any of them, but for some reason they feel like friends. They've shared something today.

Claudine's hair is wet with sweat. It's sticking to her cheeks, and feels good. Her breaths are still coming in long, luxurious pulsations, like ocean waves.

Inside, she feels a hot little spark of life. She remembers it.

Her spirit is back.

This is a small taste of Nia. It shows you what other people have gotten from it.

What do *you* need?

Physical fitness? Emotional healing? Mental clarity? Spiritual renewal?

Your body can lead the way.

Nia will make it happen.

It can start today.

THE THIRTEEN JOINTS EXERCISE

Your body is wonderfully designed and neurologically encoded to move as a whole unit. However, to move your whole body in synchronism and harmony, you must have proper mobility and stability in each joint.

Excessive muscle tension in joints reduces mobility, but insufficient muscle tension reduces *stability.* Optimal muscle tension and movement range in all thirteen major joints balances the flow of energy throughout your entire body. This is your first lesson on getting to know *your own Body's Way.* No following lesson will be more important than this one.

Here's the best, easiest way to ascertain the degree of health of all thirteen of your major joints. Simply stand up and move each joint separately to determine which joints move properly, and which feel too rigid, or too lax.

Do all of your movements within your own personalized time frame, and in

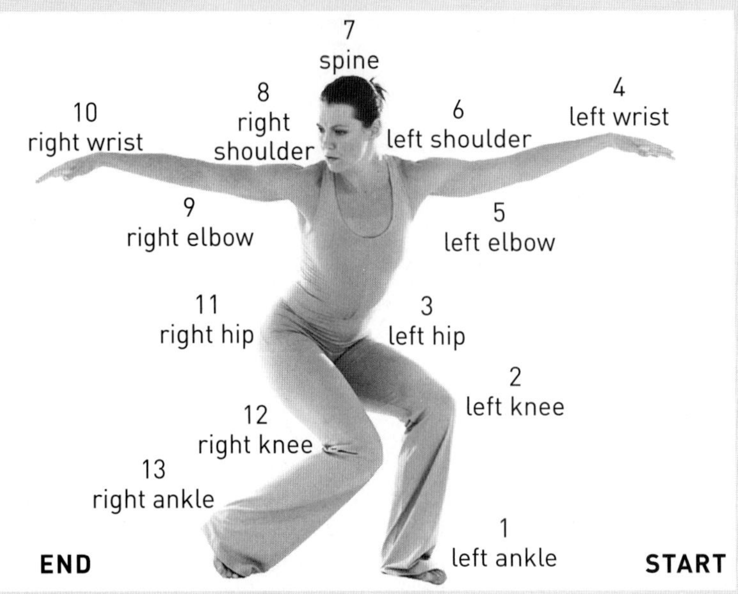

your own style—a practice that we refer to as "natural time." Here are the movements:

1. **Left ankle:** Flex, extend, and circle your foot
2. **Left knee:** Bend and extend your lower leg
3. **Left hip:** Circle your thigh around and around
4. **Left wrist:** Flex, extend, and circle your hand and fingers
5. **Left elbow:** Bend and extend your forearm
6. **Left shoulder:** Circle your upper arm around and around
7. **Spine:** Bend to both sides and to the front and back, and twist left then right
8. **Right shoulder:** Circle your upper arm around and around
9. **Right elbow:** Bend and extend your forearm
10. **Right wrist:** Flex, extend, and circle your hand and fingers
11. **Right hip:** Circle your thigh around and around
12. **Right knee:** Bend and extend your lower leg
13. **Right ankle:** Flex, extend, and circle your foot

Now ask yourself these questions: Which joints felt good? Which felt strong? Which felt too tight? Which felt too loose?

one
Beyond Exercise: Fusion Fitness

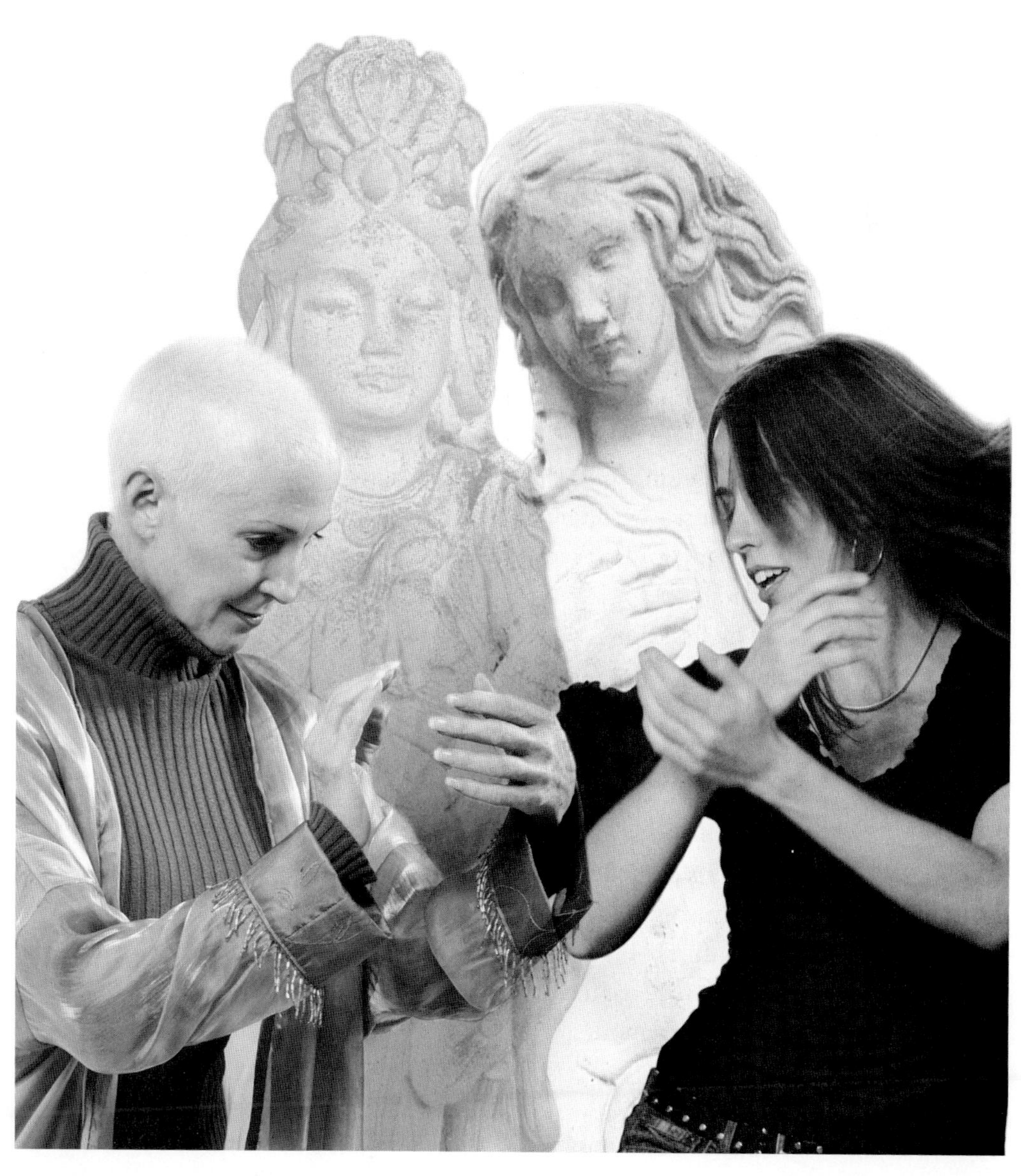

1983

"Debbie. Carlos. Let me see you move," the martial artist said to us.

We just stared at each other. Move *how?* Straight leg kick? Flat back? Cancan kick? And where was the blasting disco music to rev us up?

We began to do jumping jacks.

The sensei shook his head. "You have fifteen seconds' worth of knowledge," he said softly. "You know how to exercise, but you do not know how to *move.*"

Well. Gee. Then why were we two of the most successful aerobics teachers in California? This was way back at the height of the aerobics movement, and Debbie's fitness company had fifty teachers who together taught over a hundred classes every day.

But we had come to the sensei because we knew that something was wrong. The aerobics industry was riddled with injury, burnout, and pain. A study done around this time showed that traditional aerobics had an injury rate that hit 76 percent among teachers and 44 percent among students. Of those injuries, 82 percent were to the knee or below, indicating that the human leg just isn't built for the pounding of conventional aerobics, including long-distance jogging.

What was wrong?

We got our first feel for what was wrong that day at the sensei's martial arts dojo.

The first thing we found out was that we weren't nearly as fit as we'd thought. We were appalled, because Carlos was an indefatigable tennis teaching professional and Debbie was the diva of Bay Area fitness. However, when the sensei asked us to do some basic martial arts stances, our legs started to quiver in just a few seconds. We realized that we had strength in our large muscle groups, but were weak in the smaller stabilizer muscles that provide power and definition.

We also found that we weren't as coordinated as we'd thought. Within the confines of traditional exercises we were flexible, but when we had to simply *move,* we felt clumsy. Our heads told us to move one way, but our bodies went another. Part of the reason for this disconnect was that all our repetitive exercises had programmed us neurologically for rigid, mechanical movements, something very common among exercisers.

On that momentous day in the dojo, Debbie also became painfully aware that her style of movement had become rather hard and masculine—*yang,* in the terminology of the sensei. In trying to be fit, she'd sacrificed some of her natural physical grace.

We also found that we were *overthinking* most of our movements, which was anathema to our sensei. The whole point of martial arts is to defend yourself during an attack, and if you stop to think for even a millisecond about how to move, you're dead. That's partly why martial artists are so fluid and deft—they don't think, they just *do,* and it brings out the body's natural beauty.

Most noticeable of all, though, was that we'd both lost the *joy* of moving. As we watched our smiling sensei move with great sensual pleasure, we realized that we'd lost the childlike, playful, pleasant quality in our physical actions. For us—like so many others who struggle to be fit—movement had become *work*. It was donkey kicks. Sit-ups. Push-ups. Repetition. Drudgery. We were like wild horses, captured and domesticated, that now pulled a plow.

But what could we *do?*

If only we'd known then what we know now.

A **Nia** *Story*

RECOVERY FROM ARTHRITIS

STUDENT: Bonnie

CLASS LOCATION: Hayden, Idaho

OCCUPATION: Retired social worker

In the early 1990s, Bonnie began to suffer from severe, debilitating osteoarthritis. Her doctor recommended exercise and prescribed pain medication, but neither was effective.

"The pain was mostly in my hips," she recalls. "Then I began to also have lower back pain."

The sedentary nature of her profession exacerbated the arthritis. "When I started Nia," she says, "my hips and pelvic area felt frozen from years of sitting at a desk. I love to dance and walk for exercise, but Nia gave me the structure to explore movements I was not familiar with. For example, I began to use my upper body and arms in new ways."

When she started to do Nia, her arthritic symptoms began to improve dramatically. Her hips regained most of their former flexibility, and her entire body became more toned. She now says, "I do not experience any arthritic pain in my hips."

Even though she was receiving tangible physical benefits, her primary motivation to continue came from the fact that Nia was simply fun. "I immediately knew this was the class for me," she notes. "I loved the music. I had taken aerobics classes before and had been very turned off by the music the instructors had selected. I love to dance, and the possibility that I could dance and have such a fun workout thrilled me. I also liked my Nia teacher, Jamie. She was so comfortable in her body that I mistakenly thought she was a dancer by background and training.

"I've noticed that I can come to a Nia class feeling a little down, and within the hour my entire mood shifts. My body comes alive and is filled with energy and joy. I feel such a great physical release. My spirit soars with the rhythms of the different musical cultures of the world. I also love the integration of the various martial arts and yoga."

Despite her physical healing and spiritual growth, fun and pleasure remain the driving forces behind her ongoing practice of Nia.

"In every Nia class," she says, "I rediscover the creative child that lives within me—and I let her out to play!"

what we know now: the fundamentals of Nia

The Joy of Movement Is the Secret of Fitness. Stop exercising. Start moving. Follow the pleasure principle: If it feels good, do it; if it doesn't, stop.

When people make love, it's usually to feel good, not just to procreate, and movement is the same: People move mostly because it *feels* good. Fitness is merely a *by-product* of moving, just as procreation is a by-product of sex.

Fitness Must Address the Human Being, Not Just the Body. Exercise that's done strictly for its own physical sake, divorced from the emotions and human spirit, isn't satisfying, isn't fun, and eventually fails. To feel good enough to last a lifetime, an exercise regimen must satisfy the heart and soul.

Nia simultaneously addresses the body, mind, emotions, and spirit and puts them on the same page. Nia uses physical activity to integrate one's neurology (including the mind, emotions, and spirit), with one's outer body, or musculature. To achieve this whole-being integration, you must address the whole person, using a comprehensive, holistic exercise approach. Nia accomplishes this by combining several classic movement forms from the healing arts (including yoga), the martial arts, and dance arts.

Movement Must Be Conscious, Not Habitual. Whole-being fitness begins with heightened *awareness*—of both body and mind. To achieve this, you need to turn off the automatic pilot that so often governs your movements and thoughts. Living (and moving) by rote and routine kills consciousness and waters down the experience of life, turning people into hamsters on a treadmill.

Start focusing throughout the day on all the *physical sensations* coursing through your body, and start *moving with purpose.* Because Nia is a nonimpact program, it can be done without the protective padding of shoes. This makes people aware of exactly how they're moving, via the seven thousand nerve endings that are in each foot, and intensifies the physical and psychological feeling of being grounded. In Nia, we call the feet "the hands that touch the earth."

You should also stop performing conventional repetitive exercises, because they limit movement choices, reinforce robotic living, and often lock in mental and spiritual blocks. Constant physical repetition doesn't even build muscles, because the muscles quickly adjust to rigid, repeated movements, and muscle strength plateaus.

Use Your Body the Way It Was Designed to Be Used. Gain fitness by doing movements that shift your body's *own* weight, with varying levels of intensity, range, and speed. Replace and/or supplement repetitive jogging, jumping, and lifting with stances, postures, steps, blocks, and kicks that are compatible with your body's natural structure and that feel good. These movements will burn calories; reduce body fat; create strength and muscle definition; and promote balance, grace, flexibility, endurance, and good posture.

Use Your Body to Heal Your Mind, Emotions, and Spirit. Every muscle in the body has neuronal *nodal points,* memory receptors that are connected to the brain. These receptors help create muscle memory and help store the physical components of emotional traumas. Therefore, as you become increasingly conscious of your body, you can trigger awareness of these mind–body connectors and gain enhanced linkage to your mind and emotions.

In Nia, we use the body to heal the mind and spirit by joining muscular movement with introspection, intention, visualization, imagery, and expressiveness. Body language and verbal expression are used to help bring forgotten feelings—pleasant and unpleasant—to the foreground of consciousness. Thus Nia is commonly employed to relieve and reverse depression, anxiety, post-traumatic stress disorders, substance addictions, obsessive–compulsive disorders, and abusive behaviors. It is used in hospitals, substance-abuse centers, and even prisons.

It is also used—not incidentally—to help people who already feel good to feel even *better.*

Take the Path of Least Resistance. Contrary to conventional fitness wisdom, the *easy* way is the *natural* way. The militaristic, punishing element often found in traditional fitness is not only passé, it's not as effective. Psychologically, it creates resistance and insecurity, rather than enthusiasm and self-respect. Physically, it creates too much strain to be worth the gain.

To achieve lasting body–mind–spirit fitness on this path of least resistance, you must move in accord with what we call the *Body's Way:* the structural design of the body that dictates its proper use. Even more precisely, you must move in accord with *your own Body's Way,* because no two bodies are exactly alike.

Function follows form, and proper function of the body is always easier to perform, and is more physically rewarding, than improper function.

. . .

These few, simple concepts all seem so obvious now! However, in the mid-1980s—when, for example, virtually no one in the fitness industry was doing yoga—these ideas were widely considered far-fetched. Some experts considered them a dangerous threat to the sacrosanct no pain, no gain philosophy. They were, in fact, revolutionary, and they changed the face of fitness forever.

THE CHANGING FACE OF FITNESS

Traditional Exercise		*Nia*
Painful	----------➤	Pleasurable
Guilt driven	----------➤	Desire driven
Single-movement forms	----------➤	Fusion fitness
Stoic	----------➤	Expressive
Trains only large muscle groups	----------➤	Trains all muscle groups
Movements directed externally	----------➤	Movements directed internally, according to the Body's Way
Reinforces physical rigidity	----------➤	Creates gracefulness
Can lead to injuries	----------➤	Heals injuries
Creates muscle imbalance	----------➤	Creates muscle balance
Weakens the nervous system	----------➤	Strengthens the nervous system
Creates physical fitness	----------➤	Creates fitness of body, mind, spirit, and emotions

the revolution in fitness

These days, there's nothing strange to most sophisticated people about the concepts of mind–body fitness or cross-training or getting fit with the healing arts (such as Pilates and yoga), or even combining movement forms to create fusion-fitness methods (such as Tae-Bo and Yoga-Lates). The current widespread acceptance of these concepts might never have occurred—or may have been much delayed—if we had not inaugurated all of them during the early days of Nia.

On that first day at our sensei's martial arts studio, though, we weren't trying to revolutionize the fitness industry. We were just trying to find a way to help people get fit without back-breaking punishment. Our sensei led us in slow, controlled movements that looked easy but felt hard. By slowing down, we discovered muscles we'd never used in aerobics. We also discovered some subtle principles that had been obscured by the frenetic, whirlwind pace of conventional aerobics. For example, we found that as we shouted *Hai!* with every kick, our diaphragmatic breath tightened our abdominal muscles even better than sit-ups did. Imagine! Getting stronger abs just from breathing!

We also got a jolt of insight just by taking off our shoes to perform the martial art of tae kwon do. It was the same feeling you probably get yourself when you kick off your shoes at the end of a long day: *That* feels better! Barefoot, we could feel the exact impact of all our movements, and it forced us to stop pounding our feet into the floor as if our skeletons were made of steel.

We kept going back to the dojo and almost immediately we began to see new ripples in our abdominal muscles and more definition in our legs, hips, and buttocks. We were getting "cuts"—those fine lines that define muscles—which most athletes get only from hours in the weight room.

Suddenly, we realized how much we didn't know. It was time to hit the books. Debbie, who had a strong academic background in anatomy and physiology, was especially industrious, and spent five hours in the library every day for the next year.

We soon began to introduce the fruits of our research to our aerobics students. No more boring donkey kicks! No more searing sit-ups! Forget the leg lifts! There's a better way! And they looked at us like we'd lost our minds. Many even left our classes altogether, but it didn't matter—we knew we were on the trail of something big.

As we kept studying and experimenting, we made additions to our workout. To balance the power and volatility of tae kwon do, we added the softer martial art of t'ai chi. From the subtle movements of t'ai chi, we learned important details, such as leading with our heels, rather than our toes, when stepping. Over time, we also added aikido, a martial art that enables people to become fit without force. Aikido has the visually beautiful characteristic of turning linear movements into graceful arcs.

From our growing involvement with the martial arts community, word got around that we were doing something completely different, and students began to migrate back to our studio. We were also starting to get some important positive reviews from the leaders of San Francisco's fitness community. The most important accolade came from Dr. James Garrick, who's generally regarded as the Father of Sports Medicine. Dr. Garrick was so curious about our work that he wired Carlos with loads of electrodes, to determine the exact degree of our workout's physical exertion. The workout didn't look very hard, and, once you got accustomed to it, it didn't even feel very hard—so how could it be as effective as it seemed?

Dr. Garrick couldn't believe the results. Literally. He thought his machines were malfunctioning. So he brought Carlos back to the hospital and did it all over again. Same results. The workout hit the ideal target zone for cardiovascular exertion—without all the usual grunting and groaning and huffing and puffing.

We also caught the attention of one of San Francisco's leading chiropractors, who for the past few years had been alarmed at all the casualties hitting his office from the city's aerobics studios. He loved our approach, as did the city's leading podiatrist, who told us that our students were no longer coming to him with broken-down feet.

Our success was picking back up, and we were getting a lot of media attention for our "radical" ideas. We were even starting to influence the aerobics industry, which copied our nonimpact aerobics by introducing low-impact aerobics (and later step aerobics), definitely an improvement, but still boring.

Even so, something was bothering Carlos. One day he put it into words: "This is effective, but where is the *fun*?" Carlos has a special gift for experiencing joy, and if *he* said it wasn't fun, then it wasn't fun.

So, we asked ourselves, what's fun? Well . . . *dancing* is fun.

We now had a new project. Carlos, who was always our guinea pig, started taking every dance class in the city. Jazz dance. Modern dance. Expressive dance. Eventually, we introduced a jazz dance and a modern dance component to the workout, and our students lit up like Christmas trees! It brought out the closet dancer in every one of them, and pepped up the workout even more.

Much of the reason students loved it was because we were careful to emphasize that there was no wrong way to dance. We weren't trying to put on a Broadway musical, we were just trying to get people *moving*. When we got rid of this regimentation, we also eliminated the slew of injuries that generally plague dancers. Strict dance forms may look beautiful, but they're murder on the body. Professional dancers usually end up even more crippled than pro athletes. It's the price they pay for doing things the traditional way, instead of the Body's Way.

Then we took our freedom from regimentation even further. Instead of telling our students what steps to do, we started giving them generalized movement directions, using imagery and visualization: "Draw a rainbow in the sky!" Or "Pull bubble gum off your shoulders." "Paint a wall!" We all did our movements differently, of course, in our own Body's Way.

People were smiling without being reminded to smile and breathing without being told to breathe. They felt *good*. One student summed it all up: "I don't know if I *look* pretty doing this, but I *feel* pretty." People were playing with balance, creating shapes with their bodies, letting time slip away, and feeling sensations they'd forgotten.

The final piece of our dance component came one day after class, when we asked a beautiful sixty-year-old woman where she'd learned her exceptionally graceful, flowing movements.

"I'm an Isadora Duncan dancer," she said.

She took us to her home in the Berkeley Hills and showed us faded scrapbooks of her mother's old friend, the legendary dancer Isadora Duncan, who had revolutionized dance in the late 1800s by abandoning classical dance movements and telling women to throw away their ballet slippers and restrictive corsets to free their bodies and spirits in movement. As we paged through the scrapbooks, we realized, with a start, that Isadora Duncan was a nineteenth-century version of *us*.

When we incorporated Duncan dance into our routines, it not only increased the freedom of our workout but added emphasis on upward movements, in contrast to the gravity-based downward movements of most dance. It was light and floating and used the entire body. Duncan dance lent an expressive, spiritual element, which organically led us to Nia's final ingredient: the healing arts, including yoga.

Yoga is far more than just another tummy tightener. It has the exalted agenda of distributing nonmaterial energy, or chi, throughout the body's energy meridians and thereby helping the body, mind, spirit, and emotions to heal after the battering of daily life. We also incorporated two more of the most advanced healing arts into our workout: the Alexander Technique and the Feldenkrais Method. The Alexander Technique stresses effortless movement, which meshed perfectly with our concept of doing things the easy way (the Body's Way!). Feldenkrais teaches people how to break old physical patterns and reprogram their body's neurophysiologies. They are both Western techniques that complement the Eastern approaches of yoga and the martial arts.

We now had nine classic movement forms—three each from the martial arts, the healing arts, and the dance arts—creating a synergy that seemed to solve practically every problem we applied to it. We had moved far beyond mere physical fitness. Every year, as Nia became increasingly popular, we went deeper and deeper into the majestic realm of the body and discovered in it a wisdom and power that we hadn't known existed. As we helped students get in touch with this wisdom, we saw them fall in love with their bodies and with their bodies' abilities to self-heal. When this happened, people began to naturally use their bodies as they were meant to be used and to treat their bodies the way they were meant to be treated. With what seemed to be little effort, a great many students abandoned long-standing bad habits. They stopped overeating and bingeing. They stopped smoking and drinking compulsively. They found that they loved movement and were bored with being sedentary.

These changes showed in their bodies. In their lives. Other people noticed. Our classes became a nationwide phenomenon during the 1990s and began to be known all around the world. As word of our work spread, the fitness industry continued to respond. Low-impact aerobics became a major trend. Dance, yoga, t'ai chi, and the martial arts were recognized as viable fitness techniques. Mind–body fitness became popular, and fusion fitness was born.

However, the industry is still too fixated on fads instead of classic movement forms. It's still hung up on instant weight loss, at the expense of permanent weight loss. It's overly infatuated with how people look, rather than how they feel. It still causes far too many injuries. It's still too regimented. It's still boring. It's still too macho and masculine. And it's never really gotten past the idea that pain is necessary.

But most of our students and teachers now speak a different language of fitness. They don't talk about how their bodies look nearly as much as they talk about how their bodies feel. They don't boast about their external physical capabilities, but talk about internal strength, control, and power—mental as well as physical. They speak of being balanced and grounded, physically and emotionally. They say that they're relaxed even when they're working hard, and that they're able to change the mundane activities of living into a veritable dance of life.

More than anything else, they equate fitness with *movement,* not exercise. For them, life has become, literally and figuratively, a *moving experience* based on the Thirteen Principles that are the foundation of Nia as a fitness, personal growth, and lifestyle practice.

THE THIRTEEN PRINCIPLES OF NIA

1. **The Joy of Movement.** Joy is the primary sensation you should seek from all movement. If you momentarily lose joy, tweak your movement until joy again arises.
2. **Natural Time and the Movement Forms.** All of your Nia movements are done in your own personal, natural sense of time and include movements and energy from nine classic forms.
3. **Music and the 8BC System.** Nia is practiced to the sounds and silences of

music, using an eight-beat counting (8BC) system (1-and, 2-and, 3-and, 4-and, 5-and, . . .) to organize the movements.

4. **FreeDance.** Anything goes movement-wise. Let go of structure.
5. **Awareness and Dancing Through Life.** In Nia, you become aware that every movement in life is a dance and that every movement can be used to self-heal.
6. **The Base—Feet and Legs.** Your feet are the hands that touch the earth, and through your legs they carry the energy of the earth to your whole body.
7. **The Three Planes and Three Levels.** Every movement can be done within three planes—low, middle, and high—and can be done with three different levels of intensity. Mixing the three levels and three planes creates a wide repertoire of movement choices.
8. **The Core—Pelvis, Chest, and Head.** Your pelvis, chest, and head are the home of your emotions and your energy centers. The pelvis is a container of energy, the chest transmits and receives energy, and the head processes energy.
9. **The Upper Extremities—Arms, Hands, and Fingers.** Your arms, hands, and fingers are tools for healing, touching, directing energy, and creating connections. They are extensions of your feelings and thoughts and allow you to express yourself in personal and purposeful ways.
10. **X-Ray Anatomy.** The practice of using your eyes, your other sensory organs, and your intuition to see inside yourself is X-Ray Anatomy. You can penetrate the veil of your flesh to reveal the proper placement of your bones, tendons, ligaments, and muscles.
11. **Fitness Is the Business of the Body.** Fitness can be achieved by listening to the voices of the body, setting goals, creating plans, reaching decisions, and attaining results. As in all businesses, achieving success is a process of making changes.
12. **Continuing the Body-Mind-Spirit Education.** Healing the body is a practice that never ends. Every new workout is an opportunity to reeducate your body, mind, and spirit.
13. **Dance What You Sense.** When you experience the primary lesson of Nia—that life should be lived through sensation—you become connected.

the sixteen benefits of Nia

Nia will change your body and your life in wonderful ways. Here are the sixteen main benefits.

1. It increases the *pleasure* of living in your body.
2. It creates *weight loss* and proper weight maintenance.
3. It *strengthens muscles,* improves muscle tone, and increases muscle definition.
4. It *calms* the mind and relieves stress.
5. It improves *endurance.*
6. It increases *grace* and flexibility.
7. It *balances* the autonomic nervous system.
8. It improves *posture* and can even increase height.
9. It improves *organ function*—particularly that of the heart and lungs.
10. It enhances *sensory awareness.*
11. It heightens *sexual function.*
12. It builds reservoirs of *chi.*
13. It alleviates *emotional problems,* including depression, anxiety, post-traumatic stress disorders, obsessive–compulsive disorders, and anger-management problems.
14. It *improves circulation* of blood and improves *lymphatic drainage.*
15. It strengthens *immunity.*
16. It improves *concentration* and *cognitive function.*

two *The Body's Way*

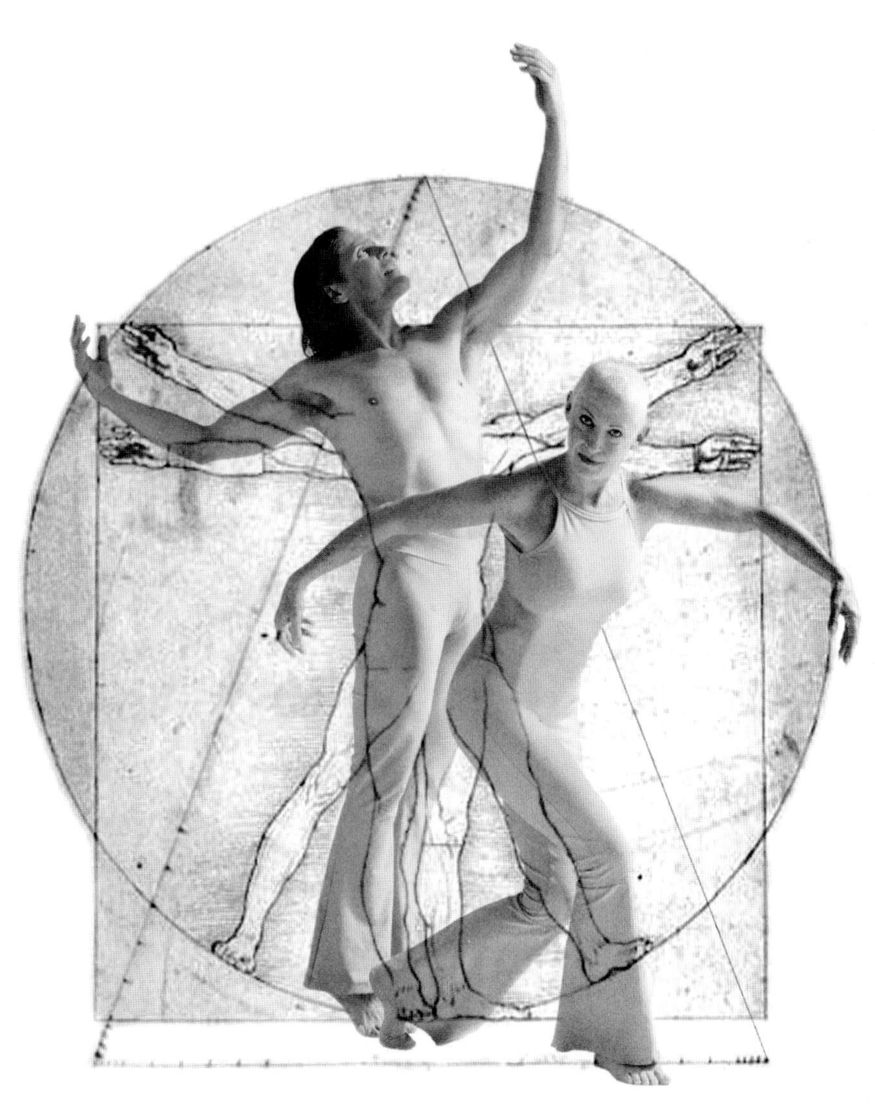

Both huddling near the back of the Nia class, moving tentatively and with pain, Janet and Laura seemed to have such different problems.

Janet was an elite athlete, a star volleyball player on her college team, but she was suffering from a rupture of her knee's anterior cruciate ligament—the dreaded *ACL tear.*

Laura was a midlife bank teller with sore feet and legs.

They looked so different. They moved so differently. Nonetheless, they both had the same essential problem: They had violated the Body's Way and were now paying the price.

Janet was known for her spectacular leaping ability, which she had first developed by playing basketball and beach volleyball with her brothers. When she'd become a competitive interscholastic volleyball player, her coaches had been delighted with the way she'd learned to jump: like a *guy,* instead of like most other female athletes. She usually landed with her knees bent, as men generally do, instead of landing relatively straight legged, as most women tend to do.

Problem, though: Janet was *not* a guy. As a woman, she had a wider pelvis than men. Because of this, the connective tissues in her knees were less able to withstand the intense stretching of a bent-knee landing than are the legs of most men. Therefore, the same movements that were successful for males had been disastrous for her.

Janet had come to a Nia class because she knew that the most successful new form of physical therapy for women with ACL tears is neuromuscular training. Seven studies, including one by the National Center for Injury Prevention and Control, have clearly indicated that neuromuscular training programs such as Nia are more effective than all other approaches at helping to heal and to prevent serious musculoskeletal injuries. Nia is successful because it not only builds muscle strength but also heightens the feedback mechanisms of muscles, nerves, and joints.

Laura, the bank teller, had the far more subtle problem of feet and leg pain, but for her it was as cataclysmic as a severe injury. Almost every day at work she experienced so much pain that she became exhausted, irritable, and unfocused. Like Janet, she had thought she was using her body properly. Every day she had stood in an erect posture, with her knees locked for added stability.

But she had not been listening to the "voice" of her knees. If she had been tuned in to the feedback mechanisms of her knees or if she had merely been more aware of the structural design of her knee joints, her knees would have told her, "I'm not *meant* to be locked tightly while you stand for long hours. I'm a hinge joint, and my shape dictates the type of use I'm meant for—agile movements." By locking her knees, Laura had actually been weakening her knee joints, and blocking the energy that naturally traveled up from her feet to her torso. When that had occurred, day after day, her entire body, and especially her legs, had become excessively fatigued and increasingly weak.

During the next few classes, we taught Laura how to distribute her weight onto her feet more evenly. She learned to place weight on the entirety of each foot—the inside and outside, the front and back, the ball and heel—and how to keep her knees loose and spring loaded, not locked but ready for action, which increases flexibility and mobility.

It took time for Laura to fully integrate a new way of standing into her body's somatic memory, or *muscle memory.* It took even longer for Janet to learn how to jump without straining her tendons and ligaments. However, when these two women did master their goals, their lives improved. Laura no longer lived in pain, and Janet no longer lived in fear of another crippling injury. *That is the power of the Body's Way.*

The Body's Way is a concept we originated ourselves, early in Nia's development. The beauty of Nia is that we always go to the intelligence of the body and ask it, "What is the Body's Way?" . . . and we listen to its inner voice.

Our first hint of the existence of this phenomenon came shortly after we began practicing martial arts in our bare feet, as is generally the custom among martial artists. We were immediately struck by how invigorating and natural it felt: Wow! This is amazing! We sought a rationale for why it felt so good and were surprised to find that even in the literature of the martial arts, very little had been written about the benefits of working out barefoot. It was simply a custom.

With no books to direct us, all we had as our guide was the design and structure of the body itself. Later we realized, of course, that this was the most profound guide of all. But in the meantime, we began to take anatomy courses. As developers of an emerging exercise system, we wanted to learn specific lessons about the relationship between the body's *structure* and its *function.* What we discovered was that, in engineering terms, "function follows form." In other words, the proper way for the body to be used followed the way it had been built. Such a simple concept!

As we refined the concept, we sought to find the most effective and powerful ways of moving, based on the body's own anatomy. For example, when we were analyzing the action of a leg kick from a one-legged stance, we discovered why it is always best to place your weight on the inside of your standing leg, instead of the outside. It's because the shin bone that's on the inside of the leg (the tibia) is thicker than the one that's on the outside (the fibula) and therefore provides better support.

From hundreds of little lessons like this, we built the system that we now call the Body's Way. *The Body's Way is a method of using the body in accord with its specific design and structure.* It involves looking at the body as it really is, instead of viewing it in an idealized, conceptualized way. Nia's Way is always in alignment with the Body's Way.

When you begin to understand the Body's Way, as you will in this chapter, you will start to forge a new relationship with your own body. You'll learn—based on the design of your body's bones, joints, muscles, and connective tissues—how to get optimum power, propulsion, fitness, and flexibility from your body, without pain. Your movement choices will change. They will no longer be based on habit but on scientific validation.

As you learn the Body's Way, you will be guided by its five most fundamental principles. You will find these principles expressed repeatedly in the next part of this chapter, in which you'll discover how the Body's Way is manifested in every major area of the body.

the five basic principles of the body's way

The Body Thrives on Dynamic Ease. Dynamic ease is the ability to perform a movement with maximum efficiency and minimal effort. When you achieve dynamic ease, you'll know it, because it creates a distinct physical sensation, a feeling of effortless power, elegance, and grace. To get a feel for dynamic ease, think back to when you learned a challenging physical task—it could be when you learned to ride a bike or ski or even type. At first, you felt weak, clumsy, intimidated, and frustrated. But you persevered until one day, suddenly: Bingo! Dynamic ease!

When you reach a state of dynamic ease, you not only achieve power and grace but also a sense of neuromuscular creativity. Dynamic ease allows you to do variations of movements without even thinking. Creativity is a natural aspect of movement, but creativity is thwarted when you have to *struggle* with a movement. People who just work, work, work at movement never experience the joy of creativity that springs naturally from dynamic ease. When you're fixated only on work, you become entrenched in the survival mode, and creativity vanishes.

The Body Demands Balance. How do we know the body demands balance? Because the body tells us so: The body *itself* is in almost perfect balance and symmetry. The body balances left and right: two arms, two legs, two eyes, two ears, two lungs, two ovaries, two testicles, two brain hemispheres, two kidneys. There is also balance among the major organs (the heart is on one side and the liver on the other) and between the upper body and the lower body.

Therefore, when you do movements, you should aspire to achieve equal balance in your movements from left to right and top to bottom. This will help promote balance in your musculature, in your skeletal system, and even in your brain and peripheral nervous system.

Furthermore, to better achieve balance, many of your movements should be circular. Circular movements are not at all common in most other exercise programs, which are generally based on linear movements. However, anytime your motion takes a curved path, it better engages your whole body, including both hemispheres of your brain. It also activates the full range of your muscle tissues, including both the small and the large fibers. In contrast, linear movements tend to work with a more limited range of muscle fibers, and generally involve more compartmentalized neurological pathways.

Balance is better.

The Body Is Balanced in Yin and Yang. Because yin and yang are balanced in the body, you must respect this balance and reflect it in the movement choices you make. We can tell that the body is made up of both yin and yang energies simply by observing the body itself. Yin—soft, "female," inward-directed energy—is constantly being manifested by the body's smooth, almost melodic movements. Yang—harder, "male," outward-directed energy—is reflected by more explosive, rhythmic movements.

Inhaling is yin; exhaling is yang. Intense activity is yang; rest is yin. Warming up is yang; cooling down is yin. All of these aspects of living and moving are indispensable and equally important. For example, how could you possibly inhale without exhaling?

Yoga is, in theory, a beautiful healing system that balances yin and yang energies within the body. In actuality, however, many Americans who practice yoga become overly yang in their movements, due to a highly physical, do-more atmosphere. Often, when people begin to practice Nia after they've received training in Americanized yoga, we need to remind them to balance their yin and yang and to take what they've learned from their yoga out onto the street. These people have trained their bodies to function in only one style, focusing on specific asanas. When our bodies become entrained to only one system, we lose the ability to adapt to the variety of rhythms and movements in real life. That's why Nia is such a wonderful complement to yoga.

The Body's Way Demands Simultaneous Mobility and Stability. Having just mobility or stability isn't enough. We know the body insists on mobility because of the abundant presence in the body of flexible joints. There are thirteen primary joint systems in the body (wrists, elbows, shoulders, hips, knees, ankles, and spine), and each was designed to provide various forms and degrees of mobility, when empowered by adjoining muscles and connective tissues. However, the same muscles, connective tissues, and joint designs also provide stability. Without stability, muscles and joints would be useless.

When we have the proper balance of stability and mobility, we have the power to move energy vertically, horizontally, and in circles, providing three-dimensional movement capabilities. This is critically important, because we live in a three-dimensional world. Some exercise programs, however, concentrate on two-dimensional movements.

Some people have too much mobility and not enough stability. An example is a baseball pitcher whose shoulder joint has been excessively stretched and stressed over long periods of time. This type of hypermobility injury is quite common among the general public these days, because—like baseball pitchers—many people make the same repetitive motions in their jobs every day and erode the stabilizing forces of their joints, muscles, ligaments, and tendons.

Other people have too much *stability,* at the expense of mobility and flexibility. This condition is extremely common among the vast number of people who sit in office chairs for many hours each day. Their joints, muscles, and connective tissues become rigid and inelastic.

Both excessive mobility and excessive stability can lead to osteoarthritis, other forms of chronic pain, injuries, and fatigue. They are both enemies of fitness—and enemies of feeling good.

The Body Itself Reveals the Body's Way. Through the language of design and through the language of feedback, the body reveals its Way. The language of design is simple: "This is how I'm built, so use me accordingly." For example, the design of the shoulder girdle tells us that the shoulder is not meant to bear heavy weights, because it is a very flexible, circular, free-moving joint. The language of feedback is equally easy to comprehend. Through neurological connections, every part of the body constantly provides you with either positive feedback or negative feedback. In their most fundamental forms, positive feedback is pleasure, and negative feedback is pain.

Negative feedback is not necessarily a bad thing; it's simply a signal to stop. When you feel pain, or any significant discomfort, you should alter your movement's intensity level or range or you should change to another movement. Forget no pain, no gain. That's an anachronism.

There is, however, a state of healthy physical stress that often precedes pain. This state, which we call *positive tension,* supports healing and builds balanced strength. In a state of positive tension, you will feel a vibration in your muscles, you will be breathing deeply, and you'll probably be sweating. You may become exhilarated, because you will feel physically challenged without feeling as if you were damaging any specific part of your body. Positive tension is much different from the feeling you get when your body is saying, "This hurts—I want to stop."

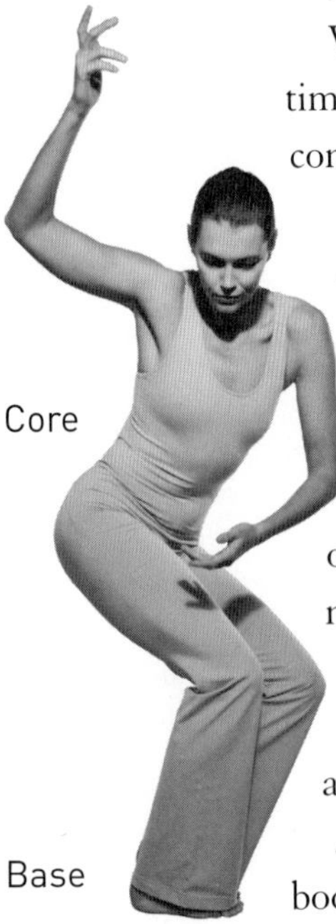

In Nia we say, "Don't go for the burn. Go for positive tension."

When people enter into a prolonged state of dynamic ease, they sometimes express this condition as "being in the zone." Professional athletes commonly reach this zone with mastery over their movements.

In contrast, we also teach Nia to many people with aggressive, type A personalities, and these people are generally too yang in their movement choices. Furthermore, people who practice certain extremely yang styles of yoga can become overly aggressive and "hard" in their movement approaches.

Nia helps people who are overly yin as well as those who are overly yang. Both can achieve balance with Nia. Its diverse menu of movement options encourages a natural harmonizing of yin and yang.

In the next sections, we discuss the three most fundamental areas of the body: the Base (feet and legs), the Core (pelvis, chest, and head), and the Upper Extremities (arms, hands, and fingers).

After you finish reading this chapter, you'll never again see or feel your body in quite the same way.

Upper Extremities

Core

Base

the base—feet and legs

Your feet, knees, and legs are, literally as well as figuratively, the Base of your body. They connect you to the earth.

Nia and the Feet

Working out in bare feet was one of the most innovative elements that Nia added to aerobic exercise—and it can be one of the most freeing and innovative elements you'll enjoy about Nia. It proved to be one of the most profound choices we made. It provided us with a way to discover our feet and to discover our energy source, the earth. It became a way to ground; to center; and to move efficiently, gracefully, and powerfully.

Balance in the whole body begins with your feet. Every imbalance in the body can be detected in the feet. Ida Rolf, the creator of Rolfing, a therapeutic practice designed to deliver postural integration, believed that to develop healthy and powerful posture and to have a strong and agile body, the feet must provide a firm, sturdy, and flexible foundation.

Like your hands, the feet are prehensile. They grasp, clutch, support, reach out, touch, and provide balance. Like the hands, the feet draw energy into the body and move it out. On the underside of the arches of your feet you have, in effect, a bubbling spring where kundalini or chi energy enters your body from the earth. Flexible feet "breathe" and take in chi. Like healthy lungs, they expand and contract as they breathe energy in and out.

The Body's Way teaches you how to properly use each foot's amazing network of thirty-three joints, twenty-six bones, more than a hundred ligaments, nineteen larger muscles and many smaller (intrinsic) muscles, and seven thousand nerve endings. Nia movement engages all parts of your feet every time you work out.

All the Nia foot motions are designed to benefit the entire body, from the ground up. They increase balance, strength, and definition, improve movement efficiency, cultivate energy, and develop awareness. The moves are all used to build strong and agile feet. They develop a firm and flexible foundation, one that is solid but adaptable. The Body's Way also shows you, through the size of various bones, the best areas of the foot on which to place weight, sink into, and push out of. For example, one large bone is the talus, located in the heel. Its thick, powerful design reminds you to rest into it, as if it were a landing pad, when you stand. This relieves pressure on the front of your foot and your toes.

One of the most important skills to develop is simply paying attention to your feet as you move. Listen to your feet. Become attentive to your Base. The more you are connected to your feet, the more power you can generate from them and the more you can express yourself through Nia movements. Having a weak connection to the earth is similar to having weak reception on a television set. The picture is unclear and lacks form. To feel the earth, you must feel your feet.

ARCHES AND ANKLES

The arches of your feet provide your entire body with strength, agility, stability, and shock absorption. The outer arch of your foot, a longitudinal arch, is defined by the bones, muscles, ligaments, and tendons extending from the outermost two toes. As you walk, this arch lifts, to establish balance. The inner arch, also a longitudinal arch, is defined by the bones, muscles, ligaments, and tendons extending from the inner three toes. Like your fingers, these toes give you stability for grounding and anchoring. It is the inner arch, along with your big toe, that makes up the major support structure for body weight. It is a flexible structure that helps you maintain an upright posture.

In addition, each foot has a transverse arch that runs across the top of your foot, much like a suspension bridge. By distributing weight over the entire base of the foot, this arch provides you with a built-in shock absorber.

Your feet support the weight of your entire body. For your body weight to be properly supported and balanced, your ankles must move freely and fluidly and have a complete range of motion. You must maintain proper strength and flexibility in your ankles to achieve abundant support. Any chronic shortening of a tendon or muscle around your ankles will decrease your power, and your ability to move freely. If your ankles are stiff, your grace, mobility, balance, and fluidity will be diminished.

Nia and the Knees

As many of you have experienced, old-fashioned aerobic education taught us merely to keep our knees over our feet. That was the extent of our sensory connection to the knees. Most of us never realized that many of the ways we were using our knees were limiting our grace and strength.

Like the hinges of a door, your knees function best when they move in a single plane, rather than slightly off to one side. Ideally, your knee and ankle joints should be aligned, both facing in exactly the same direction. The direction of your feet dramatically affects the functioning of your knees and legs. When your foot rotates to the side, your knee should also rotate. When your foot is directed forward, your knee should also point forward. If the inside of your foot isn't firmly grounded, your knee and pelvic basin rotate, stressing both the knee and the hip joints.

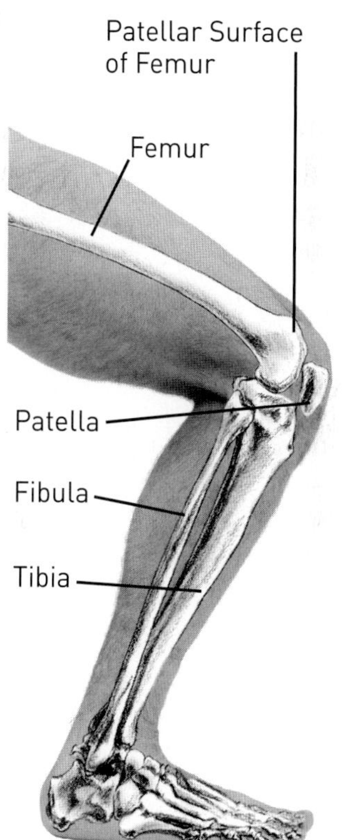

Your muscles, ligaments, tendons, connective tissue, and bones weave together to support the structure of your knees. When the knees function correctly, you experience a sense of stability, rather than tension, wobbling, or dragging to one side.

Like elbows, knees are not designed to support extreme weight, but to transfer energy from one set of bones to another. Sturdy, strong legs require flexible and pliable knees. Locking your knees compresses their cartilage and cuts off the energy flow that invigorates your legs. Locking your knees also causes you to use the bones, rather than the muscles, for support. In effect, you stand on your bones. This creates a weakening in the legs that results in muscle atrophy, and a loss of strength due to the lack of energy flow. Over an extended period of time, this results in decreased leg flexibility, power, and agility.

Nia and the Legs

Coming from a traditional fitness background, we used to think the legs ended at the top of our thighbones. However, the muscles of your legs actually extend to your waist. Your buttock muscles play a major role in moving your thighs. Thus the legs extend from the ground all the way to the top of your hip.

In Nia, we teach you to relate to your leg bones in a new way. We use the legs to dance, play, create, move, and express ourselves. They connect us to the bottom of our feet, which touch the earth.

The larger bone of the lower leg is the tibia. It is the one on the inside, closest to the center of your body, and it provides the most support. (This conforms to a general anatomical rule that *support is in the center.*) The smaller, thinner leg bone, called the fibula, is on the outside and is used for added stability. They are separate, yet like the entire body, they work together, as a functional whole.

The longest and thickest of the leg bones is the thighbone, or femur. It has a rounded end that rests in the concave hip socket. The hip joint is the strongest joint in the body. The hip is a ball-and-socket joint and is designed to allow for changes in the position of your leg. You develop strength in this joint by moving your legs while keeping the hip joint stable or by moving your pelvis while keeping the legs stable. Both ways create flexibility and strength.

The hip joint is vital in creating fluidity and power in the legs. When your hip joint is healthy, your pelvis can adjust to the movements of your thighbone. This offers you great freedom of movement. In Nia, we nurture the health of the hip joint by including pelvic moves in all of our leg movements.

The buttocks are used for support when standing and for locomotion when walking or running. When you walk, you should consciously use your buttocks to move energy through your leg bones and to relax your leg muscles. When you actively use the buttocks while walking, you eliminate the overuse and overloading of leg muscles.

Psoas Muscle

The psoas muscle, a major muscle in the groin, plays an important part in body support and coordination. Structurally, the psoas creates a bridge between the upper body and lower body. Attached to the thighbone and to the lumbar vertebrae, it has a profound effect on the leg, spine, and muscles in the body's Core. The psoas muscle must be strong and flexible. It must be balanced and well toned. Strength and flexibility in the psoas muscle are crucial to grace, agility, and power. Many experts, including the renowned Ida Rolf, say the psoas is the most important muscle in the body. When the psoas is healthy, the upper body and the lower body move with ease.

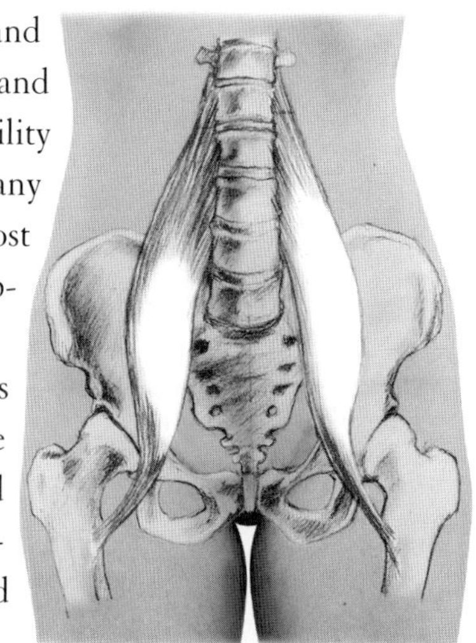

In Nia, we make a conscious mental connection to the psoas muscle. You should pay attention to what is happening in the psoas muscle when you rise and sink. Strive to lengthen and stretch it whenever possible, which will help improve your posture. Feel it stretch as you move your pelvis, thighbone, and lower back.

That is some of the science of your body's Base, but the body is more than just science. To enter fully into a new relationship with your body, you must also recognize that your body is more than mere flesh and blood—it is infused with the energies of your mind, emotions, and spirit. Your body is a holistic entity, with needs and powers all its own, and it has its own voice. This voice, in some cases, will be able to tell you more about yourself than even the voice of science can.

Now it is time to listen to the voice of your body.

The Voices of the Body's Base

The Voice of the Feet

To your physical body—I am your connection to the earth, the conduit that allows you to receive and to return earth's energy. My physical structure is alive with over seven thousand nerve endings. I am the one who encourages you to move kundalini, or chi energy, from the earth up, into, and through your body, all the way up into the heavens. I tell you where you are, how to find balance, how to step gently, and how to find grace as an upright being.

To your mental body—I send information to your brain and nervous system regarding balance and safety. If you allow me to think for you, I can tell you exactly what you need to do to create harmony in your whole body. If you awaken to my intelligence, you can relax into my vast sensation of awareness.

To your emotional body—the physical part of you that feels joy and sadness—I offer a direct line of communication that tells you exactly how you are feeling at any given moment. When you are nervous, I tap. When you're afraid, I contract. And when you feel safe, I soften and spread. I am always talking to you. I am one of the most sensitive parts of your body. Sense my changes, and discover what I am saying to you, moment to moment.

To your spiritual body—the part of you that has no boundaries—I hold the keys to the many personalities that compose you. I offer you warrior feet, mother feet, lover feet, achiever feet, and more. I can help you become any archetype that fills your form. Play with me and awaken new energies within your body.

The Voice of the Lower Leg

To your physical body—I am the lower portion of your leg bones, a fence post of stability. I have not one, but two bones to help you connect to the earth. My smaller bone, the fibula, the one on the outside, is a reminder to you to be gentle as you move to your outside. My bigger bone, the tibia, the one on the inside, reminds you that the greatest amount of support and power comes from within, from your center.

To your mental body—I help you stay connected to the left and right hemispheres of your brain. My larger bone helps connect you to your left brain, the part of you that organizes and creates structure. My smaller bone helps connect you to your right brain, your creative, softer, fluid, intuitive side. As two bones, we work together, resting alongside each other—separate, yet connected.

To your emotional body—I create a connection from the earth into your belly, the place that feeds you with nutritional and intuitive energy. I am an extension into your feelings. When you trust life, energy runs down me like raindrops falling down a windowpane. When you are afraid, energy becomes stuck around me, resulting in rigid, tight calf muscles.

To your spiritual body—I am your ethereal tree trunk. I am the physical part of your spirit that wants to tower up into the heavens, where illuminated spirit resides. As you develop trust in me, you can become light as a feather, like an angel who walks the earth.

The Voice of the Knee

To your physical body—I am a hinge joint, one of the largest joints in the body. As a valve for releasing and moving energy, I maintain a flow of energy along your leg. One piece of my bony structure looks like a cap and is actually an extension of something grander—your quadriceps femoris tendon and patellar ligament. It floats freely and is meant to move and be free. All of my movement is enabled by a slippery substance called synovial fluid, which is found where my bones meet. To the three elegant support structures that are your leg bones—the femur, tibia, and fibula—I give the freedom to bend and extend. When symmetrically balanced, your leg bones make it possible for me to stay open and move freely. When relaxed, I provide you with a dynamic energy force that allows you to gracefully spring into life. If you try to hold me rigidly, or lock me, I will complain by making your lower back or legs tense.

To your mental body—I reflect your innermost thoughts. When you think love, *I relax and soften. When you think* fear, *sometimes I lock and tighten and sometimes I become excessively loose, making you feel "weak in the knees." When you think* play, *I get excited and want to run. Be aware of me, and you will become more aware of what you are thinking.*

To your emotional body—I express your feelings. I offer you direct emotional feedback. Notice how I respond to people, situations, places, thoughts, and images. The energy in me changes as your emotions change. Allow me to communicate with you as a way to become aware of your true feelings. I offer you deep insights that need to come out. The next time you get weak in the knees, listen to what I am saying. The next time your knees shake, hear me.

To your spiritual body—I bring the expression of grace, trust, and openness. When you permit me to be relaxed, open, and free, you and I can walk the earth together in gentle harmony. When I am open and relaxed, you have access to energy within your entire body.

The Voice of the Thigh

To your physical body—I am the biggest limb above your knee. At my bottom, I am aligned more closely to your center, reminding you that center is where the strongest support comes from. I am designed to swing freely, like a pendulum, in a ball-and-socket joint. When I can move freely in your hip joint, I can move in all directions. Allow me to offer you height and extension.

To your mental body—I take what is energetically felt from below and move it up into higher states of consciousness. I receive energy from your walk, sending it into your belly, your heart, and your soul.

To your emotional body—I give rise to all feeling, and expand your energy outward. Like a river's channel, I change, and give voice to the expressive self that lies beyond the "you" that you know.

To your spiritual body—I give height to the visions of your feet. I empower your walk, because I am the backbone of your legs. I offer you the flexibility to be powerfully upright or folded and still. When you play with me, we can run wild, jump, fly, and dance.

the core: pelvis, chest, and head

People new to Nia often presume that we don't include weightlifting as part of our program of neuromuscular integration. But we do. We use the *weight of the body itself.* In particular, we use the weight of three of the primary elements of the body's Core: the pelvis, the chest, and the head.

These three body weights, plus the spine, compose the Core. These body parts act as free weights that work separately and collectively. Ideally, when walking or standing, the three body weights should balance on top of each other. When the intrinsic and extrinsic muscles and ligaments are healthy and strong, they hold the three weights in alignment and are supported by the skeleton. The alignment of the three weights also affects your general health and overall state of well-being. Every organ in your body is affected by their alignment. A head out of balance will inhibit eyesight, and add stress to the vocal chords. A chest out of alignment fatigues the body by constricting breathing, which reduces the amount of oxygen and energy available to your entire body. A pelvis out of alignment reduces leg strength and propulsive power. It also inhibits Core strength and abdominal support and creates overall body weakness, due to the immobility of the spine. To heal your body, your organs, and your spine, you need to keep the three body weights softly aligned, mobile, and in motion. When used properly, movement of the pelvis, chest, and head strengthens, stretches, and realigns the body. When functioning properly, the Core's body weights also distribute chi to all parts of the body.

Through movement, you can effectively realign these weights to improve your posture and physical functioning. By paying attention to the way you move and the way you balance these weights, you can begin to consciously re-create your body. Improving postural alignment enhances your ability to breathe more deeply and more efficiently. It also improves self-confidence and overall mental, physical, and emotional health. When the force of the three weights is integrated into your natural movements, you feel vitally alive and energetically present.

Nia and the Pelvis

The main bones of the pelvis are the left and right sides of the pelvic girdle, the sacrum, and the coccyx.

The pelvis is the bottom of the three body weights and is a base for the other two weights (the chest and head). The pelvis is said to be "the seat of your soul." It is literally what your torso sits in. When the pelvis becomes tight and constricted, your seat is an uncomfortable chair. When the pelvis is free and fluid, your seat is a royally comfortable chair.

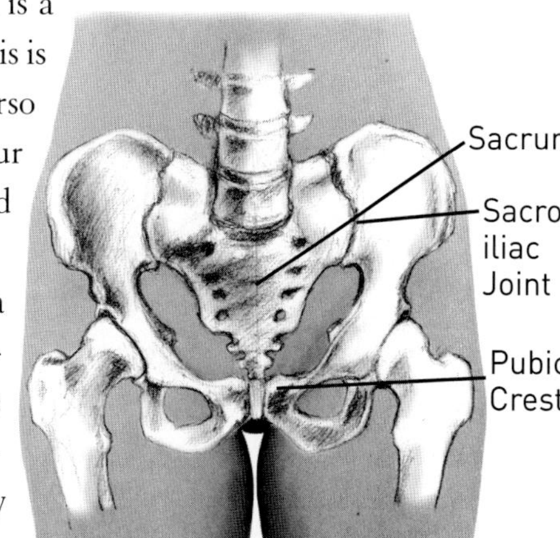

The pelvis is a bony basin that contains the abdomen. As a container, it is also a reservoir for physical, mental, emotional, and spiritual energy. In addition, the pelvis houses the sexual organs. Any movement of the pelvis can unleash primal, sexual, and sensual energy. The release of this energy can be positive or negative, depending on the emotional state of the individual. Even subtle movements can trigger emotional feelings and personal issues, including sexual trauma, self-control, desire, safety, and survival. When the sexual organs are imbalanced or restricted, the pelvis will generally be limited in freedom and expressiveness. When healthy, however, these organs help you feel physically and emotionally safe.

Denying movement to the pelvis will result in the loss of physical strength in your low back, feet, and legs. It will diminish your ability to maintain proper breathing and will also limit your overall endurance.

Any chronic tilting of the pelvic basin locks it in a frozen posture. When the pelvis tilts too far forward, your abdominal muscles and viscera press forward. If this happens, the lumbar facets of the spine hyperextend and the tailbone sticks out. This chronic tilting of the tailbone produces tightness and rigidity in the lower back and a lack of freedom in the ability to breathe and move freely. If your pelvis is out of alignment, all of its contents will be unnecessarily stressed, causing overall diminishment of function.

Look at yourself from the side in a mirror to see if you have correct alignment between the front of your pelvis at your pubic bone, and the back of your pelvis at the sacrum and coccyx. If properly aligned, there is a horizontal line between the coccyx and the pubic bone. In other words, the pelvic floor is level. If your pelvis is tilted forward, your coccyx will be higher than the pubis. If the tailbone is curled under, the pubic bone will be higher than the coccyx. If your pelvis is out of alignment, the top of the pelvis will be tilted.

Your pelvis is also a support structure that provides your body with a foundation for bearing and balancing weight. The lumbosacral joint—the joint that joins the sacrum and the lumbar vertebrae—creates a base to support upright, bipedal posture. This powerful, secure, yet movable junction is located at the back of your pelvis.

Your body may send you painful signals to indicate your pelvis is out of alignment. Pain in the hip sockets and the inability to comfortably draw your thighs up toward your chest are signs that your pelvis lacks fluidity or alignment. What keeps the pelvis and the hip joint healthy is movement—particularly movement it is *designed* to do. A wide variety of pelvic, foot, and leg movements, incorporating various ranges of motion, keeps the hip flexors and hip joint healthy.

Remember to use your pelvis in every movement of your Core. It is one of the best ways to keep your body energetically charged, your legs agile, your chest open, and your spine free. Use the pelvis as it was designed—*as a place for your soul to sit and take a load off!*

Nia and the Chest

The bones of the chest area include the sternum, the clavicles, the twelve ribs, and the thoracic spine. These bones contain and protect the vital organs, including the heart. Like an accordion, the rib cage expands and contracts, allowing energy to move in and out. When you inhale, the rib cage expands to let breath and energy in. And when you exhale, the contracting rib cage and lungs release air out. The space between your ribs is an anatomical reminder that this body weight—your chest—is meant to remain open, free, lighthearted, mobile, and accessible to energy and emotion moving in and out.

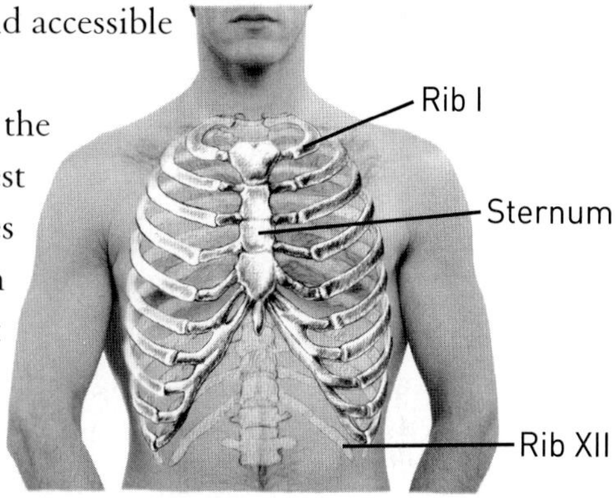

Rib I

Sternum

Rib XII

The rib cage is moved primarily by muscles in the front, back, and along the sides of your chest. Chest movement deepens diaphragmatic breath, improves energy flow, and adds flexibility to the spine (which stimulates perception of an easy feeling as the chest gains freedom). In addition, chest movement improves the function of internal organs and strengthens and relaxes the back.

In Nia, the sternum always stacks vertically above the pubic bone. Unless you are intentionally leaning, having your chest in *front* of your pubic bone places undue strain on your low back and constricts your breath. Leaning back too far, however, makes your abdomen and neck work so hard that they are consistently constricted and, as a result, grow weak. Neither option creates a sense of centeredness and comfort in the body.

Stacking the chest and head does not mean your movements will become rigid, like those of the Tin Man. Alignment promotes fluidity, not rigidity. If the chest and head stack over the pelvis, it centers your movement and eliminates strain.

Proper breathing depends on healthy chest movement. As you inhale, your lungs physically expand and your diaphragm drops toward your lower belly. The expansion of the lungs creates internal support for your back. As you exhale, your diaphragm retracts to neutral. It is the movement of the diaphragm that circulates new air and releases stale air. Like an elevator, the up-and-down action of the diaphragm allows your rib cage to expand and retract. Breathing in, receiving, the chest expands. Exhaling, giving energy, it humbles itself and softens. Giving and receiving can be studied by simply watching how you breathe.

Nia and the Head

Because it supports eight cranial bones, fourteen facial bones, and your brain, your head carries a lot of weight! You think, hear, taste, smell, kiss, and see from your head. It is a very busy place. It is a real test of balance and strength to constantly support this eight- to ten-pound weight atop your body.

The bony structure of your head houses your eyes, ears, mouth, nose, brain, tongue, and teeth. The muscles of your neck support your head and protect the cervical (neck) vertebrae. Additional protection to your neck comes from the thick muscles surrounding the bones. The muscles of your neck originate at the base of your skull and cervical spine and anchor deeply into your upper back and chest.

In Nia, when we speak of head movement, we include the movement of the eyes, ears, mouth, nose, and jaw—even the cognitive functions of the brain. The most natural way to move your head and avoid tension is to actively use your eyes to guide your head movements. When you look at something, your eyes lead your head in a natural and safe way. Your ears do the same. The eyes and ears can stimulate spontaneous movement, even in locked body parts. Using the senses to initiate movement of the head is natural and efficient. When you activate physical movement from a sensory cue, such as a desire to look in a particular direction, you decrease tension and move with greater ease.

Traditional fitness often ignores the neck and head, and this violates the Body's Way. Why does the neck require movement? Because it is one of the most mobile parts of the body. It was *built* for movement. Moving the neck and head creates their strength and flexibility. It also increases strength and ease in the upper back and chest, since neck muscles are attached there.

Even though you use your head a lot, it can be the most challenging body part to integrate into your conscious movement. Habit, social attitudes, and emotional experiences often unconsciously limit movement. However, once you begin to move your head more intelligently, it will give your body a sensory blast, and you will automatically want to move it even more.

Because head movement stirs the energy flow around the eyes, ears, and mouth, it will agitate the fluid in the inner ear, which helps the body maintain balance. If extensive head movements are new to you, the agitation can create dizziness, nausea, and fear. Over time, your body will be able to tolerate larger amounts of energy moving in and out of the head and neck. You'll be able to turn, spin, and move up and down at different speeds without getting dizzy. If you feel dizzy or nauseous when moving your head, slow down. Remember that the fluid within the inner ear is moving faster than usual, creating new pressure and greater waves of intensity. If this fluid has not moved very much recently, your body may not be able to maintain a sense of center. Go slowly.

Nia and the Spine

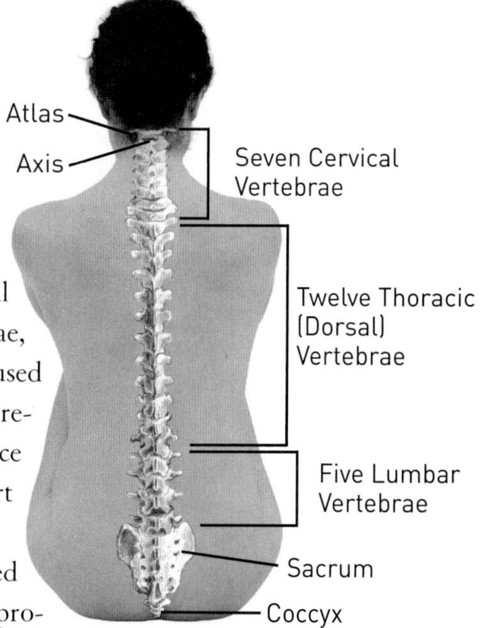

The spine is not a weight, but is still one of the primary elements of the body's Core.

The spine, consisting of twenty-six parts—seven cervical vertebrae, twelve thoracic vertebrae, five lumbar vertebrae, plus the sacrum (five fused vertebrae) and coccyx (four fused vertebrae). It is somewhat like a long strand of beads that creates a column. The spine is a carefully contoured masterpiece that not only moves but also provides a structural support system.

The vertebrae vary in size and are individually formed to bear different amounts of body weight. Each vertebra pro-

A **Nia** *Story*

FIT AND SEXY

STUDENT: Eileen

CLASS LOCATION: Saratoga, New York

OCCUPATION: Student

When Eileen began to do Nia, she just wanted to come to terms with her body, rather than to change it. "I had become convinced that my body would not be changing any time soon," she recalls. "And then Nia changed everything."

Her body began to acquire a new shape and tone, even in areas that had been particularly resistant to improvement, and it was extremely gratifying to her. As she puts it, "Any class that can help tone up that area under your arm is the *class."*

Nia changed not only how she looked but also how she perceived herself. "I am so proud of myself," she says. "I am actually loving my body now, which is something I thought would never happen. I am tuned into my body on a completely different level now."

As it does for many people, Nia had a positive impact on Eileen's sense of sexuality. "Sexually, I've opened up a lot more, in part because I'm so psyched about my body. I feel much sexier and not so self-conscious."

Similarly, she is now more in touch with her innate sensuality. "I totally pamper my body from head to toe," she says. "I love to take baths now. I have a special toning oil I made myself; I give myself massages; and I pamper my feet with foot rubs, creams, and nail polish. I am just so excited about my body!"

Eileen has more energy, a more positive outlook, more self-confidence—and a better body.

"Nia," she says, "has completely changed my life."

vides protected passage for nerves and the spinal cord to pass through, and the magnificent design of the spine makes it possible for you to stand, sit, walk, turn, bend, run, jump, and leap!

Any stiffness, thickening, or immobility of the spine results in the spine pressing itself against the soft tissue of your back muscles. This clearly impairs free and efficient movement. Any extreme or prolonged rotation of the vertebrae is equally detrimental. The rotation of one or more vertebrae, or a curvature in the spine (lordosis, kyphosis, or scoliosis), causes extreme imbalance that reduces leg power, overall body comfort, and energy.

emotions and the three body weights

For many people, movement of the pelvis, chest, or head unearths uncomfortable emotional feelings. Any postural habit that inhibits the body's natural motion also affects the flow of the emotions. The release of physical holding patterns, even small ones, can result in big emotional releases. If the emotional release is too intense, it can frighten you and cause you to contract and shut down. So go slowly and be gentle. Take gradual steps and feel for the emotional ease that tells you that you are on a safe, healing track. Guide yourself with compassion and love. Force is not the answer.

As feelings and emotions come to the surface, fear can emerge, causing you to restrict movement. This means it is time to back off. To help control the amount of energy moving, use the *volume up and volume down* control technique. If the sensations in your body feel too intense, turn down your energy and movement volume. If it feels as if you could take more emotional energy in, turn up the movement and energy volume. Regardless, remember it is always okay to stop. *You are in control.* Over time, you will find yourself able to tolerate more and more emotional energy moving within your body.

Of the three weights, the pelvis is often the one that causes the most *emotional* discomfort. This is due in part to social, moral, and personal attitudes associated with moving the pelvis. Personal experiences and beliefs that inhibit your movement may linger in your body and mind. For example, you may be limited by the belief that moving the pelvis is overtly sexual. The people who most often think this way tend to be those who have experienced some form of sexual abuse, or have been shamed in some way. They often become fearful when they connect to the sensations related to pelvic movement. Even though movement is needed to heal, they avoid it. So, go slowly. Find ways to move your pelvis in a physically and emotionally pain-free way. Experiment with different kinds of music and different kinds of movement.

The chest also holds many emotions: love, grief, joy, and sorrow. When moved consciously, the chest and rib cage can help unearth and release emotion in a healthy way. In addition, the solar plexus, located in the soft tissue just below your ribs, is also stimulated by chest movement. The solar plexus is often associated with personal power, self-confidence, and free will. Breath work, undulations, and pulsating gestures can help unlock Core energy in your solar plexus, the center of the will. Sometimes unlocking this power can be intoxicating, or even frightening. Find your own pace in releasing this force.

Emotions are also carried in and expressed by the head. Many people hold their heads rigidly, partly because the head is associated with mental intelligence. (This is only partly true, for intelligence is also found throughout your whole body, within every cell.) Unfortunately, the act of keeping your head "on straight" often encourages rigidity and truncates emotional expression. Rigidly holding the head in place, regardless of whether it is a conscious or unconscious act, actually weakens the body and dulls the senses.

For some emotionally brittle people, head movement can create the sensory feeling of being overwhelmed. If this happens to you, go slowly. Use your eyes to eliminate the sense of uprootedness that can accompany head movement. Looking keeps you fascinated by the life around you and activates natural movement of the head weight.

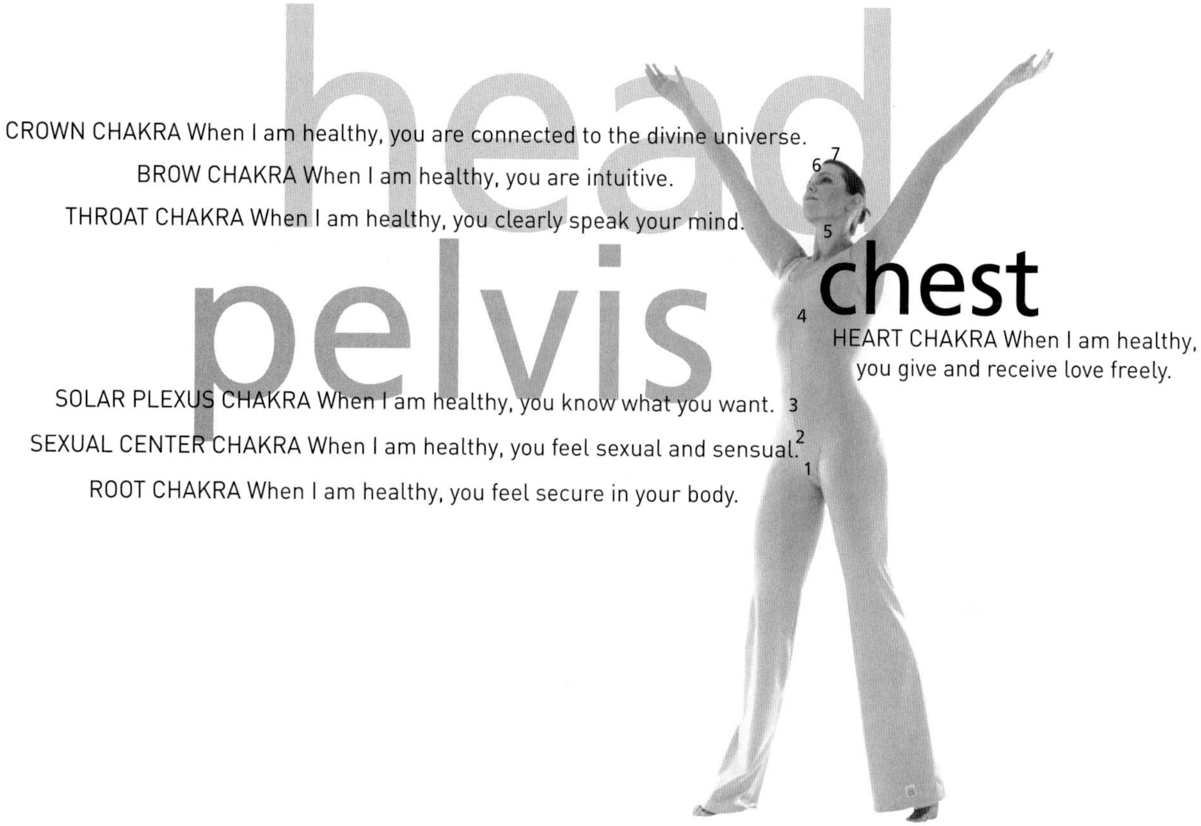

head

CROWN CHAKRA When I am healthy, you are connected to the divine universe. 7

BROW CHAKRA When I am healthy, you are intuitive. 6

THROAT CHAKRA When I am healthy, you clearly speak your mind. 5

chest

4 HEART CHAKRA When I am healthy, you give and receive love freely.

pelvis

SOLAR PLEXUS CHAKRA When I am healthy, you know what you want. 3

SEXUAL CENTER CHAKRA When I am healthy, you feel sexual and sensual. 2

ROOT CHAKRA When I am healthy, you feel secure in your body. 1

chakras and the core

Along the spine and inside the three body weights are major centers of the ethereal energy of chi. These energy centers, or chakras, are located near the major nerve plexus of the body. They are designed to move energy in and out, spinning energy clockwise and counterclockwise from the front and back of the body. Moving energy through these points increases and balances your body's energy. When your chakras are strong, balanced, and filled with energy, your body is strong—physically, mentally, and emotionally.

Moving the three body weights helps circulate the energy through these energy centers. As you move the three body weights, pay attention to individual chakras. Notice how you can become energetically and physically aware of these centers.

First Chakra—The Base or Root

The first chakra is located at the base of the spine and is physically stimulated by moving the coccyx, your tailbone. This chakra is directly affected by movement of your pelvis. When moved, it stimulates an energy exchange between the legs, coccyx, rectum, and sex organs. Move this center to develop a strong connection between your body and the earth as well as a sense of security and trust in life.

Second Chakra—The Sexual Center

The second chakra is housed in your pelvis and is affected by pelvic movement and subtle chest motions. Located at the first lumbar area, this chakra stimulates your large intestine, spleen, bladder, lower back, and sex organs. Move this chakra to develop a strong connection between your male and female sexual energy and to stimulate your powers of creation.

Third Chakra—The Solar Plexus

The third chakra, located at the mid-thoracic area near the solar plexus, is affected by movement of the pelvis, chest, and head. When moved, this chakra stimulates your heart, lungs, stomach, liver, adrenals, pancreas, kidneys, diaphragm, breasts, gallbladder, small intestines, and duodenum. Move this chakra to heighten your will, self-confidence, and personal power.

Fourth Chakra—The Heart

The fourth chakra, the heart chakra, is located at the first, second, and third thoracic vertebrae of the spine. It is affected predominantly by motions of your rib cage and chest. When moved, this chakra stimulates the

A **Nia** *Story*

RECOVERY

STUDENT: Kahlie Sue
CLASS LOCATION: Lyons, Colorado
OCCUPATION: Student

For many years, Kahlie Sue's life was haunted by bipolar disorder. The condition had caused her to self-medicate with marijuana and alcohol since the age of twelve. These substances, however, created addiction and became primary problems themselves.

To fight the disorder, Kahlie Sue was heavily medicated with conventional psychoactive drugs. "I have been on many medications," she notes, "and was once overmedicated with seventeen pills daily." These medications caused negative reactions, primarily torpor and extreme fatigue. At times, they made her feel as if she were existing in a vegetative state.

"The last medication that I was prescribed could absolutely not be used with other drugs or alcohol. I stayed with my mom the first weeks of my withdrawal. On the third day of it, she brought me to a Nia class. She made me come.

"I was in tears throughout the entire class, only to realize that it was from true release. I cried through the next two classes. After that, I cried only during the cool-down section. I don't cry much anymore, and when I do, it's from true letting go."

Nia became Kahlie Sue's most effective and enduring therapy.

"Nia has given me a venue in which I no longer have to hit a pillow in a sterile environment just to get release. Nia lets me actually work through emotions. When I was on meds, my emotions were suppressed and energy built up and caused racing thoughts, nervous tics, and compulsive outbursts.

"In Nia, though, I experience an emptying of pent-up energy. Nia is a safe environment in which I can share feelings and work out difficult issues with the help of other people's points of view, instead of being limited to just the perspectives of doctors."

"Most important," she adds, "Nia is a place to worship—not within the boundaries of any organized religion but with any higher power I choose to focus on that day."

Her work with Nia has enabled Kahlie Sue to finally understand herself. "Nia has helped me to peel away the layers and reveal my true self. After shedding these layers and remaining clean and sober, I now have the true Kahlie Sue to give to my family and friends."

Nia has, of course, also helped improve Kahlie Sue's body. She says her body now has "a glow." Her mother has also become a Nia student and has lost a considerable amount of weight. "The transformation Nia has made in my fifty-five-year-old mother is fabulous," she says.

However, Kahlie Sue's primary benefits from Nia are reflected not in her outward appearance, but in her inner life.

"Nia is a workout with your inner self," Kahlie Sue says. "It is moving meditation. Dance. Therapy. Church.

"I thank Nia for giving me a second chance."

heart, lungs, blood circulatory system, cardiac plexus, and entire chest area. Move this center to develop a connection with love, compassion, joy, and sorrow.

Fifth Chakra—The Throat

The fifth chakra, the throat chakra, is affected by head and neck movements. Located in the third cervical vertebra of the spine, this chakra stimulates the head, eyes, ears, face, and throat. Move this center to improve your ability for self-expression.

Sixth Chakra—The Brow or Third Eye

The sixth chakra, the brow chakra, is located at the first cervical vertebra of the spine, or bridge of the nose. When moved, this chakra stimulates the head, face, eyes, ears, throat, pituitary gland, lower brain, and nervous system. Move this center to develop a connection to your intuition.

Seventh Chakra—The Crown

The seventh chakra, the crown chakra, has no spinal contact at all. It is located above the crown of your head and is affected by your intention and your conscious connection to things beyond the physical realm. Physically centered at the point of your pineal gland, the seventh chakra stimulates the upper brain development of spiritual energy, and creates a connection between your physical and ethereal bodies. Move this center to develop a connection between you and divine energy.

The Voices of the Body's Core

The Voice of the Pelvis

To your physical body—I offer a basin, a bony container to hold the sacred parts of you that can create and bear life. My bones are a container meant to be filled with your essence. My tissues are soft. They are meant to be loved, respected, and nurtured by you. My movement is meant to be free like a butterfly. I am open so you can let life in. I connect you to your deepest desires, to the parts of you that seduce life. Move me, and dance the motion of love and freedom. Awaken the sexual and primal energy that lies waiting to be freed from within me.

To your mental body—I offer a conscious soul, the seat of your soul. Blending my energy and sensation with your desire and your will doubles your power. If you let me, I can speak to you, guiding you from a high place where your emotional charge and energy move you, but do not run you.

To your emotional body—I am a strong magnet, a force that grounds desires and dreams. Fill me with your sexual and sensual desire, to become powerful and strong.

To your spiritual body—I offer the freedom of flight. Move me and light up your cerebrospinal fluid. Feel the flow of this electromagnetically charged lava enlivening you. Move me and become unbound, expressive, and vital. I am the seed, touched by the hand of woman and man.

The Voice of the Chest

To your physical body—I offer protection for your heart. I govern the space where love and heart power grow. By design, I am open to the light; yet, like a birdcage, I protect something sacred and precious, your heart and lungs, the internal organs that make you a human. Through my openings, pulses the sound of life heard as a beat, the eternal rhythm of life.

To your mental body—I provide a path to your heart. My way of directing and thinking is linked to your breath and to the lover within. I am fuller at the bottom, making way for kundalini to rise and meet with the prana mind.

To your emotional body—I provide a home for feelings of love, sadness, grief, and joy. I am the transmission of energy through your flesh.

To your spiritual body—I awaken the expressive self. I am the vibration, the volcano of love and passion that flows into the world. I hold within me the child's heart, the heart that loves without condition. Move me, and rattle the insides of human memory.

The Voice of the Head

To your physical body—I am a container, the protector of your brain. My bony cap is an envelope whose jagged lines connect many thin bones. My jagged edges are a reminder that electrical energy is mind energy. Settle into my vase, where your thoughts and dreams dance within.

To your mental body—I am the place where cognition dances and imagination plays. Passion and excitation move me. My mobility becomes your freedom.

To your emotional body—I can take you into and out of your body, by pulling you up into the consciousness of mind. Let me flow, and you will deepen your mind-body connection. Feel me, and let go of thoughts.

To your spiritual body—I am an open vessel. I am the channel into your creative, intuitive, and thinking selves. I bring light and power into your upright being. I allow you to see with the eyes of the divine.

The Voice of the Spine

To your physical body—I am the internal structure of the trunk that allows movement. Long and flexible, I remind you to move from within, like a strand of pearls. My spiny protrusions, like thorns on a rosebush, extend from your back into spaces behind you. My energy centers, along the back of you, cascade your energy down into the earth.

To your mental body—I provide assistance in sensing spatial balance. I talk to all other parts of you, reminding you where center is: within. I am the one who can elegantly direct all running, dancing, and leaping. Listen to the voice of my mind, the mind of flexibility and direction. I support you with movable love.

To your emotional body—I provide a backbone. I make it possible for you to feel life with the utmost intensity. I ground the flow of emotion so you can remain upright, even in the most distressing of circumstances. I am to you what the stem is to the flower. I feed you, nourish you, and give birth to new buds as you open up to your feelings.

To your spiritual body—I provide support, regardless of how you may try to avoid me. I talk to you and remind you that love, pleasure, and ease are the paths of least resistance. My task is to align you with heaven and earth. I unite you with all that is. Love me, and I will guide you with the grace and power of an eagle.

the upper extremities: arms, hands and fingers

Reflecting the body's exquisite balance, the arms, hands, and fingers of the Upper Extremities are the perfect counterpoint to the legs, feet, and toes of the Base. However, you've probably seen people who had very little neuromuscular coordination between their Upper Extremities and their Base: Their arms probably seemed to be going in one direction, while their legs went in another. Nia corrects this disconnect. It unites the Upper Extremities, the Base, and the Core. In so doing, it helps create complete human beings.

Nia and the Arms, Hands, and Fingers

Your hands and arms are the messengers of your heart. Their movement gives voice to the silent world inside you. Every gesture expresses a part of you. Hands and arms feel and heal.

As a child, when you were afraid, your hands came to your face. When you needed love, you put your thumb in your mouth. When you wanted Mommy and Daddy, you reached out for them. However, over time, reaching out into the world may have lost its joy. Maybe no one was ever there to touch. Your environment, and the way you have responded to it, has embedded movement patterns into your arms and hands. Nia helps you break limiting patterns, and reconnect to the natural process of exploring the world and expressing yourself with your arms, hands, and fingers. It is easy, fun, playful, and efficient.

Like your feet, your arms and hands have their own sense organs that inform you about pain and pleasure. The hands have energy portals that move chi in and out of the body, and they have proprioceptors that are highly sensitive to physical sensation. These proprioceptors receive information about your internal body conditions. They tell you if you need to pull back or move more slowly and gently. They also communicate via sensation. Pain and pleasure, comfort and discomfort are their voices. As you move your hands and arms, the proprioceptors send information to your nervous system.

Since the hands have the capacity to gather so much information, in Nia, we use them extensively. Some schools of fitness rely on hard linear arm work and ignore the hand. Nia, however, combines both linear and fluid arm movements, as well as hand movements. The key to establishing fluidity and power comes from using the hands and arms together, in a natural and free way. Nia uses the joints of the fingers, wrists, and elbows as gateways to move energy. Opening and closing these joints "milks" the muscles and stimulates active communication between sensory organs and the nervous system. The more relaxed and efficient your movement, the better the communication. Furthermore, the better the communication, the more relaxation you experience in your movement.

In Nia, we often use imagery to initiate arm movements. We encourage people to pretend they're pulling strings, opening doors, wiping mirrors, tossing salads, or chopping wood. These visualizations trigger natural arm motions, which helps create a balanced energy flow. For example, if your body thinks it is actually going to lift a rock, it prepares for the lift by grounding and dropping energy. The Core of the body then engages, creating a natural, internal support structure in which to move the arms and hands. Using your hands to feel and sense will do far more for your arms than mechanical, repetitive movements. Visualizations create an engaging, familiar experience that fosters greater ease.

We also use many different kinds of arm and hand movements. Small delicate movements create dexterity and develop coordination. Larger movements help your hands, arms, and upper back muscles to become strong, defined, and flexible. Martial arts and jazzy movements require more precision, energy, practice, mental focus, and somatic attention. Combined, they allow you to gain muscle definition, flexibility, and strength without the use of external weights. You gain definition not by pumping iron but by moving the bones, joints, muscles, and connective tissues.

In Nia, we also link arm movements to emotion. Emotion is an effective way to stimulate movement of the hands and arms. Any reach, block, or strike is a direct response to a thought, intent, desire, or emotion. They are *real* expressions of what you feel.

Like lungs, the hands breathe. They breathe chi. They can spray and splash chi energy as if the fingers were shaking and releasing water. Closing the hands pulls energy into the arms and body, while opening the hands expands and releases energy. They can be used to consciously direct the flow of vital energy to a specific area that needs healing. From our study of aikido, we learned that the arms can "spiral" energy. All energy spirals begin with the hand, and move into the forearm. In fact, the forearm contains the only two bones in the body that spiral.

Your fingers, like wands, are magical tools. Each one can individually direct and move energy along particular meridians. In Nia, you vary the energy flow through the arm by using all five fingers, either one at a time or together. Moving finger by finger, you wake up the intrinsic muscles of the hands and arms. By visualizing, you can enhance the way you direct energy through your fingers.

Never dangle your arms aimlessly, unless it is intentional. Keep the arms and hands alive and engaged. This keeps a steady and constant flow of chi moving. In Nia, every hand and arm gesture counts. Nothing is random. Every gesture has meaning.

Nia and the Shoulder Girdle

The bones of the shoulder girdle support the movement of your arms and hands. These bones are the clavicles and scapula. The shoulder includes the shoulder girdle, the front, back, and sides of the body. The freer the shoulder girdle, the freer the arms and the more room for expression.

Anatomically, the upper arm bone actually floats—it is not anchored into a ball-and-socket joint (as the leg bone is to the hip). There is simply a gentle indentation where the bone rests. The support comes from muscles that are underneath, around, and inside the shoulder. This tells us that the design of the shoulder is intended to support free movement, with the shoulders floating.

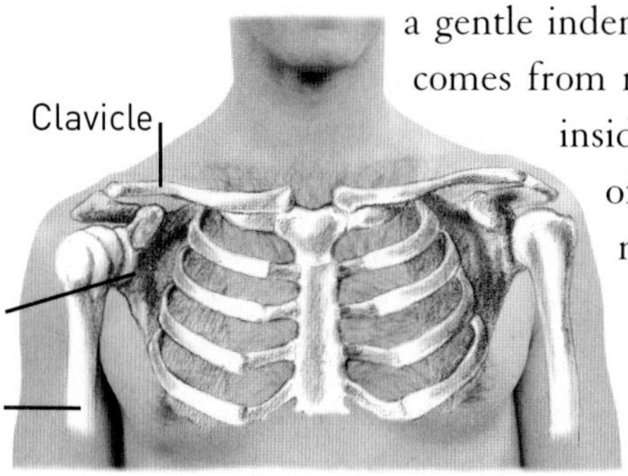

A flexible shoulder girdle will support fluidity in your upper body and along your spine. If the shoulder is locked, your body will feel stiff and rigid. This rigidity places stress in the neck, head, and shoulders. This, in turn, weakens the amount of energy and power you can move through the upper body, arms, and hands.

Rhomboid Muscles

Among the most important muscles of the Upper Extremities are the rhomboid muscles. Your rhomboids are located between your shoulder blades. They help draw the base of the shoulder blades in toward the midline of the body. If your rhomboids don't release, your movement will be restricted, and every time you lift your arm, your whole shoulder will go with it, straining your neck. Once they open, your arms can move freely, while your shoulder blades remain stable on the back. To get a sense of your rhomboids, draw your shoulder blades together and notice how they come close together at the back of your body. Now, open and stretch the rhomboids by giving yourself a strong hug. Notice how this releases the area between the shoulder blades, much like stretching the fabric at the back of your shirt. To contract the rhomboids, place your elbows behind you, and squeeze your shoulder blades gently together. Feel the front of your body stretch. Opposing movements allow for both expansion and contraction of the muscles, and pump fresh blood and chi through the muscles.

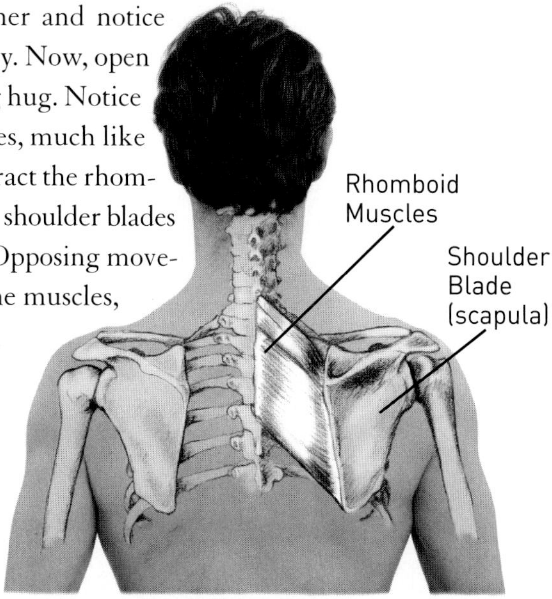

Rhomboid Muscles

Shoulder Blade (scapula)

Arm and Hand Movement

In Nia, after each arm movement, the arms return to the Core, or *neutral.* Physically, neutral is where the shoulder girdle is relaxed and the upper arm bones hang, vertically aligned to the earth. With every repetition, you have a new opportunity to execute the movement with greater skill, emotion, and power. Returning to the Core of the body helps you experience internal support for your movement. With each repetition, your awareness grows. In neutral, you can rest and recharge before moving again. We call this *coming back to neutral.* In neutral you gain energy and power by moving from a place of relaxation. This creates power and ease in your movement.

Another unique aspect of Nia is its emphasis on palm direction. The direction of your palms plays a key role in the way your shoulder joint opens or closes. For example, let your hands hang at your sides and turn the palms to face forward. Notice how the shoulder joint is open in the front, and closed in the back. Take a deep breath. This effectively and easily supports your arms when lifting them above your head or creating circular motions. Then, for contrast, turn the front of your palms to face behind you. The shoulder joint is closed in the front and open in the back. Take a deep breath. Any different? This limits your ability to breathe, to circle the arms around the shoulder joint or to effectively direct energy into the heavens. A closed joint limits your ability to deliver power.

Now, place the palm of your left hand against the front of your right shoulder and allow your right arm to hang. Turn the palm of your right hand in and out. Feel the opening and closing in the front of your shoulder joint as you turn the palm. Which position facilitates deeper breathing?

Voices of the Upper Extremities

The Voice of the Arms and Hands

To your physical body—I offer you a way to touch, hug, and love. When you desire, I open like a fan and reach out to fulfill your wishes. When you are scared, I hold you. When you need love, I touch you. Use me, and discover the joy of play: throwing, grabbing, scooping, and pushing. I am alive. Awaken to my endless possibilities.

To your mental body—I offer a way to outwardly express what you are thinking and imagining. When your thoughts are free, I am open and relaxed, available to sensations of life. When your thoughts are rigid and fearful, I become tight and bound. When your thoughts are free to move, I expand and dream. I am agile, strong, and powerfully available to help you create.

To your emotional body—I offer visual aids for expressing what you feel. As you open to what is moving inside of you, I respond, without needing any thought. I speak without words. I am clear, direct, and exact. I do not lie. I cannot.

To your spiritual body—I offer ways to experience becoming the angel, the warrior, the goddess or god. My energy is magic, and fills you with the power of lightning, to become strong, or liquid, to become full and soft. My divine essence allows you to hold space for yourself and for others, through the magic of touch.

The Voice of the Shoulder Girdle

To your physical body—I offer you wings. Use me to feel free, not bound or rigid in your arms. By design, I am light, movable. Dance with me and sense effortless action. Breathe fully and give flight to your shoulder blades.

To your mental body—I offer you a way to pull your thoughts back or release them. Allow my wings to tenderly embrace you. Trust that my movement, empowered by your imagination, has the intelligence to heal.

A **Nia** *Story*

FROM FAT TO FIT

STUDENT: Helen

CLASS LOCATION: Houston, Texas

OCCUPATION: Teacher

Helen stepped out of her size-eighteen pants one night, looked in a mirror, and stopped dead in her tracks. "What happened to my body?" she asked herself.

She had been so busy establishing her career as a stockbroker that she'd slid into bad habits: late, heavy meals with clients; no exercise; and compulsive eating.

"I'd be so exhausted after work that I'd make a beeline for the couch, stare numbly at the TV, and stuff my mouth without thinking. In the morning, I'd panic just thinking about dragging myself through another day. What had happened to the lively woman who, only a year earlier, had been able to breeze through twelve-hour workdays with ease? How did she turn into such a tired wreck?"

Helen had gone from a size twelve to a size eighteen and had forty pounds of fat layered onto her once-lithe body.

"I signed up for an aerobics class, but two minutes into the first routine, I was panting and perspiring, and knew I'd never be able to keep up. I ran out of the room, humiliated.

"Out in the hallway, I heard music coming from the studio next door, an odd mix of jazz, reggae, and classical. Curious, I went inside, and there were about a hundred people—some of them much heavier than me—dancing and gliding to the beat of a Nia class.

"The instructor was saying, 'Imagine the floor is a sea of electrical sockets and every time you take a step, you're plugging in your foot and drawing energy!' I stood in the back of the class, and in spite of myself, I closed my eyes and swayed to the music. By the time the class was over, I felt more energetic than I had in months, mostly just from watching.

"When I got home, I did what I've always done; I headed to the couch. But I had too much energy to sit still. The next morning, I actually found myself looking forward to the day ahead. If just one Nia class could make me feel this good, I knew I wanted more.

"Soon I was doing Nia every day, and the weight came off. Within a year, I went from being burned out and overweight to enjoying simple pleasures like dancing, exercising, and going to parties. It was at one of these parties that I met my husband, Joe, and fell in love.

"Now, six years later, I'm more successful than ever. I'm a Black Belt Nia trainer. I've lost forty pounds, and Joe and I have a beautiful little girl.

"Sure, I'm still busy, but I'm no longer tired. Thanks to Nia, my life has meaning."

To your emotional body—I am an extension of your feelings. When you desire a hug, it is I who wraps and entwines you in self-love. I help you respond to the outside world and protect you from harm.

To your spiritual body—I remind you of your birthright to give and to receive. Through my wings, receive earth and heaven energy. Soar with me, making every hand, arm, shoulder, and shoulder blade action one of peace and harmony.

the body's way

This is the Body's Way. It is the way the body is designed to function. But is it the way *your* body functions? Chances are, probably not—at least not at this time. Not yet.

Your body likely functions in its own unique, personalized way—*your* Body's Way—and that is what we'll look at next, as you continue your quest for healing and fitness.

three
Your Body's Way

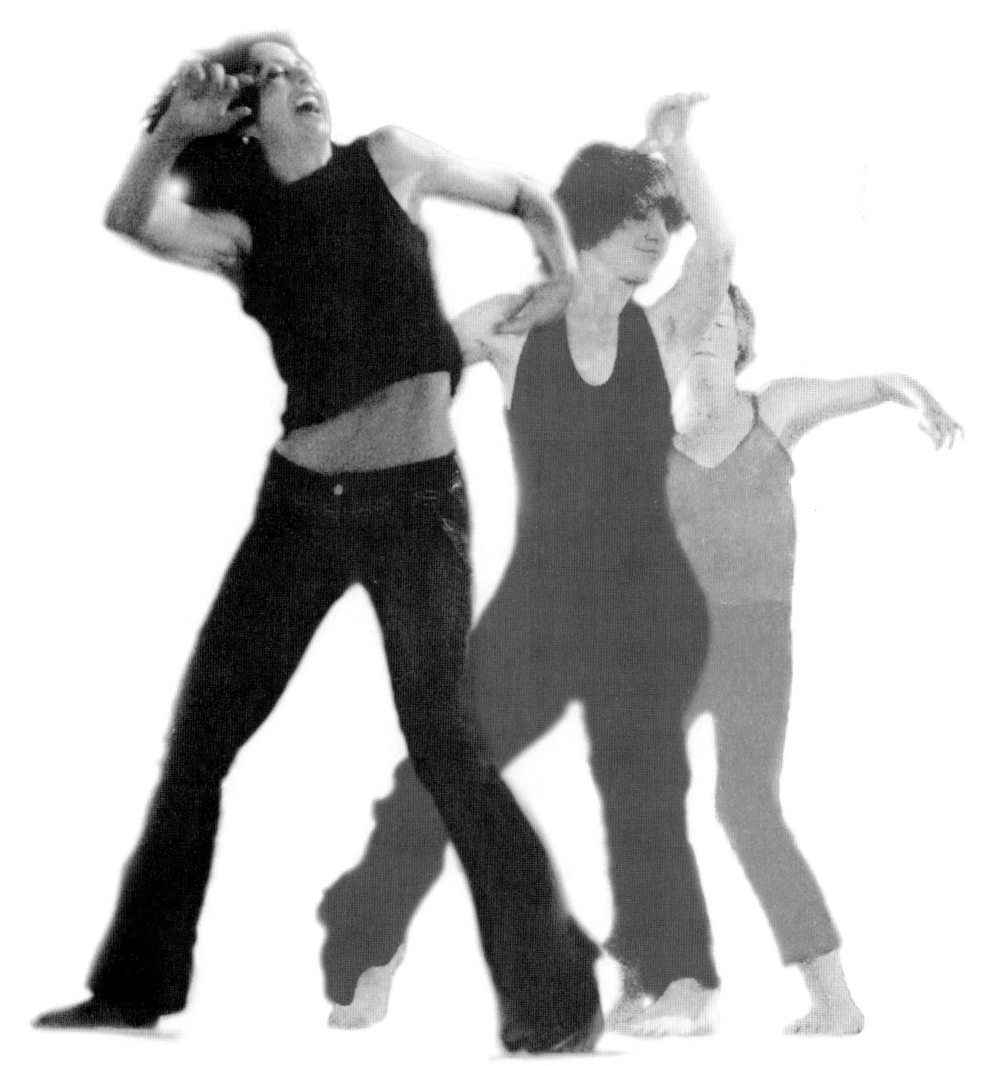

Every Nia student wants to always function in perfect accord with the Body's Way. But no one can—not all the time.

Why?

Because rarely is anyone structurally perfect.

The Body's Way represents the absolute pinnacle of proper physical function. It means using the body with faultless efficiency and dynamic ease. It means achieving consummate balance, the perfect mix of mobility and stability, and an unparalleled blend of yin and yang energies. Mastering the Body's Way is a fantastic goal; but like all other forms of perfection, this goal is unattainable for many people, much of the time.

Therefore, in Nia, we emphasize moving in accord with not only the Body's Way, but also with *your* Body's Way.

Your Body's Way is the current design and function of your own body.

Every body is somewhat different, so your Body's Way is somewhat different from that of any other body on earth. In Nia, we start with *your* Body's Way and try to gradually merge it with *the* Body's Way.

Often, Nia students come extremely close to achieving the Body's Way in almost all of their movements. Even more often, they regularly achieve the Body's Way in some of their movements but fall short in others. This does not mean that these students are failing. It simply means that the Body's Way is an ongoing process and that Nia is an ongoing practice.

Your Body's Way has been influenced by a number of factors, many of which were probably quite negative. As a child you probably experienced the flood of energy that's common among kids and felt like being active during most of your waking hours. However, if you were like most children, your parents and teachers frequently told you to sit still and be quiet. If so, this enforced inactivity was largely a mistake. Children—and adults, too—are *physically designed for movement.* If this were not true, we wouldn't have mobile joints, pliable muscles, and motor nerves. The human body was *built* for motion—and emotion.

As we leave childhood—with its endless hours of sitting at school desks—other negative forces take over. For most of us, the worst force fighting the Body's Way is our job. Too often, we either get stuck behind desks or get trapped in jobs that require frequent physical repetition.

Desk jobs are far too sedentary, and jobs based on physical repetition cause overuse injuries such as carpal tunnel syndrome and chronic back pain. For about forty hours every week, many of us find ourselves doing work that takes us further and further from the Body's Way.

Often we try to compensate for the physical abuse of our working lives by exercising. We think exercise will make us limber, strong, and youthfully exuberant again. However, many people find conventional exercise to be emotionally stultifying and brutally repetitive—and it often actually exacerbates the existing insults against the body. In effect, people rotate from assembly-line jobs to assembly-line workouts. Imbalances are burned into the body's neural networks and are imprinted on muscles, bones, and connective tissues.

Other factors also influence the all-too-common departure from the Body's Way. One major factor is attitude. Rigid, uptight thinking often results in rigid, uptight bodies. In addition, poor sleeping habits, including not getting enough sleep or even sleeping on an unsuitable mattress, can take a toll on the body. So does bad nutrition. The most frequent form of bad nutrition is simply eating too much, which causes the body to sag beneath the onerous burden of excessive weight. However, the body can also be hurt by insufficient intake of various nutrients, such as calcium and magnesium, which keep bones strong and muscles and ligaments flexible.

The Body's Way is also assaulted by accidents, illnesses, and injuries. Sometimes these forces are subtle and take a gradual toll. Other times they're cataclysmic.

So, after surviving all these negative factors, what's left? A broken body, beyond repair? No—just *your* body, with the signature weaknesses, strengths, and "design modifications" that have come to make up your Body's Way.

If you're similar to most people, your Body's Way is probably characterized by problems in five primary places: knees, hips, lower back, neck, and shoulders. These are the overly abused trouble spots that commonly suffer from the chronic movement mistakes that may have become a part of your Body's Way.

Fortunately, people often gain almost immediate relief in these common trouble spots when they begin to practice Nia. For example, in one recent Nia class, a new student made progress in just a matter of minutes. She was a young woman who had been suffering from almost constant tension in her neck and shoulders. We convinced her of the importance of keeping her jaw muscles relaxed and showed her how to direct all of her arm movements with her palms—as *you* will soon learn to do. At the end of the class, she was ecstatic and said her neck and shoulders felt better than they had in years.

This success could not have happened, however, if we had simply insisted that she start moving her arms in just "the right way." She had not yet established the neurological connections that would have made this possible. Instead, with our coaching, she first identified her *own* Body's Way—the way of moving in which she felt most comfortable—and then modified it into a style that was more consistent with the Body's Way.

In this chapter, we'll coach you on how to discover your Body's Way, so that you can begin to shift *your* Body's Way to *the* Body's Way.

This shift will not occur all at once, in all parts of your body. Instead, it will happen in stages and will probably be confined to separate areas and individual movements. Over time, each of these different improvements will be integrated into the entirety of your body, mind, spirit, and emotions.

In fact, your rate and degree of progress will be governed completely by *you,* as you set goals and then achieve them. The goals you set will all be grounded in your Body's Way and will move toward *the* Body's Way. As you set these goals, it's important to make them achievable and realistic. Successes don't have to be spectacular to be important. Often, success that is built by increments is more enduring than sudden success. In fact, our most fundamental beliefs about self-healing are

- *Small is big.*
- *Less is more.*

Let's say that you have set a goal for yourself, based on your Body's Way, of improving your hip mobility. That's a realistic goal and an important one. As you create incremental successes, you will find yourself going through five distinct phases of self-healing. Here are the five stages you'll experience on your way to reaching this goal.

the five stages of self-healing

Inspired by Stanley Keleman's book *Emotional Anatomy,* we incorporated the following process of healing as an integral part of Nia practice and training. It is a way to accept and value where you are and safely guide yourself along the path toward self-healing.

Embryonic. In the embryonic stage, you inaugurate change by listening to the voice of your hip, with its language of pleasure and pain. The discomfort you feel in your hip joint when you try to move your leg tells you that the joint is insufficiently mobile and needs self-healing.

You consider the design of the hip joint. It's a ball-and-socket joint, which tells you that it is built to allow your pelvis to move freely, your femur to swivel, and your body to squat down and rise up effortlessly. However, in the embryonic stage, you can't achieve this. Obviously, there is a big gap between your Body's Way and the Body's Way.

The first, embryonic step you'll take in closing this gap is to simply explore the condition of your hip. Pay attention to the things that make it feel more flexible, more comfortable, and stronger. Don't force anything. *Just be aware.*

Creeping. The second stage of self-healing, creeping, requires consciously guiding your hip movements in new, healthier patterns that support you in moving more freely. Maybe this will mean softening and seeking more flexibility in the hip joint, or it could mean the opposite—the need to tighten and strengthen the hip joint. It all depends on your Body's Way.

Crawling. In the crawling stage, you continue to explore, venturing into new movement territories and taking occasional minor risks. You consciously change the range of motion, so you begin to discover new skills, such as the ability to squat and rise more effortlessly, and change the direction of your feet, which makes moving the thighbone in the hip joint more efficient.

Standing. You are no longer exploring when you reach the fourth stage, standing. You are enjoying the benefits of your heightened attention and your actions. You keep challenging yourself, pushing back the edge of risk as you gain strength and flexibility. You sink more deeply as you move and play with your ability to balance.

Walking. At the walking stage, you have reached your goal. You can move freely. Your femur can swivel pain free in the hip joint. You can squat down and rise up in comfort. Your hip joint has achieved significantly more mobility (or stability), and this feels good. You take time to enjoy it. Once you arrive at the fifth stage and have achieved your goal, you set another. This time it may be the ability to squat down and rise up faster and with more power, improving speed as well as range of motion. Every time you set a new goal, you move inexorably toward the Body's Way.

As people move through these five stages again and again and progress from success to success, they invariably begin to look better. Often, they lose fat and gain muscle. Other times, they become notably more graceful and exude more confidence and self-esteem in their body language. Of course, everyone likes looking better. Ironically, though, the natural desire to look better can be a major obstacle to improvement.

A **Nia** *Story*

I FEEL LIKE A KID AGAIN!

STUDENT: Lynda

CLASS LOCATION: Tempe, Arizona

OCCUPATION: University Health Educator

After taking just two Nia classes, and then the Nia White Belt Intensive Student-Teacher Training, Lynda wanted to quit her fitness job and become a Nia teacher. Nia had changed the way she saw the world.

The first change in her perspective was the way she perceived exercise. Before Nia, she had worked hard at being fit, to the point of developing an exercise addiction, abusing and injuring her body. She *liked the results of exercising—her* body *didn't. "I was out of balance, not listening to my body. Nia has shaken up my beliefs about traditional fitness," she says. "I now prefer listening to my body and moving in a way that fits my energy that moment, rather than pushing, forcing, and pounding during workouts. I realized that I had a lot of ideas that were based on what I had learned from experts, but now I view my* body *as the expert. I honor what my body needs."*

Nia also changed the way she perceived herself. "I changed how I defined myself," she recalls. "The artistic, creative, and expressive parts of me are now present in the world. Emotionally, Nia has reconnected me to the joy of being alive and enhanced my self-awareness. It brought out the kid inside me."

Because Lynda is now forthright about who she truly is, she has gained deeper intimacy with others. "Nia has helped me be more present in my friendships," she says. "Instead of hiding parts of myself, I am letting friends see who I am and what I really think and feel. Doing Nia has also made me more playful in my relationship with my husband. I now see myself as a beautiful, powerful, sexual woman. For me, Nia is about being truly present in the world and being myself 100 percent of the time. No more censoring and hiding!"

Nia has even changed elements of her basic personality. "I used to get stressed out a lot," Lynda recalls, "and have wicked outbursts of anger, with temper tantrums. Since my Nia White Belt training, though, the need to express myself this way has disappeared. Nia grounds me in the present moment, and I find this calming and centering. I focus on sensing the present and enjoying my daily life."

Most of all, Nia has changed the way she sees her own body. "I feel so beautiful doing Nia—and I feel beautiful afterward. Fat days just don't happen anymore!"

Nia and body image

An older woman came to a Nia class in Portland, Oregon, and while she was chatting with Carlos before the class, she said, "I want to change my thighs."

"Do you like your thighs?" Carlos asked.

She looked at him as if he were from another planet.

Nevertheless, she began attending classes on a regular basis, and eventually Carlos convinced her to start wearing shorts to class to reveal her thighs, instead of wearing a long, loose skirt. It was hard for the student to do this; but as soon as she did, she began to *accept* her thighs, just as they were. She realized that her thighs were a part of her—not punishment from heaven above—and that to hate them was to hate herself. When she finally accepted her thighs, and herself, *then* she really began to change.

Many people think that change can come only from *dis*satisfaction, but it's the other way around. As long as you refuse to accept yourself, you'll stay stuck in the low-energy, black hole of self-doubt. But if you can find things you like about yourself, you'll get a new rush of energy and a new burst of confidence and ambition. Self-hate is self-defeating, but self-acceptance is empowering.

Unfortunately, many people, particularly women, become mired down by the terrible inertia that arises from not liking their own bodies. At its worst, this attitude becomes the diagnosable phenomenon of body dysmorphic disorder. Nia, however, creates the opposite effect—a "body euphoric" phenomenon.

One of the ways we do this is by focusing on the immediate pleasure of physical sensation, rather than on image-oriented goals that cannot be reached until far into the future. We teach people to *enjoy* their bodies and to savor how good their bodies feel. Once students begin to enjoy how their bodies feel, it's usually easy for them to start to love their bodies, flaws and all.

Furthermore, we teach people to look at themselves from a whole new perspective, using a technique we call *X-Ray Anatomy.* This technique is far more advanced than the conventional assessment of "How fat am I?" or "How strong am I?"

X-Ray Anatomy can change the way you see yourself.

x-ray anatomy

The body's surface tells a story about what lies within, physically as well as emotionally. You can access this information with X-Ray Anatomy and use it to realign and heal your body.

The purpose of X-Ray Anatomy is to help you see beneath your skin, using your eyes, intuition, and imagination. When you perform the technique correctly, it will allow you to discover where your bones sit and how muscles and connective tissues rest over the bones. With the information you gather from X-Ray Anatomy, you can properly strengthen and stretch muscles and connective tissues to achieve correct balance and alignment.

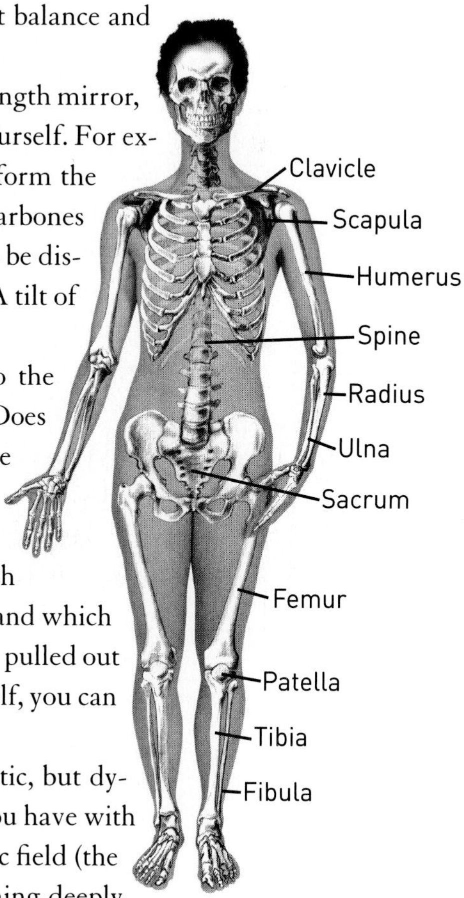

To perform X-Ray Anatomy, stand in front of a full-length mirror, preferably with most or all of your clothing off. Study yourself. For example, look at your clavicle bones (collarbones), which form the front part of your shoulder girdle. Ideally, your collarbones should be perfectly level. Are they? If not, what seems to be disrupting their position? Tight muscles in the shoulders? A tilt of the spine?

Focus on other body parts, such as your knees. Do the kneecaps turn in, turn out, or tilt? Look at your hips. Does your pelvis tilt, front or back? Is one hip higher than the other? How are your arms hanging? Are they in front of your body? Too far out from the sides?

Merely by looking at yourself, you can determine which muscles are too tight or too lax, which muscles lack tone, and which muscles or connective tissues are causing your bones to be pulled out of alignment. After you've gained this insight into yourself, you can use the knowledge to change the ways you move.

Keep in mind that alignment and posture are not static, but dynamic. They are maintained through the relationships you have with gravity (the "down" forces), and with the electromagnetic field (the "up and out" forces). Through movement and by breathing deeply and fully, you can help your bones and joints slip into proper alignment, so that your bones can do the job they were designed to do: to maintain the proper internal space that is necessary for the body to function efficiently. Your bones provide the framework for maintaining that space.

With X-Ray Anatomy, you can easily see the vertical and horizontal lines that reflect the internal placement of your bones and joints. Using this information, you can determine which of your muscles are too tight or too loose. Then, you can begin the process of self-healing, through movement. You can use the Nia moves, and your Nia workout—as well as the daily movements in your own life—to help bring your body back into proper alignment.

X-RAY ANATOMY 101

When your bones and joints are in alignment:

1. They provide you with both stability and mobility.
2. They make it possible for your bones, joints, muscles, ligaments, and tendons to work in proper coordination with your nervous system, providing you with a neurophysical structure that moves efficiently.
3. They use the internal, small, intrinsic muscles the way they were designed to be used—for internal stability and support; this is exactly what you need in order to move efficiently and to avoid overuse of the external, larger, superficial muscles.
4. They use the external, larger, superficial muscles the way they were designed to be used—for external gross mobility and stability.
5. They support the necessary relationship between the vertical and the horizontal flow of energy, which supports you in moving dynamically, with less physical effort and strain.
6. They help you achieve dynamic posture, which balances internal pressures with external environmental pressures.
7. They help you identify the sensations of proper bone and joint alignment, making it possible for you to break bad movement habits and to choose better ways of moving.

witnessing

Have you ever stood in front of a mirror and really looked at yourself objectively? As you look at yourself—whether during a session of X-Ray Anatomy or at other times—it's very helpful to implement another Nia technique: Witnessing.

Often it's difficult to be completely objective about your own body. We all tend to be our own toughest critics. However, you will never gain true, realistic information about your own body until you are able to see yourself as you really are. You've got to turn off your self-critical inner dialogue. You can't let fears about your own image make you look *worse* to yourself than you actually are, and you can't let vanity trick you into thinking you look *better* than you really do.

Witnessing involves not only assessing yourself visually but also focusing on how you feel. When you are doing a movement and you see that your arms are too high, you need to connect that information with how it feels. This enables you to fully integrate the new knowledge into your mind and body.

Witnessing creates awareness during exercise, which is one of the most vital components of Nia. Awareness, in Nia, is the starting point of all action.

natural time

Have you ever been in an exercise or yoga class and felt you couldn't keep up or simply felt out of sync? Nia has one more individualizing element that helps people remain aware and stay in the here and now while they work out. We call this element *Natural Time.* Natural Time is different from standard, by-the-clock, mechanical time. Mechanical time is absolutely uniform among all people, during all activities. Natural Time, however, is relative from one person to the next and from one activity to the next. It is based on the fact that different people operate at different speeds, and perceive the world according to varying time frames. Thus *Natural Time is your time.*

It is critically important for you to perform your Nia workout according to your own Natural Time. If you try to speed up or slow down the pace of your movements to match a contrived ideal, your movements will no longer be individualized and in accord with your Body's Way.

When you move in harmony with Natural Time, you will often find yourself moving slowly as you learn new movements. This slow pace will allow you to build proper neural connections and muscular coordination as you master the movements. If you rush through new movements in mechanical time, however, you will build faulty neural networks, which create improper muscle memories. As these incorrect neural networks and somatic memories become established, you might often *feel* as if you were doing a movement correctly, even though you're really not. Therefore, it's important to learn all new movements in Natural Time, and to *later* accelerate them. After all, *speed is the illusion of mastery.*

One of the advantages of doing movements in Natural Time is that it decreases the amount of thinking that you must do as you move. If you're rushing through your movements at a pace that's too fast or to keep up with the music or with those around you, you'll find yourself thinking too much in an effort to coordinate your movements: "Left, right, one, two—whoops!" This inner dialogue only makes coordination more difficult. It separates the body and mind. Natural Time doesn't require an inner dialogue. Rather, it's instinctual, you do it because it feels right.

discovering your body's way

Now it's time for you to heighten your own physical awareness and to more fully understand your Body's Way.

To help you do this, we have devised a series of checklists that help you explore the mobility and stability of your joints, your levels of body awareness, Sensory IQ, and your energy type as they relate to the different forms of Nia movement. Once you complete these self-exploratory checklists, you'll probably know more about your Body's Way than you ever have before. And you'll be better able to adapt the workout in Chapter 5 to your own physical and sensory needs.

Mobility and Stability

The Body's Way reminds us that healthy joints require toned surrounding muscles. Good muscle tone keeps your joints and bones aligned and your muscles responsive to the demands for mobility and stability. To check out your body's joint mobility and stability, use the "Joint Mobility and Stability Guide," as well as sensation, to find out which joints are too tight or too loose. Then record your findings in the "Joint Mobility and Stability Results" chart. The sensation of too tight means you've lost mobility and can't fully move the joint the way it was designed to move. This indicates you need to do some self-healing by loosening things up. The sensation of too loose means you don't have enough positive tension—the kind of tension that provides strength and stability. If you lack stability, you'll need to do some self-healing by tightening things up.

As you work your way through the guide, record your findings in the results chart by checking the appropriate box. Do both your right and your left sides and choose among "full mobility" (F), "moderate mobility" (M), and "slight mobility" (S). In general, *Full* indicates that you have 90 to 100 percent of the ideal range of motion and means your joint is healthy. *Moderate* indicates you have 50 to 90 percent of full range of motion. *Slight* indicates that you have less than 50 percent of the full range of motion.

Once you've completed the test, feel free to move on without much concern for joints you've marked "full." For joints you've marked "moderate," you'll need to exercise with greater care. For joints marked "slight," you should move ahead cautiously.

The Ankle

Full mobility means your ankle joint can fully open up in the back and close in the front (to flex your foot up toward your shinbone) and circle in both directions. It also means you can stretch the muscles in the front of your shin and contract your calf muscles (to point your toe all the way downward).

Mobility Test *Lift your leg slightly off the floor and flex your foot up and down. Next, circle your foot in both directions, sensing for mobility in your ankle joint. Repeat while standing on the other leg.*

Full stability means your ankle joint can support you in rising up and down on your toes, without wobbling in or out to the sides. Instability is the feeling of your feet grabbing the floor, your toes pulling in and overly contracting the muscles of your feet.

Stability Test *While standing, slowly rise onto the balls of both feet, bringing both heels high off the ground. Sustain elevated balance. Then slowly lower both heels back down, sensing for stability in your ankle joints as you stop moving.*

The Knee

Full mobility means your knee joint can close enough to bring your heel up and close to your buttocks. It also means your knee joint can open all the way, contracting your quadriceps (front of thigh muscles) and stretching your hamstrings (back of thigh muscles).

Mobility Test *Lift your leg off the floor so that you can freely bend and extend your lower leg, sensing for mobility in your knee joint. Repeat while standing on the other leg.*

Full stability means your knee joint can support you in moving and stopping without locking or tensing. Instability is the feeling of your knees pushing back and overly contracting your thigh muscles.

Stability Test *Walk briskly around the room and stop suddenly, several times, sensing for stability in your knee joints.*

The Hip

Full mobility means your hip joint can freely move your thigh and pelvis, making it easy to lift and lower your leg, turn your toes (in, out, or parallel), walk with grace, run with ease, sink and rise effortlessly, and move your pelvis freely.

Mobility Test

Stand with your feet wider than hip width, and your knees slightly bent. Circle your pelvis in both directions, as though using a hula hoop, with minimal knee movement. Next, lift one foot off the floor and circle your thigh. Then turn your toes in, out, and parallel, moving from the hip joint, to assess your mobility. Repeat while standing on the other leg.

Full stability means your hip joint can fully support you in balancing, walking, sinking, and rising. Instability is the feeling of your hips being out of control.

Stability Test

Walk freely around the room and stop suddenly. Pause, balancing on one foot, as you sense the stability in your hip joint. Repeat and balance on the other foot.

The Wrist

Full mobility means your wrist joint can flex and pull your fingers up and back. It can also extend your palm forward, pointing your fingers down. You can also fluidly circle your hand in both directions.

Mobility Test

Circle your hand in both directions. Next, flex your hand with your palm facing away from you, and gently pull your fingers up and back toward you. Next, bend your palm forward, pointing your fingers down. Now gently pull your fingers toward you, noticing the mobility in your wrist.

Full stability means your wrist joint can support you in starting and stopping motions, as in catching a ball, and in holding, balancing, and bearing body weight, as in a handstand or holding on to a handrail. Instability is the feeling of your wrists collapsing.

Stability Test

Wave your hand aggressively, then suddenly stop your hand and forearm from moving. Sense for stability in your wrist as you stop moving.

The Elbows

Full mobility means your elbow joint can open up to extend your forearm in a straight line. It can also close, bringing your hand up to your shoulder. Full mobility also means you can freely shake the muscles in your forearm and hand.

Mobility Test *With your arm hanging down at the side of your body and with your palm facing front, bring your hand up toward the same shoulder. Next move your hand back down, opening up the inside of your elbow. You should be able to open and close all the way. Repeat with the other arm.*

Full stability means your elbow joint can suddenly stop any hand and arm motion. It can also support body weight. Instability is the feeling of your elbows giving out.

Stability Test *Point out into space with your index finger and extend your entire arm. Sense for stability in your elbow joint as you sustain your reach into space. Repeat with the other arm.*

The Shoulder

Full mobility means your shoulder joint can support your upper arm in moving in all directions.

Mobility Test *Freely move your upper arm in all directions: up, down, front, back, and all around. Sense for mobility in your shoulder joint and notice any resistance. Repeat with the other shoulder.*

Full stability means your shoulder joint can support your hands and arms in starting and stopping motions and in supporting body weight. Instability is the feeling that your shoulders are incapable of providing support and power to your arms and hands.

Stability Test *With your hand, throw an imaginary ball up into space. Next, thrust your arm and hand up in front of you, as a shield. Sense for stability in your shoulder joint as you stop moving. Repeat with the other shoulder.*

The Spine

Full mobility means that your spine can support you in moving off your standard vertical alignment—folding, opening, bending, extending, and twisting. It can change shape easily and return to a relaxed and powerful state of vertical alignment.

Bend forward, rounding your spine, and hang. Next, stand tall and look up at the ceiling, extending and lengthening your spine. Then stand tall and twist from left to right. Now bend side to side. Sense for mobility in your spine. *Mobility Test*

Full stability means your spine can support you from the inside out to lift, lower, bend, twist, push, and pull. Instability is the feeling that your spine is weak and vulnerable.

With your hands holding on to an imaginary blanket, shake the blanket several times, sensing for stability in your spine as you stop moving. *Stability Test*

JOINT MOBILITY AND STABILITY RESULTS

	*Mobility**			*Stability**		
Joint	*F*	*M*	*S*	*F*	*M*	*S*
Left ankle						
Right ankle						
Left knee						
Right knee						
Left hip						
Right hip						
Left wrist						
Right wrist						
Left elbow						
Right elbow						
Left shoulder						
Right shoulder						
Spine						

* *F*, full; *M*, moderate; *S*, slight.

Body Awareness

Do you, like so many people, essentially sleepwalk through the physical aspects of your life, unaware of your movements from moment to moment? If so, you should try to become more aware of your physical actions, since awareness—based on sensation—is the first step toward improvement.

The "Body Awareness Checklist" will help you monitor your awareness. If you answer never to any of these statements, work on increasing your attention to these physical acts. Wake up! Get into your body! Become aware!

BODY AWARENESS CHECKLIST

Body Area	*Always*	*Sometimes*	*Never*
1. I am aware of my feet, and the exact direction they point in as I walk.			
2. I am aware of my pelvis moving when I walk.			
3. I am aware of my spine moving as I walk.			
4. I am aware of my head moving as I walk.			
5. I am aware of where I look with my eyes when I walk.			
6. I am aware of the vibration in my chest when I talk.			
7. I am aware of the tone of my voice.			
8. I am aware of my facial expressions.			
9. I am aware of my hands when I hold a fork, knife, or spoon.			
10. I am aware of the texture of the food I eat.			
11. I am aware of the physical feeling of being full.			
12. I am aware of the water touching my body when I shower.			

A **Nia** *Story*

HEALING FIBROMYALGIA

STUDENT: Sandy

CLASS LOCATION: Thornhill, Ontario

OCCUPATION: Nia Teacher

"It is a cliché," Sandy notes, "to say that Nia changed my life—but that's the truth!"

Since childhood, Sandy had been very athletic. She'd participated in a variety of sports and outdoor activities, as both a player and a coach. In July 1994, though, she suddenly became quite ill, with symptoms of severe muscle pain and weakness.

After several harrowing weeks of diagnostic workups, her physicians concluded that she had contracted fibromyalgia, a generally intractable chronic condition that causes excruciating, widespread muscle pain.

"My doctor," she recalls, "was wise enough to tell me that conventional medicine would probably not help me. She said that each individual must explore every available option." Thus Sandy began a long and difficult process of medical exploration. During this period, she was frequently incapacitated by the pain and fatigue caused by fibromyalgia, which cannot be effectively treated with conventional medical care.

"The prospect of being a virtual prisoner in my body was terrifying to me," she recalls. "It took nearly two years of experimentation and severe disability before I discovered Nia.

"As soon as I set foot in my very first class," she notes, "I was mesmerized. My first reaction was utter amazement that I was even able to complete the class without totally exhausting myself. For the first time in many months, I was able to receive pleasure from physical activity."

Soon, Sandy was attending three classes every week, a physical feat that previously would have been impossible. "In the beginning," she says, "I virtually had to learn how to walk all over again, and in time I rebuilt and reshaped my entire physical structure. I became convinced that this opportunity to re-create my physical being was truly a gift. Not many people get a second chance."

As Sandy's involvement with Nia progressed, she began to experience not only physical improvement but also mental, emotional, and spiritual growth. "I gradually developed a heightened awareness," she says. "The attention I gave to my mental, emotional, and spiritual selves was a unique experience for me. Each realm seemed to take on a life of its own, and after a while I learned how to live among all of them together."

Nia has also had a great impact on her family life. "At the time I became ill," Sandy recalls, "my three kids were still quite young, and I was scared, frustrated, and depressed at my state of affairs. I could do very little for them." Now, that frustration is over. "These days, there are very few times I cannot participate in my life to the extent I want."

Sensory IQ

Just as your brain has a cognitive IQ, your body has a Sensory IQ, which is a measure of how adroit you are at noticing physical sensation. Whereas body awareness relates to knowing and understanding how your body is moving in space, Sensory IQ relates to understanding and recognizing physical sensations, such as pleasure and pain.

It should be easy for people to be aware of the physical sensations of pleasure and pain, but many people are not. People often become, in effect, divorced from their own bodies. They repress pleasure and ignore pain, often under the misguided assumption that they're being strong. Alienation from your own body is not a sign of strength. It's a weakness.

The checklist on page 85 will help you become more aware of your pleasures and pains and be better able to identify your trouble spots. You are going to rate the pleasure and pain you feel day to day in different parts of your body. *Slight* means the sensation you feel of pain or pleasure is minor and transient. *Moderate* indicates a mid-range level of sensation—stronger, fuller, deeper, and longer lasting. *Acute* indicates a high level of sensation—very strong, very full, very deep, and essentially constant.

Based on your answers, you'll either celebrate the parts of your body where you feel pleasure or, using the Nia workout, you'll change what you do in order to reduce or eliminate pain.

SENSORY IQ CHECKLIST						
Body Area	***Painful***			***Pleasurable***		
	Slight	*Moderate*	*Acute*	*Slight*	*Moderate*	*Acute*
Feet						
Ankles						
Calves						
Shins						
Knees						
Thighs						
Hamstrings						
Hips						
Abdomen						
Lower back						
Middle back						
Upper back						
Rib cage						
Chest						
Spine						
Neck						
Head						
Shoulders						
Upper arms						
Elbows						
Forearms						
Wrists						
Hands						

Your Pleasure Journal

The power of journaling is that you become a conscious observer of your own experience. Taking time to journal helps you to explore your private consciousness, and to reflect upon your experience. Journaling is a mind-body-emotion connection that gives you time to relive and reflect, and to gain new insights and understanding. We suggest you make writing a part of your practice. Feel free to journal as part of the process of practicing the fifty-two moves and working out. Journal every day or once a week. Any type of diary or composition book will do. From time to time, reread what you have written to acknowledge and track your changes and growth.

Pleasure is a gift of the body. Although fun is most often associated with an activity, pleasure is associated with the body. To know physical pleasure is to know your body, yourself, and the world around you. Choosing pleasure cultivates personal awareness, creativity, the willingness to let go, and the freedom to become whole.

In Nia, pleasure is a sensation you seek in order to become spontaneous, feel joy, self-heal, get fit, stay healthy, find meaning, and be expressive. Pleasure keeps you choosing what is right for yourself and for your body in each moment.

The questions that follow are designed to help you discover what gives your body, mind, emotions, and spirit pleasure. Like most people, you are probably excellent at knowing what you don't like but rarely take the time to discover what you *do* like. Learning what gives you pleasure can be your guide on the journey from the world of pain to the world of joy.

As you continue to practice Nia, you will probably find that you will be able to add items to your Pleasure Journal.

- What kind of movement does my body love and get pleasure from?
- What parts of my body receive pleasure most easily?
- What kind of touch gives me pleasure?
- What gives my feet pleasure?
- What gives my head and neck pleasure?

- What gives my back pleasure?
- What kind of exercise gives me pleasure?
- What speed of movement gives me pleasure?
- What kind of music gives me pleasure?
- What scents give me pleasure?
- What foods give me pleasure?
- What shapes and images give me pleasure?
- What colors give me pleasure?
- What temperature gives me pleasure?
- What clothes give me pleasure?
- What people give me pleasure?
- How do I define pleasure for my body?
- How do I define pleasure for my mind?
- How do I define pleasure for my emotions?
- How do I define pleasure for my spirit?

discover your energy type

You've probably heard the expressions type A and type B personalities. They refer to a person's general energy type—either energetic or calm. This labeling system sometimes helps people better balance their personalities, slowing down a little or becoming somewhat more aggressive. In Nia, we have a rather more sophisticated system of energy typing. We base it around the nine classic Nia movement forms, which are described below. For example, we might say that you have a predominantly "t'ai chi personality" or a predominantly "jazz dance personality," because each of the nine movement forms can be accurate descriptors of basic personality traits, or energy types.

The Nine Basic Movement Forms of Nia

The Martial Arts

1. *T'ai chi* is a "slow dance" that focuses on efficiency of movement. T'ai chi movements are all centered around the body's inner core. They create grace and strengthen the mind–body connection.
2. *Tae kwon do* is an aggressive, physically demanding martial art that employs powerful kicks, blocks, and punches. Its stances and kicks are the cornerstones of Nia leg work and create physical strength and psychological confidence. It is the dance of precision.
3. *Aikido,* which emphasizes harmony in movement, focuses on finding resolution in conflict, through the blending of apparent opposites. Using spiral motions to create force, it evokes connectedness, gracefulness, and wisdom. It is harmonious spherical motion.

The Dance Arts

4. *Jazz dance* is all about fun, showmanship, and expression. It develops rhythm, coordination, and cardiovascular fitness. By replacing the rigid movements of traditional exercise with jazz movements, Nia facilitates the dialogue between the brain's two hemispheres.
5. *Modern dance* is creating shapes in space. With its emphasis on dropping and then recovering the body's own weight, it's an elegant way to direct muscle loading.
6. *Duncan dance* is free-spirited, honest movement. The most liberated, self-directed form of dance, it develops gracefulness, strength, flexibility, balance, and expressiveness. It can be as easy or as physically demanding as desired.

The Healing Arts

7. Moshe Feldenkrais teachings are about the conscious sensation of movement. This nonworkout movement reprograms the nervous system to change physical habits. By enabling people to become aware of subtle physical movements, it increases control over voluntary action. Moshe Feldenkrais described its linkage of mind and body by saying that it "straightens out kinks in the brain."

8. The *Alexander Technique* is movement from the top. It places primary attention on the position of the head, especially its carriage by the neck and shoulders, because so many people store tension there. It also emphasizes paying more attention to the quality of movements than the quantity.
9. *Yoga* is all about conscious connection. It's an inner-directed dance of bone alignment that allows the joints to achieve maximum efficiency. By redistributing chi energy, it increases awareness, relaxation, and balance.

Use the "Nia Energy Type Questionnaires" to evaluate your own energy type. You may find that several different types seem to fit you and that others are more foreign to your nature. Simply check true or false to each statement, then count the number of each answer to find out if you are somewhat—or strongly—predisposed to any of the energy types. If you're weak in any one type, you'll want to focus on its traits, particularly during your Nia workouts, in order to better balance yourself.

NIA ENERGY TYPE QUESTIONNAIRES

The Martial Arts

T'ai Chi	*True*	*False*
I am often soft, relaxed, and internally calm.		
I move through life tenderly.		
In confrontations, I am fluid, like water, and yet I remain strong and grounded.		
My emotions are mindful and balanced, respecting the world around me.		
I am internally harmonized, and I value equality in all things.		
I am deeply rooted, and I seek oneness and connection with everything.		
I am efficient, strong, agile, and compassionate, and I move through life in effortless, natural ways.		
I generally feel patient, focused, meditative, and graceful.		
I breathe with great ease.		
Totals		

Mostly true: *Your energy personality type gravitates to the martial art* t'ai chi. *To balance these soft attributes, you should also practice tae kwon do to incorporate precision and aikido to incorporate harmonious spherical motion into your movement and life.*

Mostly false: *You need to add more of this energy personality type, incorporating more of the slow dance into your workouts and life.*

Tae Kwon Do	***True***	***False***
In life I respond like an antagonist and defend myself by attacking.		
I react in sharp, masculine, and protective ways, thrusting my energy out to be seen and felt.		
I am keenly aware, and I live in a survival mode, always ready.		
I love speed and power.		
My way to move through life is to start and stop, to be forceful, cutting, direct, and quick.		
My voice and body gestures tend to blast.		
I am physical, conscious, precise, focused, and directed in my life, getting what I want through hard work and precision.		
I move quickly and intentionally, without hesitation, and work toward a goal.		
I stand in a strong base, and my words are exact and powerful.		
Totals		

Mostly true: *Your energy personality type gravitates to the martial art* tae kwon do. *To balance these harder, more forceful attributes, you should also practice t'ai chi to incorporate the slow dance and aikido to incorporate harmonious spherical motion into your movement and life.*

Mostly false: *You need to add more of this energy personality type, incorporating more precision into your workouts and life.*

Aikido	*True*	*False*
In life, I am all about win–win.		
I enter into rooms with a sense of oneness, connected energetically to the world.		
I breathe and move as a continuous, flowing, spiral of energy.		
I recycle my energy, never wasting time.		
I always center myself and speak and move from a place of center.		
I move with grace and seamless dynamics, turning lines into circles.		
I speak with conscious intent and focus.		
I am cooperative, peaceful, and powerful.		
I yield my position to include others and bend, swirl, and adapt—going with the flow.		
Totals		

Mostly true: *Your energy personality type gravitates to the martial art* aikido. *To balance these harmonious attributes, you should also practice t'ai chi to incorporate the slow dance, and tae kwon do to incorporate precision into your movement and life.*

Mostly false: *You need to add more of this energy personality type, incorporating more harmonious, circular motions into your workouts and life.*

The Dance Arts

Jazz Dance	*True*	*False*
I am all about the snap, crackle, and pop in life.		
I am interpretive and playful, and parts of my life are wild.		
I often express myself in jazzy, soulful, vital, happy ways.		
I am impulsive, lusty, sassy, demonstrative, showy, alive, fun, and electrifying to my friends.		
I love to shimmy, get dressed for the party, and be uninhibited.		
I share my smiles with the world.		
I love movements that are short and fast, choppy, linear, and percussive.		
I love rhythmic, asymmetrical, upbeat, and sensual actions.		
I contract, isolate, burst out, give my total attention, and want to be seen and heard.		
Totals		

Mostly true: *Your energy personality type gravitates to the art of* jazz dance. *To balance these fun, expressive attributes, you should also practice* Duncan dance *to incorporate free-spirited, honest motion and* modern dance *to incorporate more shapes and contrasts into your movements and life.*

Mostly false: *You need to add more of this energy personality type, incorporating more fun and showmanship into your workouts and life.*

Modern Dance	***True***	***False***
I can be very moody and serious, and enjoy emotional expression and drama.		
I move between feeling free, and bound in life.		
I am very introspective, and go inside to be expressive.		
I can be very on balance, and then fall off balance.		
I love playing with extremes and contrasts.		
I love not only form but formlessness.		
I react and recover with ease.		
I am wildly emotional and change shape easily.		
I love contrasts, gravity, surprise, and the start and stop of life, as well as moments of continuity.		
Totals		

Mostly true: *Your energy personality type gravitates to the art of* modern dance. *To balance these changing and on/off-balance attributes, you should also practice* jazz dance *to incorporate fun, showmanship, and expression along with* Duncan dance *to incorporate free-spirited, honest expression into your movements and life.*

Mostly false: *You need to add more of this energy personality type, incorporating more of the dance of creating shapes in space into your workouts and life.*

Duncan Dance	*True*	*False*
I am all about the soul, and in life I move in childlike ways.		
I am a free spirit, angelic in heart and mind and free with my body gestures.		
I flow spontaneously through my life.		
I love things that are natural, like walking, running, playing, and skipping.		
I am social, interactive, hopeful, and positive.		
I am almost always joyful.		
I am a fairy-like dreamer who creates and re-creates new experiences for myself and others.		
I love to relate to life through my primal body, an inner core of love and joy.		
I love smoothly sliding waltzes, a bouncing polka, melodic phrases, childlike gestures, imaginary scenes, and any creative process.		
Totals		

Mostly true: *Your energy personality type gravitates to the art of* Duncan dance. *To balance these childlike and free attributes, you should also practice jazz dance to incorporate fun and showmanship and modern dance to incorporate more shapes and contrasts into your movements and life.*

Mostly false: *You need to add more of this energy personality type, incorporating more free-spirited, honest expression into your workouts and life.*

The Healing Arts

Teachings of Moshe Feldenkrais	*True*	*False*
I am all about sensation.		
I am somatic. I love the body, the corporeal, the physical.		
I am very individualistic.		
I live life as a functioning, animalistic being.		
I feel and perceive life and others in a tactile way.		
I relate to things both modern and ancient.		
I am reflective and create patterns in time.		
I am healthy and love anything that is healing.		
I know how to adapt, adjust, get body centered, and assimilate.		
Totals		

Mostly true: *Your energy personality type gravitates to the teachings of Moshe Feldenkrais. To balance these conscious and sensory-based attributes, you should also practice the Alexander Technique to initiate movement from the head and yoga to incorporate the conscious alignment of bones and joints into your movements and life.*

Mostly false: *You need to add more of this energy personality type, incorporating more of the conscious dance of sensation into your workouts and life.*

Alexander Technique	***True***	***False***
I am subtle and gentle.		
I explore life with ease and flexibility.		
I love freedom, sensing space, perceiving, and transforming.		
I am physical, emotional, imaginative, natural, resourceful, and unbound.		
My communication methods include being available, accessible, conscious, and aware.		
I seek the simple, useful, authentic, and organic ways.		
I am keenly aware of my balance and posture as I move through life.		
I am aware of myself as a physical, emotional, and mentally integrated being.		
I am kinesthetic, and love touch. Living in a body feels easy and pleasurable.		
Totals		

Mostly true: *Your energy personality type gravitates to the healing art of the* Alexander Technique. *To balance this, you should also practice the teachings of Moshe Feldenkrais to incorporate the conscious awareness of sensation and yoga to incorporate the conscious alignment of bones and joints into your movements and life.*

Mostly false: *You need to add more of this energy personality type, initiating more movement from the head into your workouts and life.*

Yoga	***True***	***False***
I love physical human structure, and relate to bones and alignment with great excitement.		
The sensation of counterforces and postures drives me to achieve greater physical awareness.		
I can be gentle, powerful, focused, conscious, and receptive.		
My focus in life includes unity, oneness, and balance.		
My energy reflects harmony and an internal, effortless endurance.		
I am guided by light and have the ability to sustain.		
I love lying down, sitting, being prone, and playing with backbend motions.		
I speak of spiritual, expansive, supportive ways of living and being.		
I am about peace and stillness, and I am committed to preserving my body's ability to be open, soft, and supple.		
Totals		

Mostly true: *Your energy personality type gravitates to the healing art of* yoga. *To balance this, you should also practice the teachings of Moshe Feldenkrais and incorporate the conscious awareness of sensation along with the Alexander Technique to initiate movement from the head into your movements and life.*

Mostly false: *You need to add more of this energy personality type, incorporating more of the conscious alignment of bones and joints dance into your workouts and life.*

By now, you should know your own body better than ever before.
It's time to use it!
Move on—to the "moves chapter"!

four

The Basics: All the Nia Moves

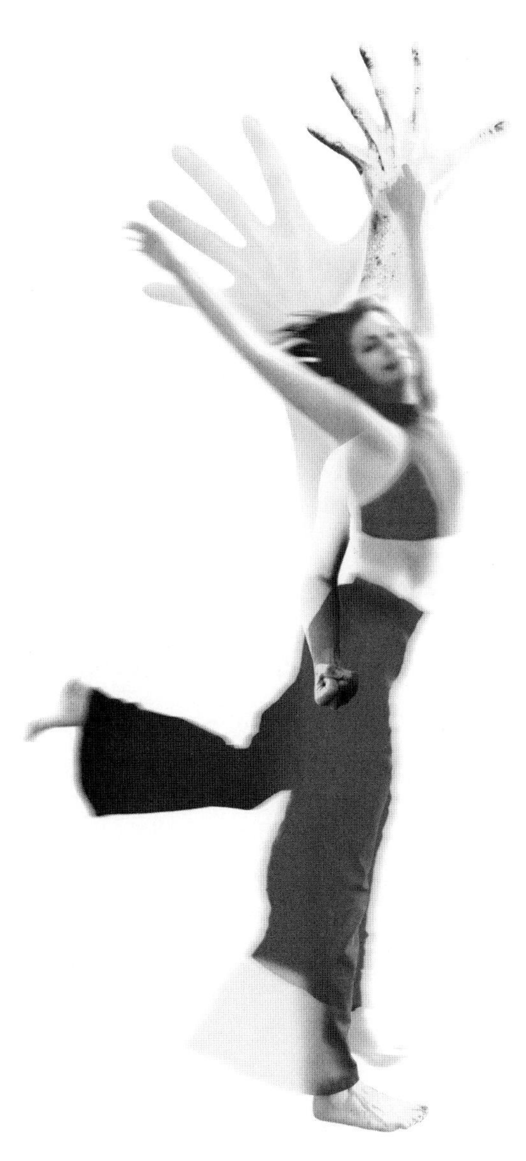

In this chapter, you will find all of the Nia moves that we do in both the Classic and the Athletic Nia workouts. These fifty-two moves are the building blocks of all Nia workouts. Before you begin to do the workout (in Chapter 5), you should practice the individual moves and become comfortable with them. None is difficult, but some may feel a bit awkward when you first experience them.

The Nia moves are designed to deliver fitness results, but as you've already seen from many of the Nia stories, they also fill therapeutic needs. You can use them—as many other people have—to self-heal and to live more easily with developmental disabilities, respiratory diseases, arthritis, Parkinson's disease, osteoporosis, heart disease, and diabetes and to assist with cancer recovery, drug rehabilitation, musculoskeletal rehabilitation, and overcoming self-defeating behaviors (such as overeating, bulimia, anorexia, and negative self-talk).

The moves are broken into three basic categories, corresponding to the three essential areas of the body: the Base, the Core, and the Upper Extremities. Within each of these three basic categories are different types of moves that affect specific body parts. For example, the moves for the Base include moves specifically for the feet as well as various stances, steps, and kicks.

THE FIFTY-TWO NIA MOVES

The Base

Feet

1. Heel Lead
2. Whole Foot
3. Ball of the Foot
4. Relevé
5. Rock Around the Clock
6. Squish Walk
7. Duck Walk
8. Toes In, Out, Parallel

Stances

9. Closed Stance
10. Open Stance
11. "A" Stance
12. Riding (Sumo) Stance
13. Bow Stance
14. Cat Stance

Steps

15. Sink and Pivot Table Wipe
16. Stepping Back onto the Ball of Your Foot
17. Cross Front
18. Cross Behind
19. Traveling in Directions
20. Lateral Traveling
21. Cha-Cha-Cha
22. Slow Clock
23. Fast Clock

Kicks

24. Front Kick
25. Side Kick
26. Back Kick
27. Knee Sweep

The Core

Pelvis

28. Pelvic Circles
29. Hip Bumps

Chest

30. Chest Isolations
31. Shimmy
32. Undulation
33. Spinal Roll

Head

34. Head and Eye Movements

The Upper Extremities

Arms

35. Blocks
36. Punches
37. Elbow Strikes

Hands

38. Touching
39. Fist
40. Pumps
41. Strikes
42. Chop Cut
43. Webbed Spaces
44. Palm Directions

Fingers

45. Finger Extensions
46. Finger Flicks
47. Creepy Crawlers
48. Spear Fingers
49. Catching Flies
50. Claw Hand
51. Power Finger Crossover
52. Balance Finger

Fifty-two moves may seem like a lot to learn, but wait until you see how simple most of these moves are! Some aren't much more complicated than just standing up. You may be thinking: "Standing up? That's not an exercise!" But it is. If you don't think so, ask someone who has to stand up at work all day.

The purpose of these moves is to help you develop a movement vocabulary you can use in life to self-heal and in your workouts to get the most benefits. The moves address all parts of the body. Practicing them one by one will train your mind and body and prepare you to move with greater confidence.

the three stages of practice

We've designed three stages of practice to help you learn and embody the moves. Practice each move one at a time and repeat sixteen times in each stage.

1. ***Learn the Move.*** In this stage, say the name of the move and use the text and photo cues to become consciously aware of how to do each move. You'll be *thinking* about it, so it might feel somewhat mechanical, which is okay at this point.
2. ***Move the Move.*** As you continue to practice the move, gain a whole body *feeling* for it. In this stage you'll feel freer, be thinking less, and should feel more natural with the move—less mechanical. Your whole body will be involved, even though you are isolating a body part.
3. ***Energize the Move.*** Now that you're moving as a whole, it's time to integrate the energy of the movement forms (dance, martial, or healing arts). Choose a different form each time you practice a Nia move and integrate its energy into the move to bring it to life.

As you practice each move, get to know your own body. Notice how you feel from moment to moment. Observe what moves you can easily do and which ones are more challenging.

The more you practice the moves, the more efficient and skillful you'll become at self-healing and working out. You can even use these moves throughout the day. Practice foot moves while waiting in line, waiting for water to boil, or waiting for the elevator to arrive. Practice other moves while walking to your car, before bed, when you wake up, or at lunch. Soon you'll find that your body begins to move more freely and naturally, of its own accord, even when you're not working out.

Even as you begin to incorporate the Nia Workout into your life, you should return to this chapter on a regular basis to continue self-healing and improve your craft and technique.

ENERGIZE THE MOVES

- ***T'ai chi:*** Flowing, tender, fluid. Float like a balloon, and move like a willow tree in the wind.
- ***Tae kwon do:*** Sharp, powerful, active. Move with confidence, and feel your own speed and strength.
- ***Aikido:*** Harmonizing, peaceful, cooperative. Connect and blend with everything around you.
- ***Jazz dance:*** Playful, peppy, sexy. Move with pizzazz and express your most passionate emotions.
- ***Modern dance:*** Languid, moody, balanced. Create different shapes with your body. Play with balance and contrasts.
- ***Duncan dance:*** Soulful, spontaneous, unbounded. Move like a child enchanted by life.
- ***Teachings of Moshe Feldenkrais:*** Reflective, healing, conscious. Move with sensory awareness and feel life as it happens.
- ***Alexander Technique:*** Transformative, exploratory, natural. Move as a whole person, connected up and balanced.
- ***Yoga:*** Timeless, linked, expansive. Move in ways that link your body, mind, and spirit to the outer world.

the art of sensing: the five sensations

So is it enough just to practice the moves or is there something more you can do when practicing and working out to get results? Yes, there's sensing.

Sensing is what you do to know whether or not you are actually getting the results you want. What you want to sense is the sensation of strength, flexibility, mobility, agility, and stability. These are the five sensations responsible for maintaining functional fitness, which is the dynamic interaction of all five sensations that results in balance and harmony. So what do these five sensations feel like, and how will you know when you're there?

In Chapter Three you had your first taste of sensing when you discovered the sensations of mobility and stability, two of the five sensations. You learned to feel the sensation of too loose and too tight. Now you're going to learn how to train yourself to trigger all five sensations. Each sensation is unique with qualities you can learn to recognize in your own body. Sensing precisely what you feel at any given moment during a Nia movement is a superb way to become your own best teacher and conscious personal trainer. Your sensations will tell you exactly how to move; you just need to know what to "sense" for.

Sensing for Strength

- Strength is sensed as energy moving inward.
- Strength is the sensation of sustaining power.
- Strength is sensed as a vibration of positive tension in the muscles.
- Strength feels like a warm power along the bone that contracts the belly of the muscle without pulling unequally in any direction.
- Dynamic strength—the perfect balance of power and grace—is sensed as relaxation, not tension.
- Losing strength is sensed as quivering of the muscle, pain, and fatigue and as a diminishment of balance, grace, speed, and coordination.

Sensing for Flexibility

- Flexibility is sensed as energy moving outward.
- Flexibility is sensed as an elastic quality of muscles and joints.
- Flexibility is sensed as a warm stretch of the muscle, without a sense of tension.
- Dynamic flexibility—the perfect balance of contraction and release—is sensed as opening and lengthening.
- Losing flexibility is sensed as heaviness, rigidity, stiffness, cramping, and fatigue.

Sensing for Mobility

- Mobility is sensed as energy in constant motion.
- Mobility is sensed as a continuous energy flow and excitation of the nerves around the joints.
- Dynamic mobility—the perfect balance between excitation and relaxation—is sensed as youthful freedom.
- Losing mobility is sensed as tightness, discomfort, and loss of power.

Sensing for Agility

- Agility is sensed as a shifting of dynamic tension.
- Agility is sensed as a feeling of pushing and pulling.
- Agility is sensed as the ability to easily start and stop movement.
- Dynamic agility—the perfect balance of movement and stillness—is sensed as a balance between yin and yang.
- Losing agility is sensed as a diminishment of response, speed, and control.

Sensing for Stability

- Stability is sensed as a calmness in the muscles, combined with readiness for action.
- Stability is maintained by equalizing muscular contraction and relaxation.
- Stability is sensed as a harmony between the muscles and joints.
- Dynamic stability—the perfect balance of opposites—is sensed as powerful peace.
- Losing stability is sensed as weakness and a loss of balance and support.

NIA TIPS FOR BEGINNERS

1. ***Train yourself.*** Push away all your thoughts and worries as you exercise. Talk to yourself, like a personal trainer. Use verbal guidance to remain focused on what you are doing and how you are doing it. Use self-talk to coach your physical body into moving more efficiently and sensing more pleasure.
2. ***Begin small.*** At first, don't reach out, sink, or rise too far. Build muscle strength and joint mobility slowly.
3. ***Pick up your feet.*** To protect your knees, don't drag your feet. Instead, pick up your feet and place them in the direction you want to go.
4. ***Sit back.*** When you lower your body, sit back as if you were sitting down in a chair, moving your buttocks back behind you and away from your knees.
5. ***Dress to move.*** When you dance, wear anything that makes you feel free, comfortable, and excited to move. Yoga clothing, street or exercise wear, even a skirt changes the way you move and feel and work out.
6. ***Go barefooted.*** Unless you need shoes for medical purposes, take off your shoes and let the bottoms of your feet send information back to your brain so your body can move safely and efficiently.
7. ***Start easy.*** Let your body slowly acclimate and adjust to Nia movement. Allow yourself the freedom to enjoy being a beginner. Keep your interest and fascination up and criticism and judgment down. Be gentle, be pa-

tient, and allow yourself to move through levels and stay on plateaus—this is the way to master and enjoy Nia.

8. ***Strive for balance.*** Don't strain; listen to your body's signals and move in a smooth, relaxed way that doesn't make you breathless or fatigued. If your body does not relate well to a movement, adjust and move within your own comfort zone to put positive, loving information into the muscle memory.
9. ***Find your rhythm.*** Get in as much nonstop movement as possible by finding your own pace. This may mean working slower and longer, rather than faster and harder.
10. ***Express yourself.*** Make the movements an expression of you—this is *your* workout. Express your own unique rhythm and body language and use your emotions to fine-tune your physical body. Be jazzy, luscious, lyrical, snappy, or sensual. Most of all, be yourself and have fun.
11. ***Belly breathe.*** When you inhale, smell the moment, and feel your belly expand, then your ribs and chest filling. Exhale, placing the tip of your tongue directly behind your top teeth, which naturally supports belly breathing.
12. ***Use your whole body.*** Connect with every part of your body and move as if your body were your ballroom dance partner.
13. ***Balance your fitness program.*** Combine a good diet with internal and external exercises. With enough sleep, proper nutrition, and exercise, you will see and feel results far beyond changing the shape of your body.

moving with Nia

To move with Nia safely and efficiently, incorporate these tips into your practice and workouts.

- Use visual imagery to make movements feel natural. As you do the various Nia moves, you'll notice that many of them feel like normal, everyday motions—because they are! To help make these movements easier to remember and to better integrate your body with your mind, it's helpful to visualize the movements as familiar physical tasks. We provide visualization cues for many of the exercises. For example, kicking a ball, walking through thick mud, throwing a ball, turning a doorknob, wiping a table, or stretching like a cat.

- Combine small movements with large movements. To experience dynamic ease, practice each movement in small and large ranges of motion. Small movements engage the intrinsic muscles, the ones closest to the bone that provide stability. Large movements engage the superficial muscles, the ones on top that provide more power.
- Use your Base, Core, Upper Extremities, breath, and voice to add energy and power to your moves.
- Use a variety of speeds. The more speed variety you feed your body, the stronger and more adaptable you become.
- Use your joints to move energy. Sense your joints opening and closing to keep energy flowing and your body in motion.
- Use breath to start and stop the flow of energy. Exhale longer to sustain endurance and balance. To harmonize your breath with body motion, synchronize the speed of your in–out breath with the speed of your movement.
- Add intensity to your movements by sinking lower and rising higher.
- Shift your body weight—don't drop it—as if you were moving along a curve similar to that of a *Smile Line.*
- Add emotion to every motion. When you become personally motivated, involved, and interested in what you do, more of you is involved in working out. This means more bang for your buck and a greater return for your energy investment.
- Use your fingers and hands to express how movements make you feel. Engaging the fingers and hands activates brain activity, engages the emotional body, and physically keeps tension out of the neck and shoulders.
- Use your voice as you move, to activate your abdominal muscles. The most efficient way to involve your abdominal muscles is to make sound, which engages them effortlessly to provide you with support from the inside out.
- Lead your head movements with your eye movements. Because the head is the heaviest weight of the three weights of the body, moving

it energetically is the most efficient. When the eyes are engaged in looking, tracking, and focusing, the head follows and is supported from the inside out. This is the safest way to move the head weight.

Now it's time to start moving! All by yourself! No class. No leader. It's easier than you think. This book lets you become your own teacher—or, in the language of Nia, your own *conscious personal trainer.*

HEEL LEAD

Maintain vertical alignment

Allow your hands and arms
to move naturally
Wag your tail
to integrate
the spine
Step, leading with your heel

Lift your toes to shift body weight fluidly

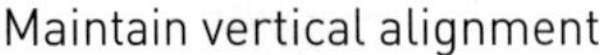

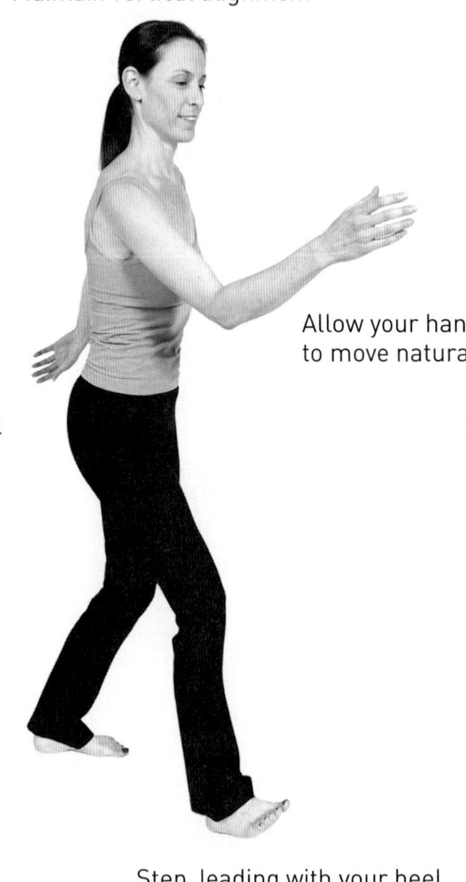

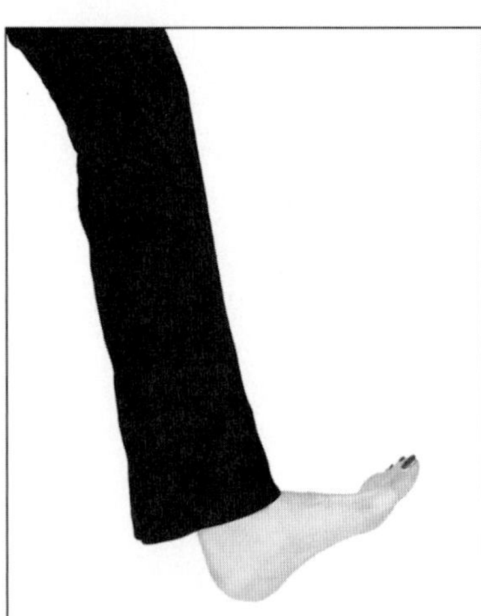

BENEFITS: Practicing the Heel Lead develops good body skills, so that, regardless of your activity choice, you gain body control.

Step directly forward or diagonally in a normal walking step. Lead with your heel, and focus on the sequence of heel . . . ball . . . toes as you shift your body weight. Use the heel lead for walking freely and expressively. As you walk, sound the word *relax* very calmly. Imagine that your foot is fifty times its size. Focusing on this move will improve the way you walk, and nurture your Base with every step you take.

WHOLE FOOT

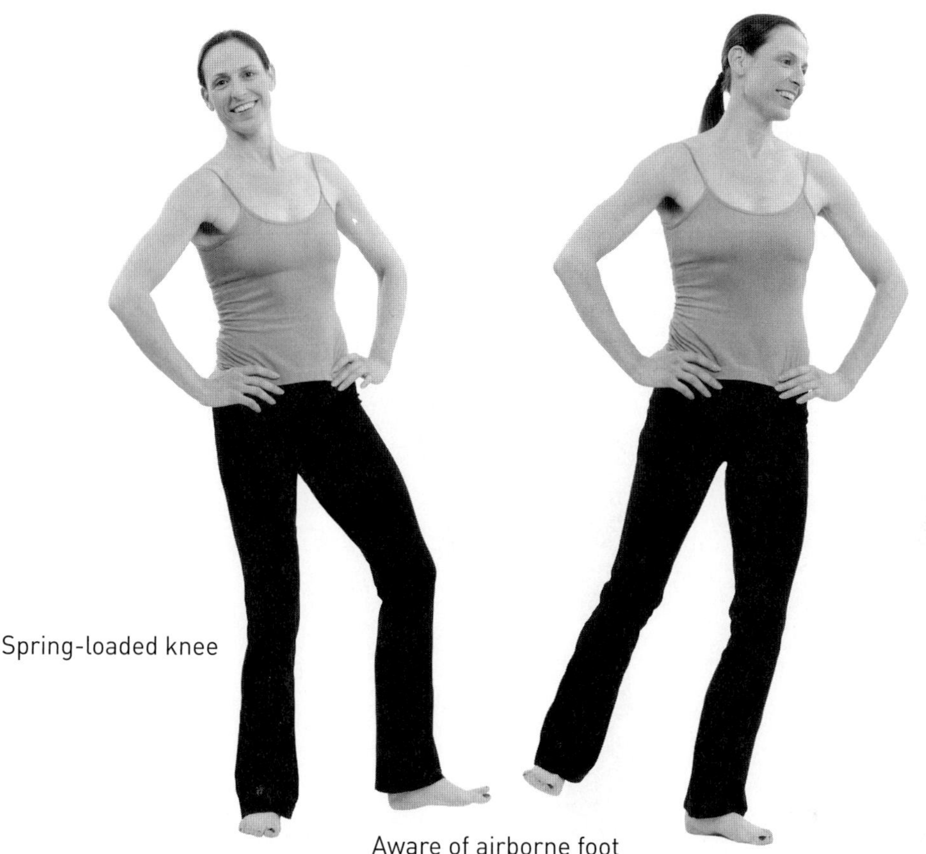

Spring-loaded knee

Aware of airborne foot

Settle into the edges of your foot

BENEFITS: Practicing Whole Foot stimulates sensation in the foot and ankle, making it possible for you to move in agile and safe ways.

Instead of leading with your heel, as you would in a normal walking motion, walk, step, or land on your whole foot. Sense your entire foot as the foundation of your body. Be aware of three points on the bottom of your foot—the center of your heel, the inner edge of the ball of your foot, and the outer edge of your foot. Sound the word *melt* or *root* to emphasize deep-rooted grounding. Imagine leaving an imprint of your foot in the sand. This is a great move for feeling grounded.

BALL OF THE FOOT

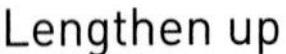

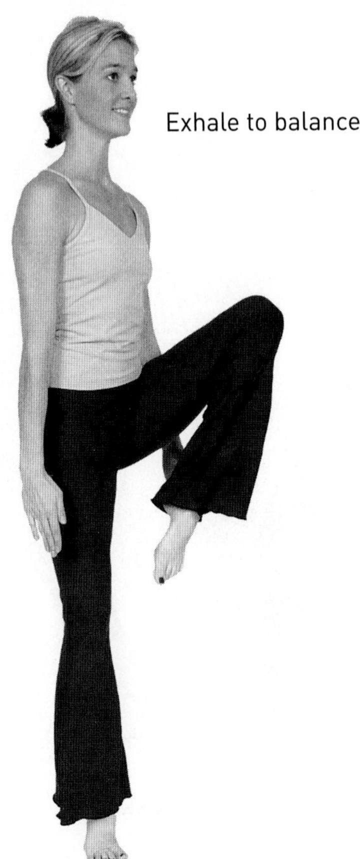

Press into the earth

BENEFITS: Practicing Ball of the Foot improves your ability to move quickly and with more agility.

Stand as if you were in high heels, and march in place, stepping directly onto the balls of your feet, and keeping your heels off the floor. Keep your toes relaxed and stretched forward. Boldly sound the word *stick* to accentuate the feeling of balance. Use this move to help heal your feet and ankles and improve your posture.

RELEVÉ

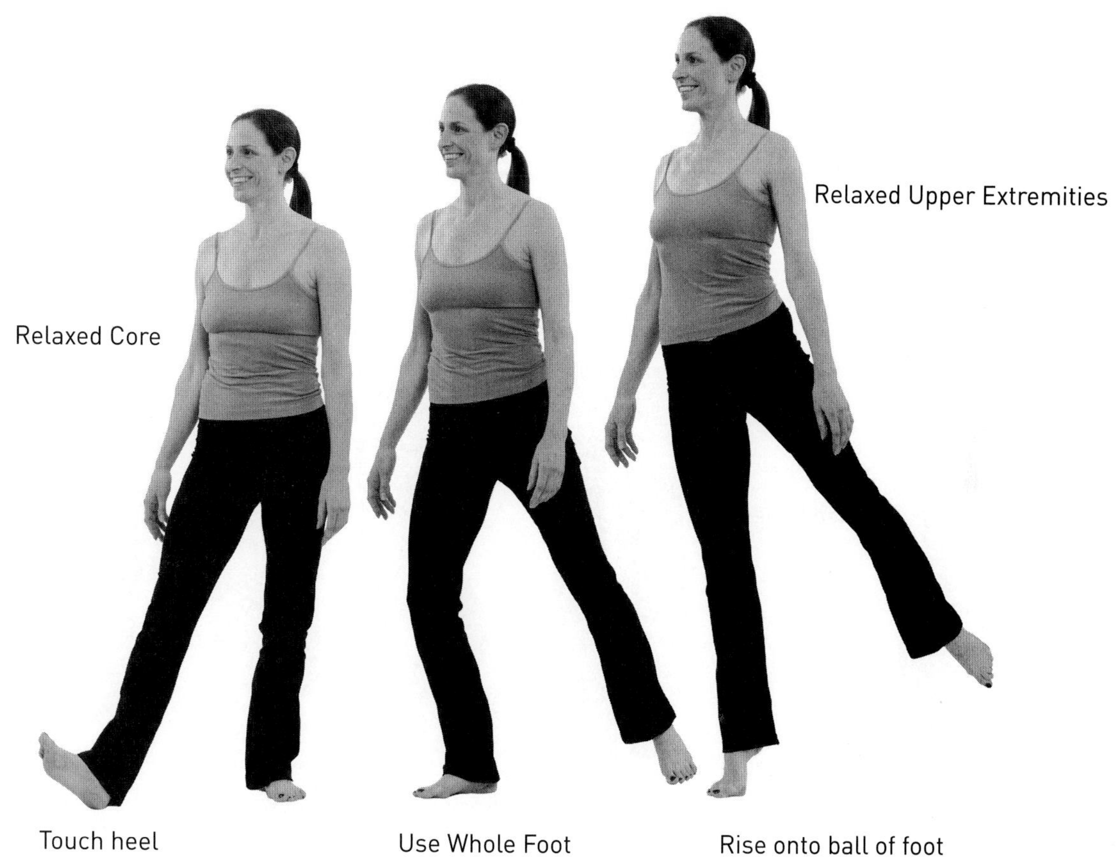

BENEFITS: Practicing Relevé improves agility, speed, and whole-body coordination so you can safely stop and start on a dime.

Roll up on to the balls of your feet, leading with your heels. Use this to develop agility and a sense of lightness. Lovingly sound the word *light* as you do this move.

ROCK AROUND THE CLOCK

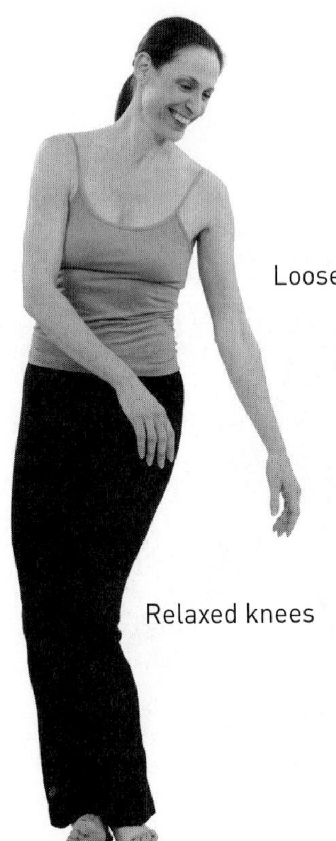

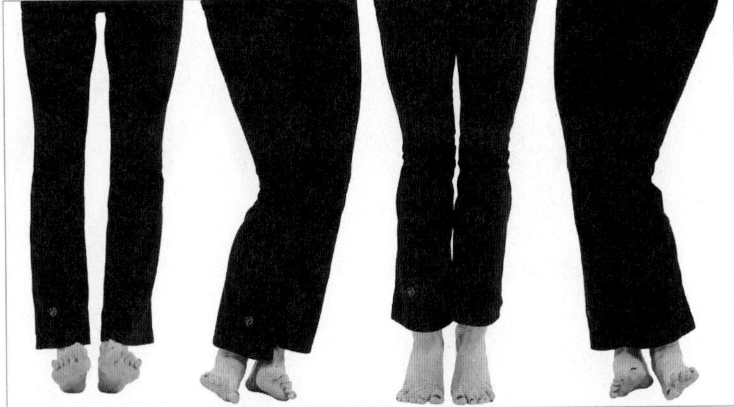

Rock back lifting toes | Rock right shifting weight | Rock front lifting heels | Rock left shifting weight

BENEFITS: Practicing Rock Around the Clock improves agility in your feet and ankles, so that regardless of the locomotion speed, you have control.

Standing with your feet slightly apart and no wider than hip width, roll around the outside edges of your feet sensing the edges of the back, right, front, and left sides. Sound the word *wow* to heighten the sense of playfulness and imagine balancing and rolling on top of a ball, in a hula-hoop motion. Now repeat in the other direction.

SQUISH WALK

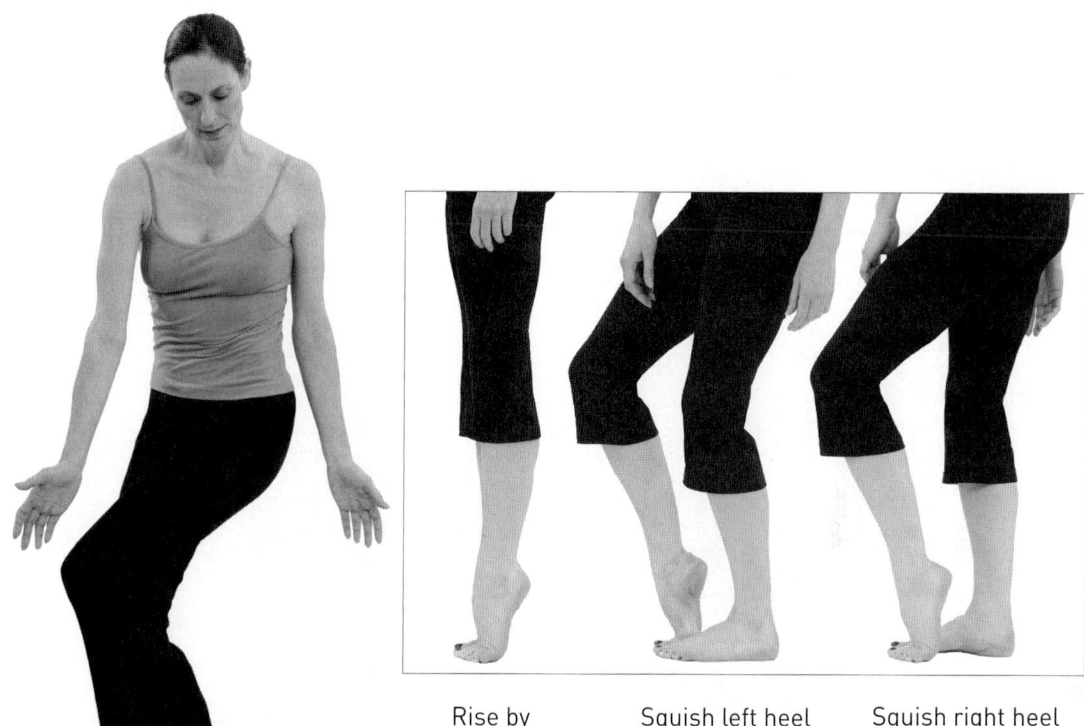

Sink into Whole Foot

Rise by pressing down

Squish left heel down slowly

Squish right heel down slowly

BENEFITS: Practicing Squish Walk improves strength and flexibility in the lower leg, foot, and ankle, which helps you move safely with different speeds and intensities.

Standing with your feet hip width apart, rise up onto the balls of your feet. Now, bring one heel down at a time (alternating), and imagine that you are squeezing juice out of an orange under that heel. Happily sound the word *squish* as you step down, to accentuate the quality of slow compression. This is excellent for improving balance, posture, range of motion, and stability in the feet and ankles.

DUCK WALK

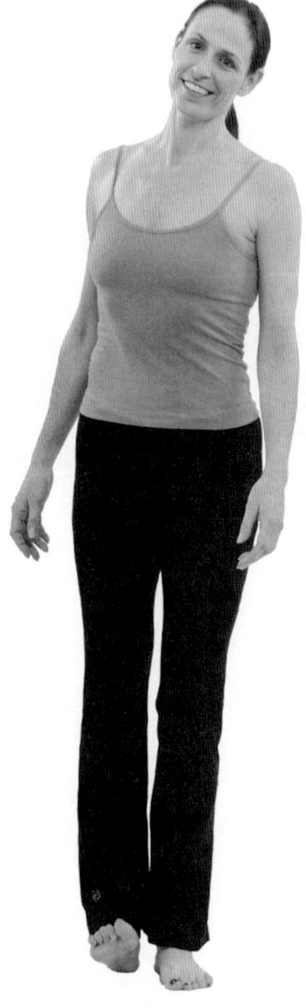

Hips remain under chest

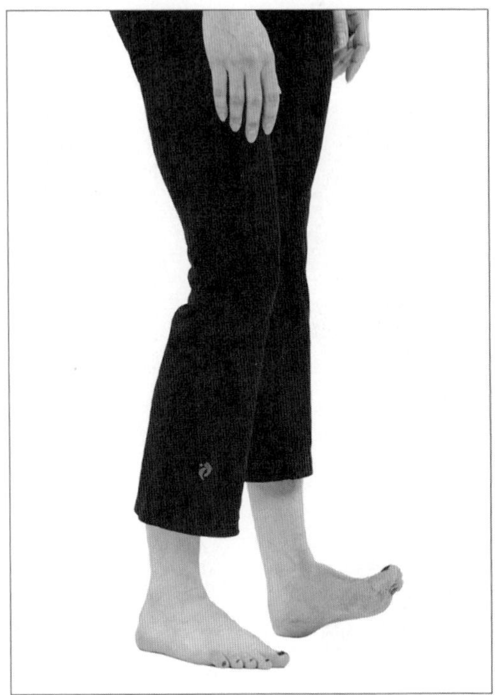

> BENEFITS: Practicing Duck Walk improves your ability to start and stop in a stress-free way.

Standing with your feet slightly apart and no wider than hip width, alternately lift and then lower the toes and balls of each foot, as if you were slapping the ground to splash water in a puddle. To get into the mood, sound the word *quack!* This is excellent for the calves and shins.

TOES IN, OUT, PARALLEL

Move from the hip joint

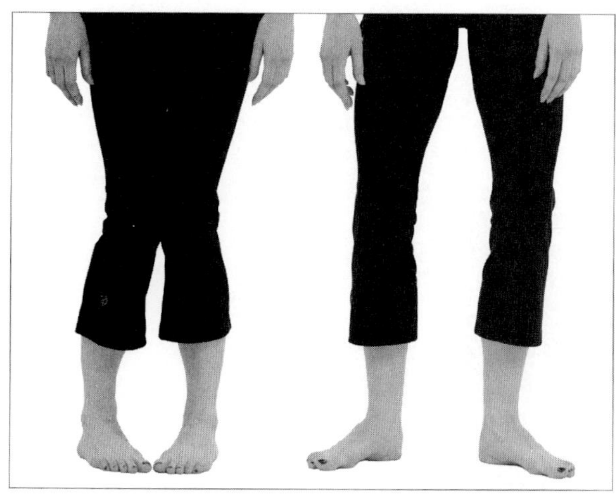

In Out

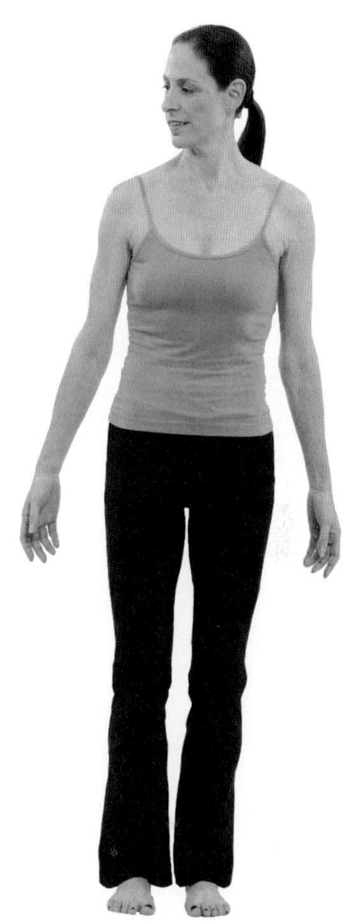

Parallel

BENEFITS: Practicing Toes In, Out, Parallel improves mobility in your ankle, knee, and hip joints, making locomotion more comfortable and dynamic.

In this move, you point your toes in different directions. First, place your feet parallel to each other. Then, turn them in, as if you are "pigeon-toed"; then turn them out or away from each other. Practice walking, pointing your toes in each direction. Imagine your feet as windshield wipers and firmly sound *in, out, parallel* to increase your mindfulness. This move improves hip mobility and stability, which in turn improves power, speed, and reflex responses of the legs.

CLOSED STANCE

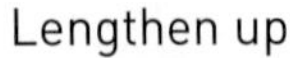

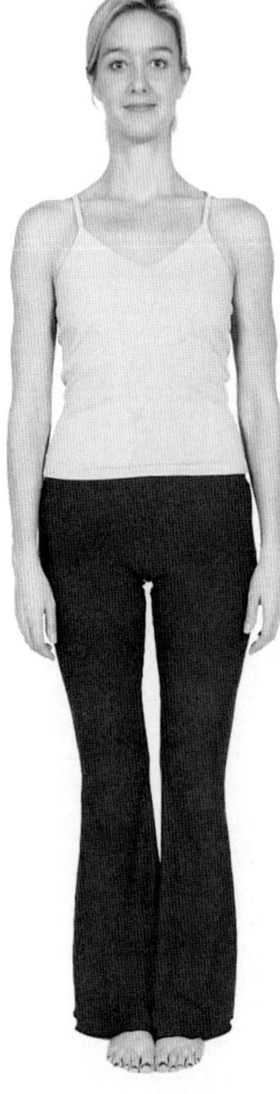

Arms hang

Toes touch, heels slightly apart

> BENEFITS: Practicing Closed Stance trains the upper body to work efficiently with the lower body.

Stand in place, with your big toes touching and your heels slightly apart. Keep your feet and knees relaxed, and your spine tall. Practice by walking a few steps, then stopping in Closed Stance. Imagine that you are a deeply rooted tree. Sense your entire skeleton, and sound the vowel *o* to create volume in your chest cavity.

OPEN STANCE

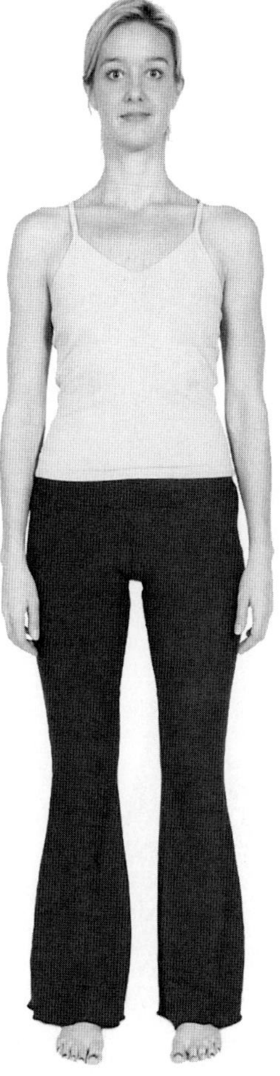

BENEFITS: Practicing Open Stance improves hip-joint strength and flexibility, for increased comfort in moving.

Stand in place, with your feet hip width apart, and your toes pointed directly forward. Keep your feet relaxed and parallel and keep your knees flexible, or spring loaded. This will help your balance. Practice by walking a few steps, then stopping in Open Stance. Imagine that you are standing on two railroad tracks. As you do it, sound *balance* or *ground.*

"A" STANCE

Energy up and out

Relaxed Core and Upper Extremities
Feet parallel

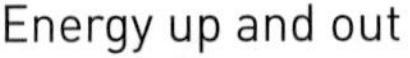

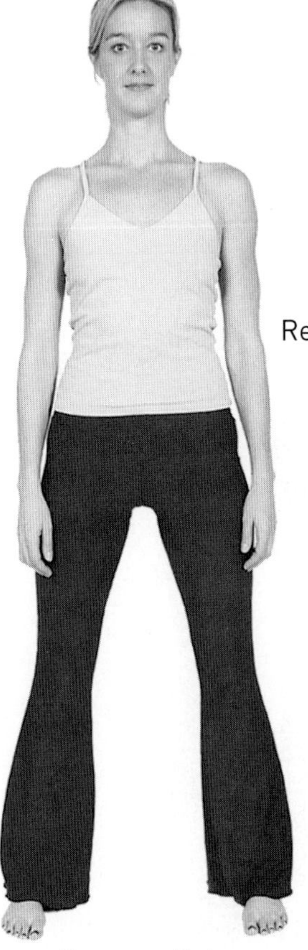

BENEFITS: Practicing "A" Stance improves hip flexibility and leg strength, which improves agility and mobility.

Stand in place, with your legs wider than hip distance, as if creating the letter A. Keep your knees spring loaded, relaxed, or soft. Practice by walking a few steps, then stopping in "A" Stance. This stance is effective for improving breathing. As you do this move, make the sound *aaaaahh!* until your body says, "Let's *inhale* now, and smell the moment!"

RIDING (SUMO) STANCE

Three body weights aligned
Engage your hands and arms
Feet parallel

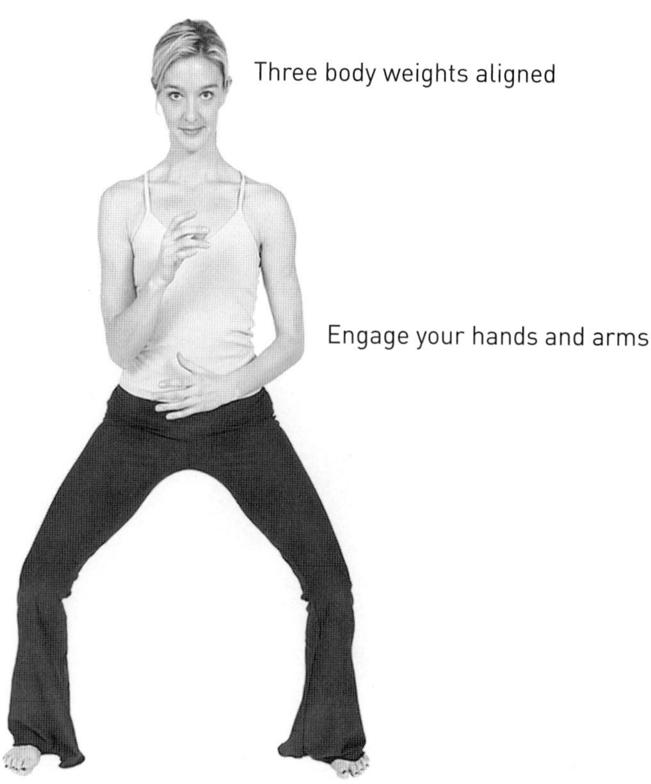

BENEFITS: Practicing Riding (Sumo) Stance is excellent conditioning for all the muscles of the legs—the foundation that makes it possible for you to move around.

Stand in place, with your knees slightly bent and your feet apart, as if you were riding a horse. Practice by walking a few steps, then stopping in Sumo Stance. This stance triggers a natural desire for deeper breathing. Sound *ha!* explosively to release muscle tension.

BOW STANCE

Engage hands and arms
Vertical thighbone
Back heel high
Press into back ball of the foot
Press down into whole front foot

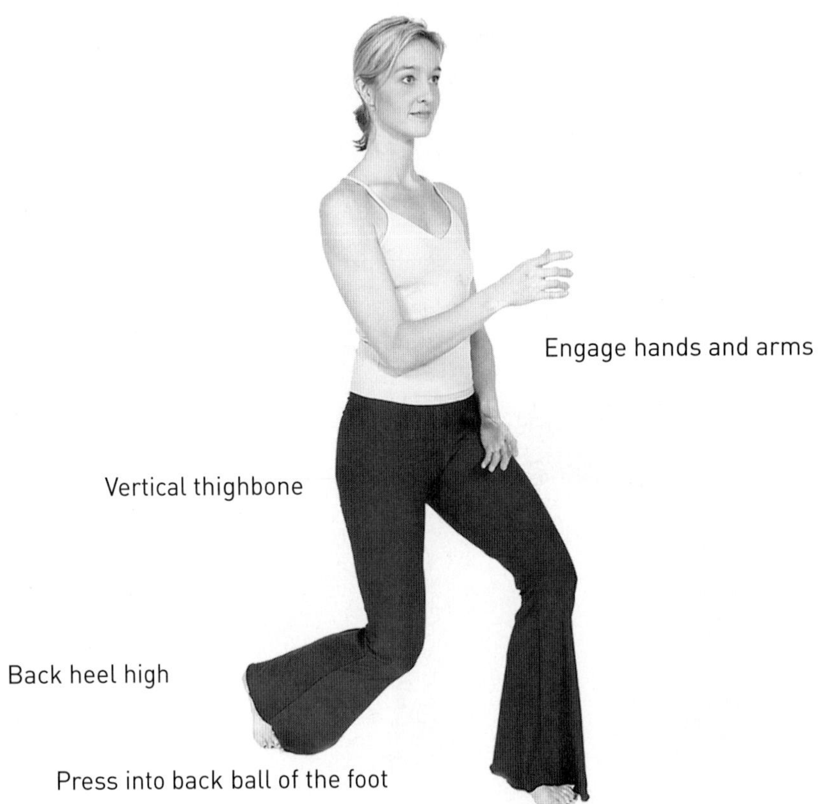

BENEFITS: Practicing Bow Stance is excellent conditioning for walking and for dealing with changes in levels, as you descend and ascend, changing the body's center of gravity.

Stand in place, with your feet hip width apart, in Open Stance, then step back onto the ball of one foot, as if that leg were a bow drawing back. Maintain your balance by keeping both knees slightly bent and your back heel high. This move builds powerful agility. As you step back onto the ball of your foot, land and stick, powerfully sounding the vowel *u*. Return to Open Stance and repeat on the other side. Alternate sides.

CAT STANCE

Elbows down, hands and arms engaged
Press foot against leg
Rest into Whole Foot

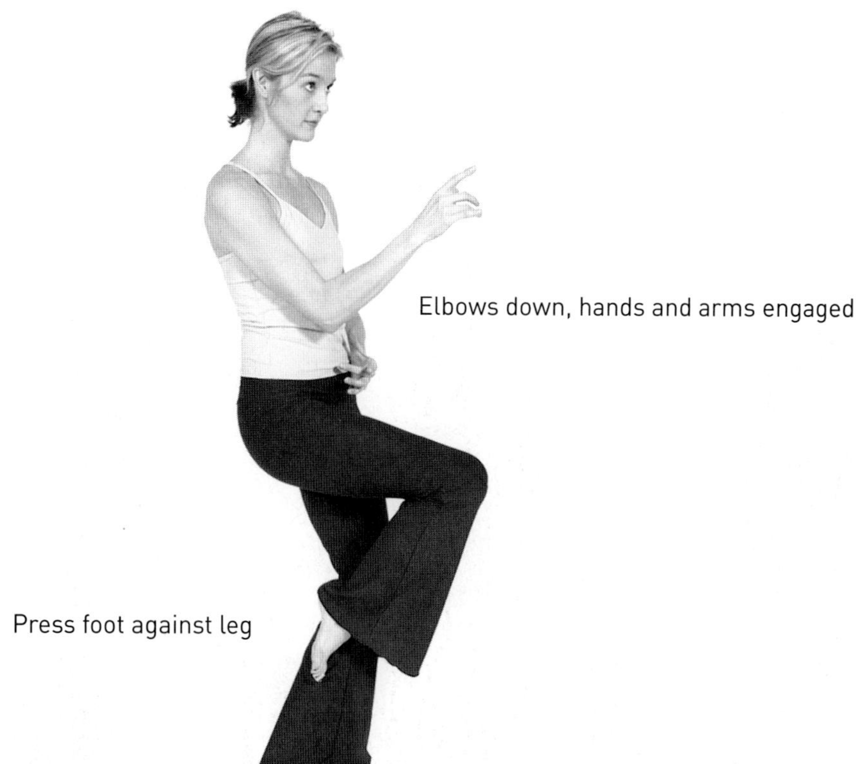

BENEFITS: Practicing Cat Stance improves balance, which improves your ability to move at various speeds.

Stand in place, on one foot, and balance yourself as if you were poised to pounce. Keep the knee and hip joint of your supporting leg soft and spring loaded, and keep your hips level. This develops agility for all of the movements that require balancing on one leg. To support your balance, sound *woooo* in a sustained exhale. Alternate sides.

SINK AND PIVOT TABLE WIPE

Follow hand
Engage opposite hand for balance
Release hip joint
Vertical shin bone
Pivot and place

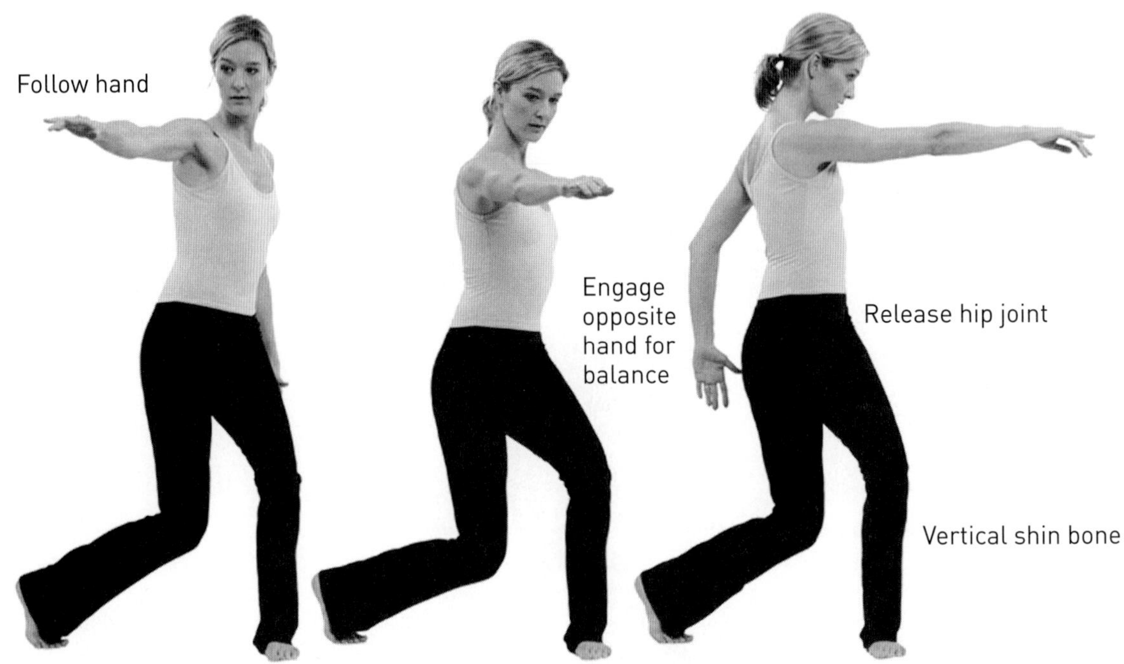

BENEFITS: Practicing Sink and Pivot Table Wipe keeps the feet, ankles, knees, and hip joints agile and the upper body mobile.

Standing in "A" Stance make a quarter turn to the right, bending at the knees and sinking slightly, and picking up your left foot and pivoting your left thigh as you place the ball of your left foot on the ground. At the same time, use your left hand to wipe off an imaginary table, moving your hand from behind you to the front. Alternate sides. Sound the word *whoosh* to integrate upper and lower body.

STEPPING BACK ONTO THE BALL OF YOUR FOOT

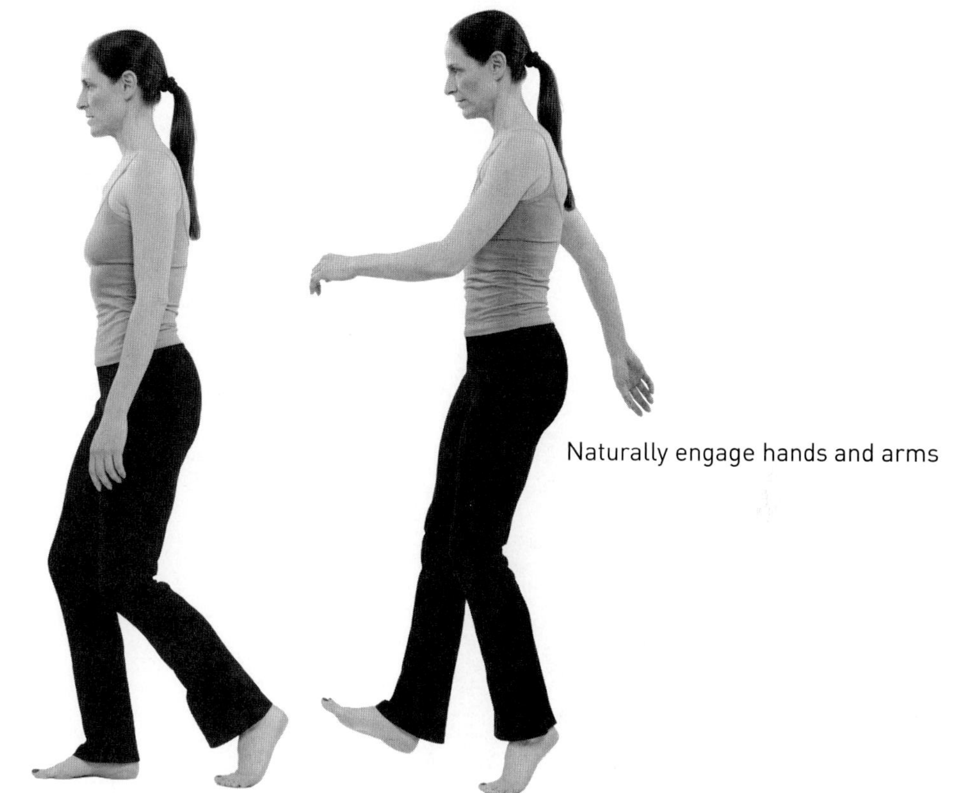

Naturally engage hands and arms

Whole Foot Press into ball Step back onto the ball

BENEFITS: Practicing Stepping Back onto the Ball of Your Foot improves mobility and stability in the foot and ankle, which helps you move with precision and sensitivity.

Standing in Open Stance, step back directly onto the ball of one foot, keeping your heel high. Practice walking around the room, stopping and stepping back, and then rising onto the ball of your foot. Keep your head, chest, and pelvis upright, and imagine that the ball of your foot is your whole foot. Sound the word *onto* to improve balance. Alternate sides.

CROSS FRONT

Look in the direction you move
Free and natural arm motion
Cross over

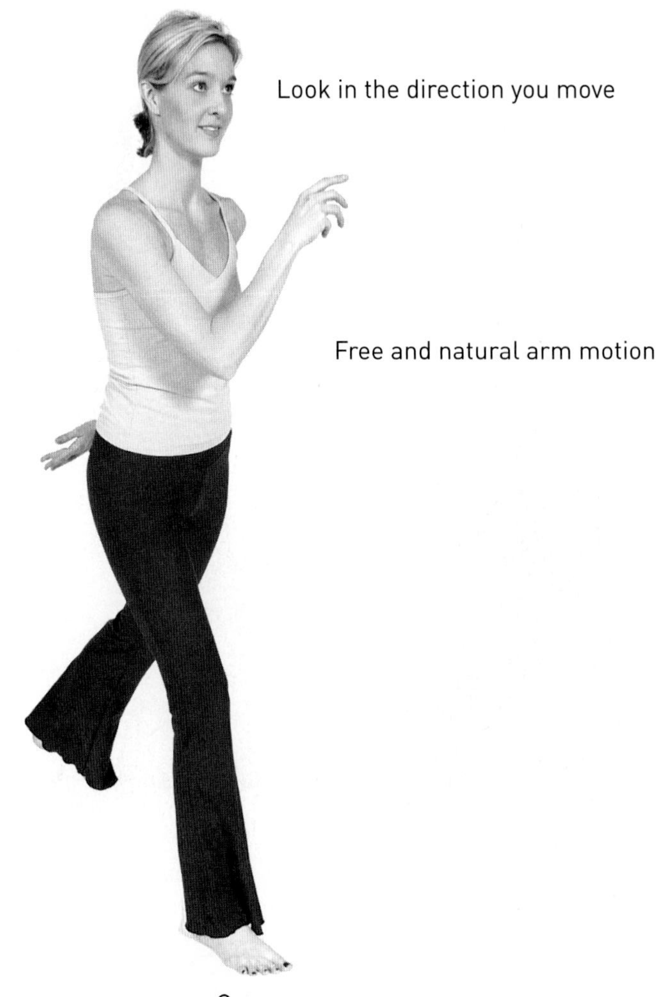

BENEFITS: Practicing Cross Front strengthens your inner thigh muscles, which helps you develop greater stability when stopping suddenly.

Standing in Open Stance, step out diagonally and face the corner, pointing both feet in the direction you want to go. Let your arms and hands swing freely, as if energetically walking. Imagine responding to someone calling your name as you change directions. Sound the word *corner* to mindfully guide your body. Alternate sides.

CROSS BEHIND

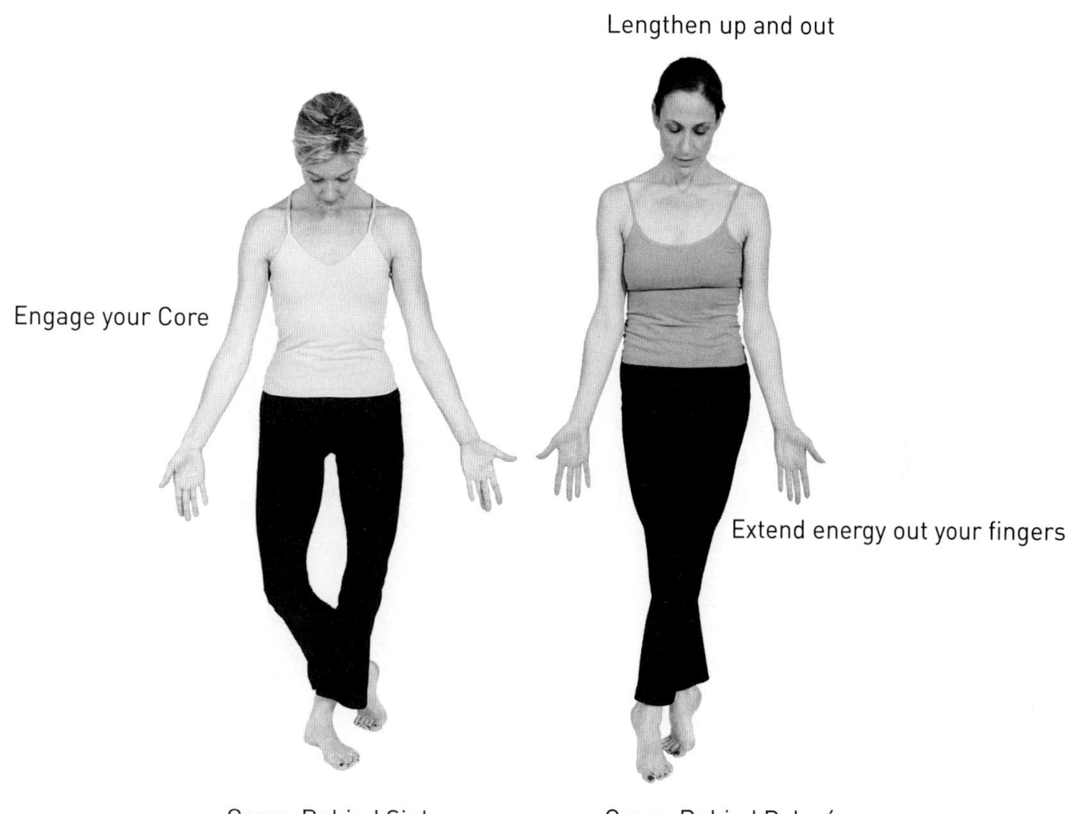

Cross-Behind Sink

Cross-Behind Relevé

BENEFITS: Practicing Cross Behind develops mobility and stability in your legs, which helps you move more efficiently.

Standing in Open Stance, step back and onto the ball of your left foot, crossing your ankles as if making a small "x." Keep your back heel high, and practice alternating sides. Now, step back crossing your ankles, and this time rise up onto the balls of both feet. Maintain your small "x" by keeping both feet under your hips. To guide your alignment, sound *cross.* Alternate sides.

TRAVELING IN DIRECTIONS

Look where you go
Integrate your upper and lower body
Step out freely

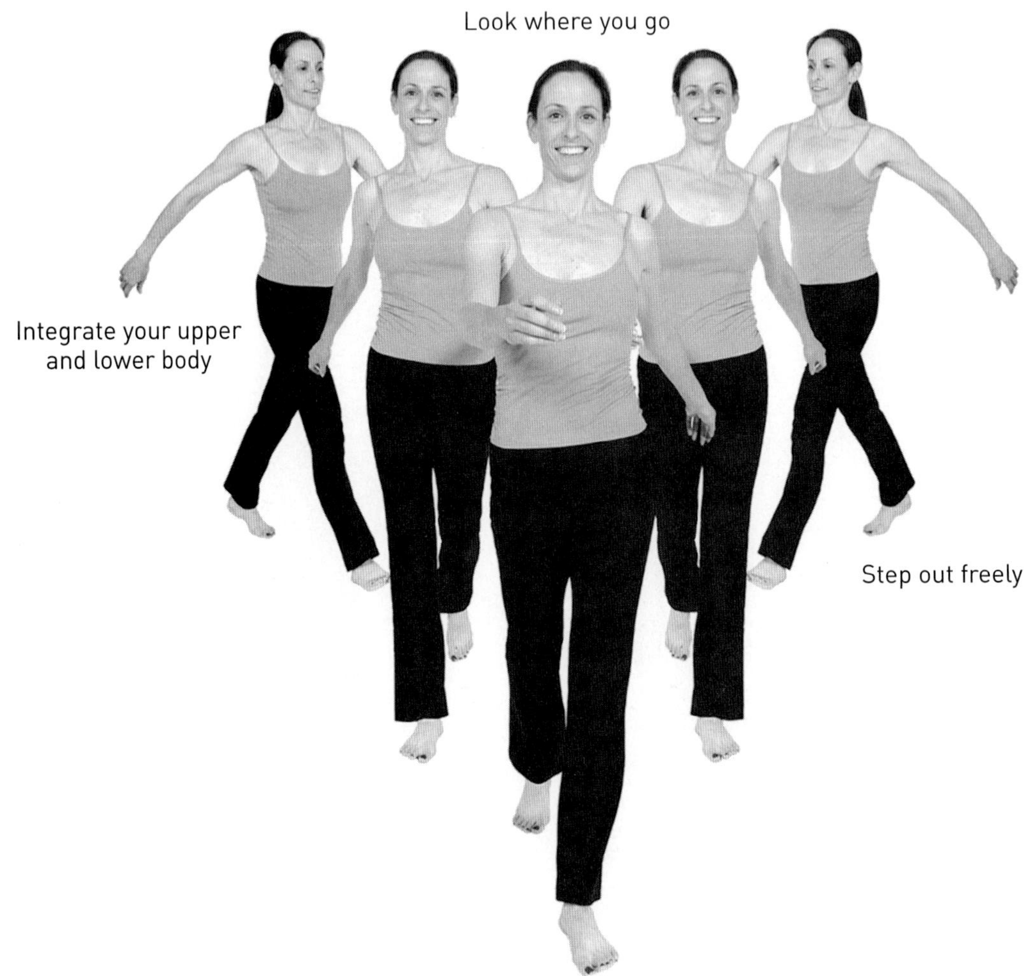

BENEFITS: Practicing Traveling in Directions keeps your body agile for moving through space in all directions, able to change direction with ease.

Move through the room and consciously change directions every few paces. As you change direction, move the position of your entire body at once. Think about the move before you make it, to heighten your brain–body hook-up. With determination, sound the word *change* as you do the move. Lead each change of direction with your eyes.

LATERAL TRAVELING

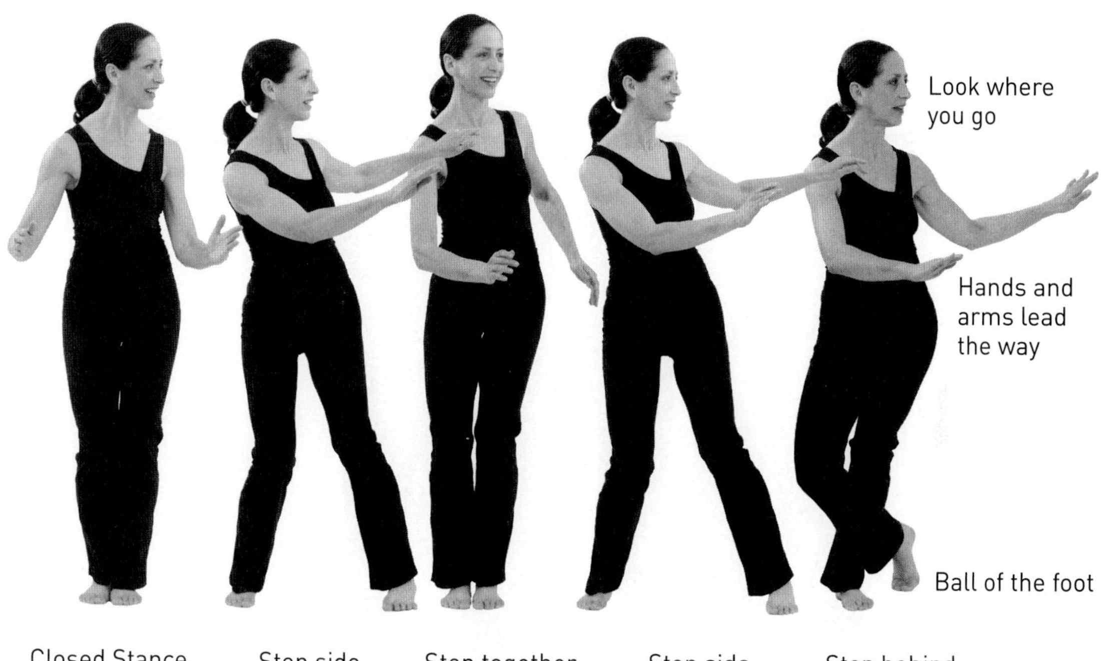

BENEFITS: Practicing Lateral Traveling improves your ability to move from left to right in a relaxed way.

Begin in a Closed Stance. You're going to repeatedly step to one side, practicing these two stepping motions. 1) step side, step together, step side; and 2) step side, step behind, step side, a move similar to the "grapevine." For both variations, extend your hands and arms in the same direction in which you are moving. When you step behind, step onto the back ball of the foot and keep your knees spring loaded and your spine vertical. To help get the feel of the motion, imagine you are a dancer and sound the word *side.* Work with various speeds to develop power and agility. Alternate sides.

CHA-CHA-CHA

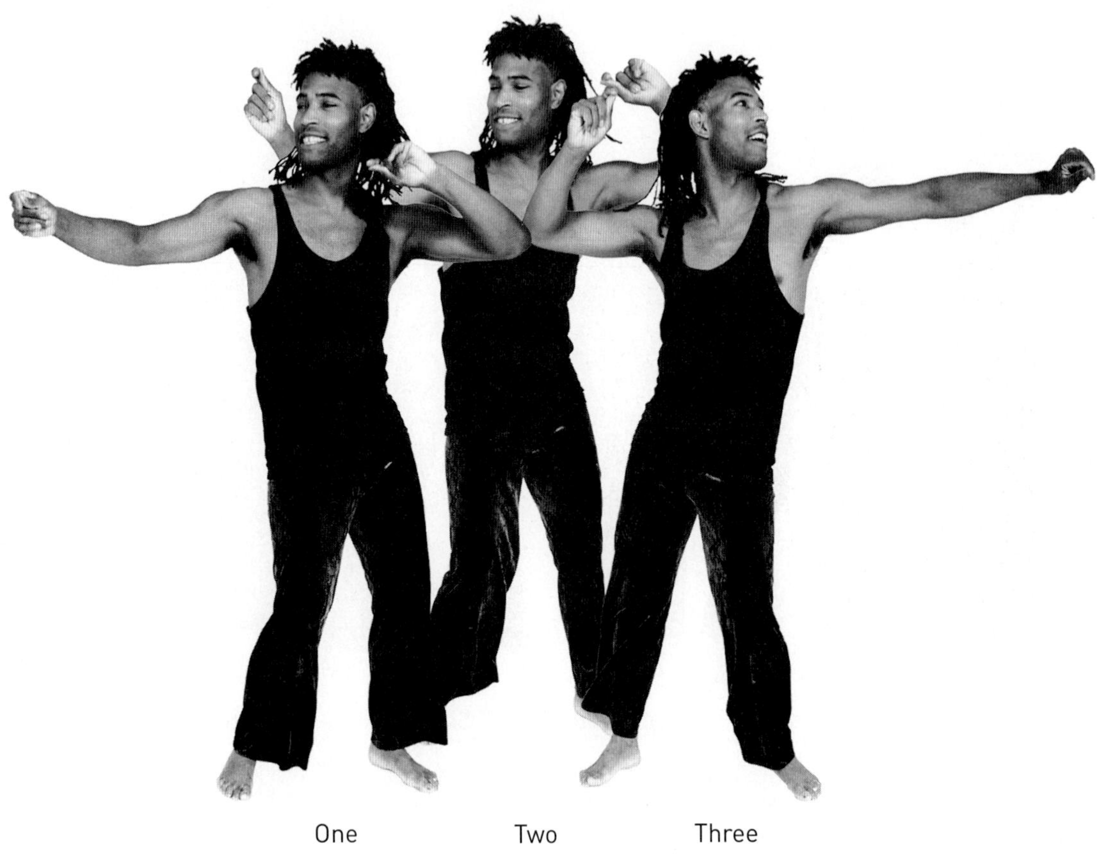

One Two Three

BENEFITS: Practicing Cha-Cha-Cha is good coordination training.

Cha-Cha-Cha is like the cha-cha dance step. In place, step left-right-left, then right-left-right, in a one-two-three count. Keep your feet close to the ground. Feel free to use your hands and arms to express yourself in many playful ways. To help keep your rhythm, sound *cha-cha-cha*. This helps develop athletic skill, lower-body speed, and coordination.

SLOW CLOCK

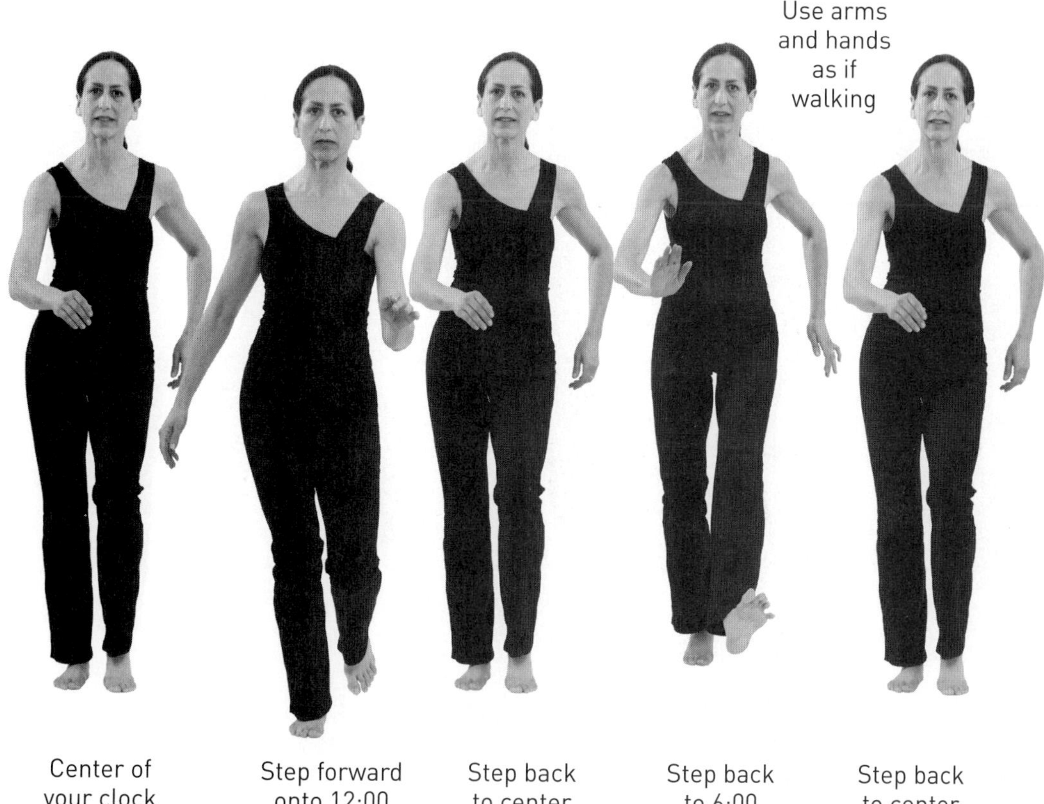

BENEFITS: Practicing Slow Clock teaches you to sense moving from center as the way to monitor relaxation in the body.

Begin by marching in place, in the center of an imaginary clock on the floor. Starting with your left foot, march at a rhythmic pace and on 1, step to the front with your left foot landing on 12:00; then back to the center of your clock. Then step back to 6:00 and back to center. "Slow" clock refers to always returning to center after stepping to any number. Sound *12:00, center, 6:00, center* as you move, and then try stepping to other numbers. This move adds precision and grace. Alternate sides.

FAST CLOCK

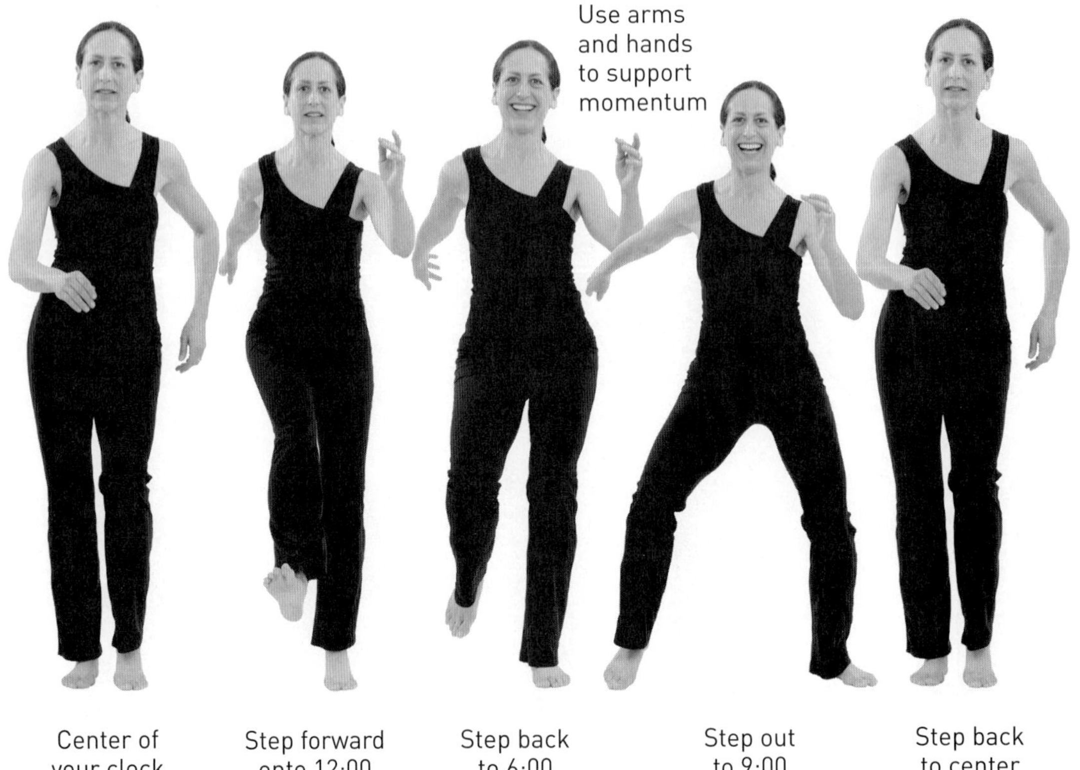

Center of your clock | Step forward onto 12:00 | Step back to 6:00 | Step out to 9:00 | Step back to center

BENEFITS: Practicing Fast Clock improves your stamina, agility, coordination, and ability to move and breathe faster.

This is similar to the Slow Clock, but this time you'll be stepping from one number to the other, combining two or more numbers before returning to center. Begin by marching in place in the center of an imaginary clock on the floor. Maintain a rhythmic pace, and on 1, step to the front with your left foot, landing on 12:00; then with your left foot, step over the center of your clock and onto 6:00, as if stepping over a puddle; then with your left foot, step over the center of your clock and out onto 9:00; then step back to the center of your clock. The moving leg steps to a number while the other leg steps in the center of your clock. Now change sides, leading with your right foot, stepping to 12:00, 6:00, and 3:00. Sound *12:00, 6:00, 3:00, center* as you move. Alternate sides.

FRONT KICK

Use hands for stability
Look where you kick
Relaxed knee
Ready Position
Balance on Whole Foot
Push down to power your kick

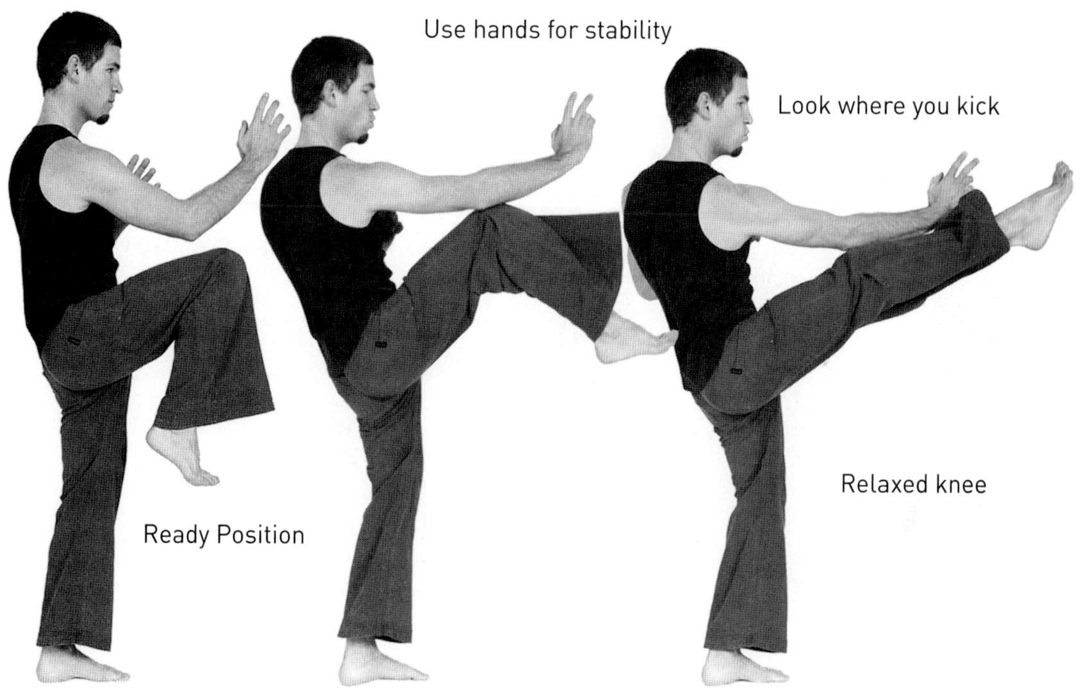

BENEFITS: Practicing Front Kick is excellent training for grounding explosive movements in a balanced way.

Lift your thigh, tucking your heel in toward your buttocks into Ready Position. Look in the direction you intend to kick, and with your hands at heart level and your palms flexed, kick your foot out and to the front. Push down into the earth with the supporting foot, and use your hands and arms to maintain vertical alignment and balance. As you kick front, keep the front of your thigh facing the ceiling, and keep the knee of your supporting leg unlocked and spring loaded. Start with a low kick, then work higher. Imagine kicking a balloon. This move will build balance, coordination, confidence, and strength. As your kicks gain power, shift from sounding *purr* to *pow!* Alternate sides.

SIDE KICK

Look
side
Engage
Core
Elbows in and down
Press out to extend
Shift into your
supporting leg
Ready Position,
heel to buttocks
Turn toes out to kick higher

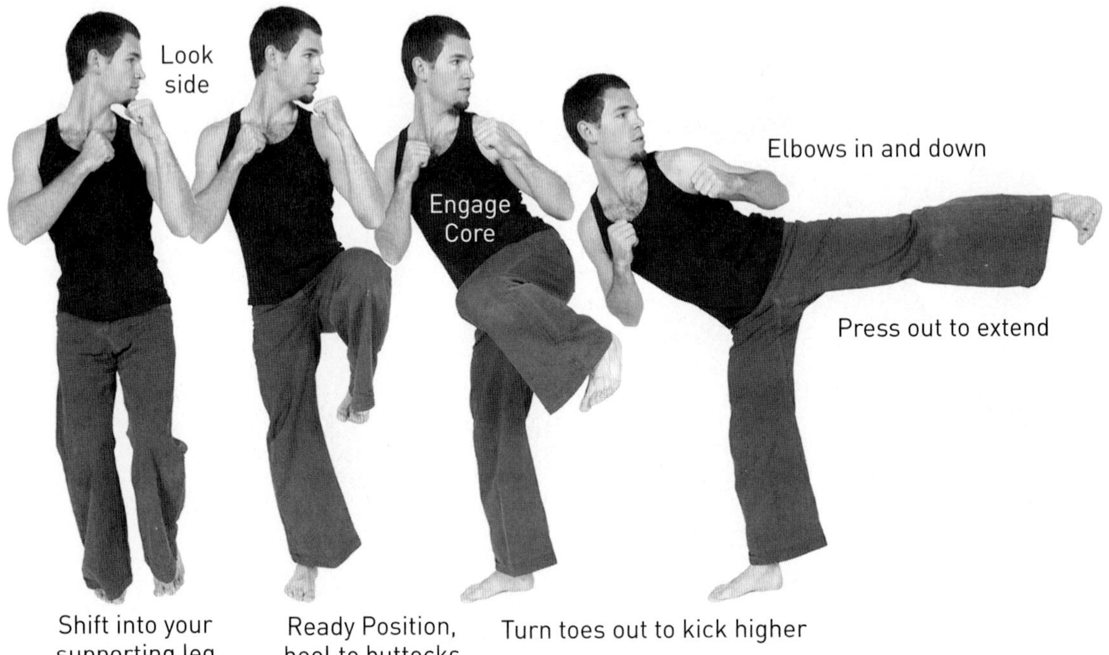

BENEFITS: Practicing the Side Kick is excellent conditioning for the buttock muscles, which powers your leg and kicking motions from behind and underneath.

Pull your heel up and back toward your buttocks as you did in Front Kick, into Ready Position. Then kick to the side, with the side of your thigh facing toward the ceiling. Keep the knee of your supporting leg unlocked and spring loaded. Imagine pushing a boulder. To kick higher, turn out the foot and toes of the supporting leg first. This opens up the hip joint and allows higher kicks. Sound the word *yes* or *no* with each kick. Alternate sides.

BACK KICK

Look behind to rotate
Elbows down and into your body
Ready Position
Use Whole Foot for power
Press down to power your kick

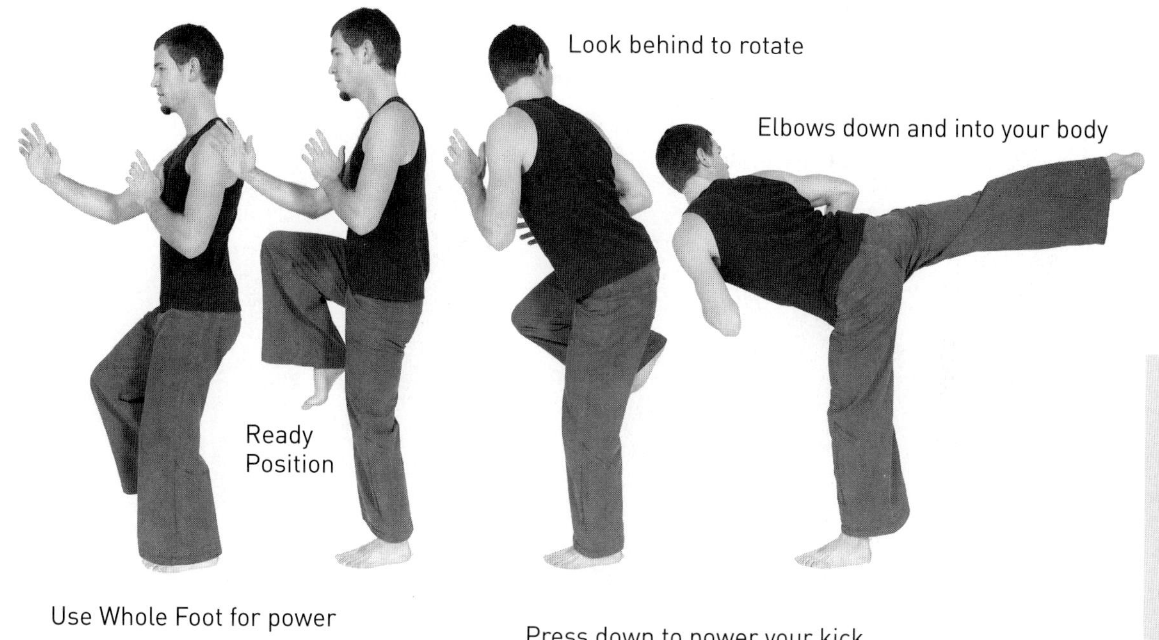

BENEFITS: Practicing Back Kick is excellent conditioning for the muscles along the back side of your body.

Pull your heel up and back toward your buttocks into Ready Position, then kick backward, in a motion similar to a mule kick. As you kick, keep the knee of your supporting leg unlocked and spring loaded, using your hands and arms for balance. Imagine you are leaving a footprint on the wall behind you. To challenge your sense of balance, look backward as you kick. To kick high, rotate on the supporting leg's hip joint. To bolster your balance, sound the word *wheeee!* Alternate sides.

KNEE SWEEP

Ready Position, palms up, elbows back
Knee in
Knee up
Hand pushes knee out to the side
Knee out
Sumo Stance

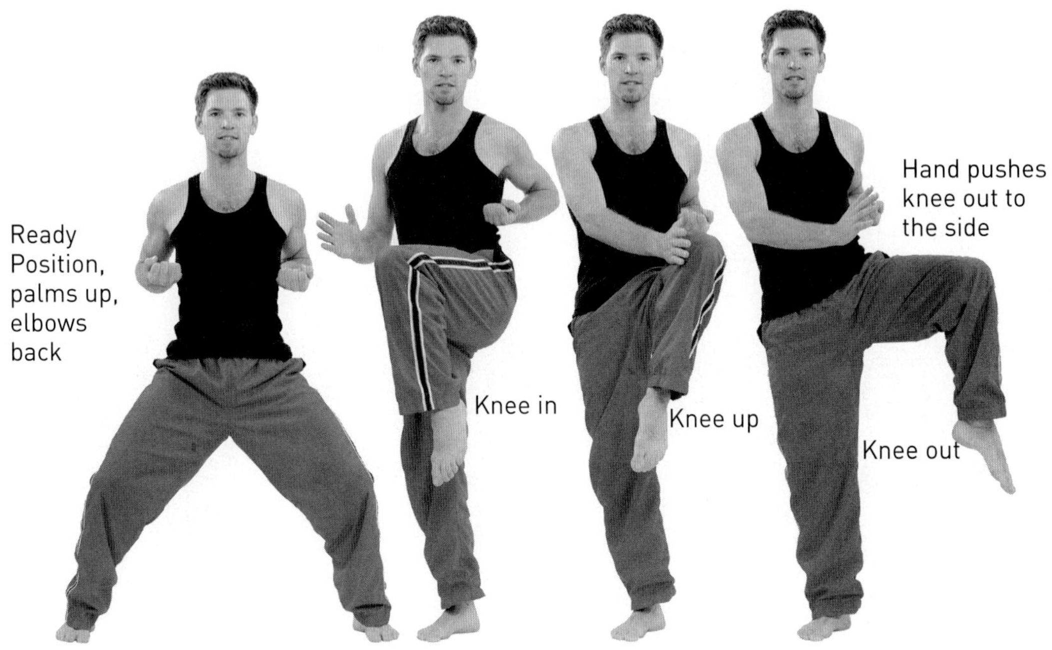

BENEFITS: Practicing Knee Sweep improves stability and agility in the hip joint and will help you develop power in your whole body.

Bring one of your knees up and across your body and, with your opposite hand, push your knee and sweep it out to the side, as if you were stepping over a big box. Then lower your foot to the ground. Walk around the room, pretending to step over boxes of different heights. Keep the knee of your supporting leg spring loaded. To maintain dynamic ease, sound *sweeep!* Alternate sides.

PELVIC CIRCLES

Express yourself
with your arms
and your hands
Push your
pelvis to circle
Lift one heel to
circle deeper

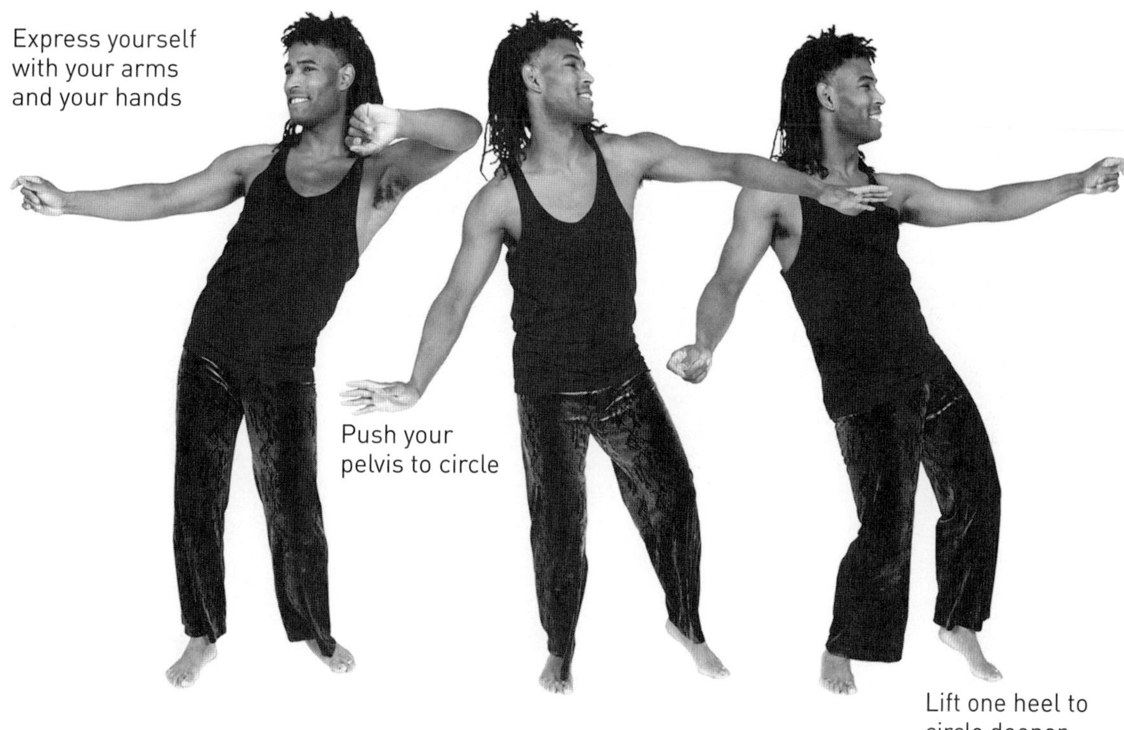

BENEFITS: Practicing Pelvic Circles strengthens your back and Core, so that all upright locomotion is dynamic and free. This move will help bring up energy from your lower chakras and will strengthen your abdominal muscles.

Stand in "A" Stance and circle your hips in a fluid motion, as if you were playing with a hula hoop. Sense the motion of the ball of your hip joints rotating in their sockets. Circle in both directions to maintain relaxed mobility, and sound *ahhh!* Alternate directions.

HIP BUMPS

Freely use your hands and arms

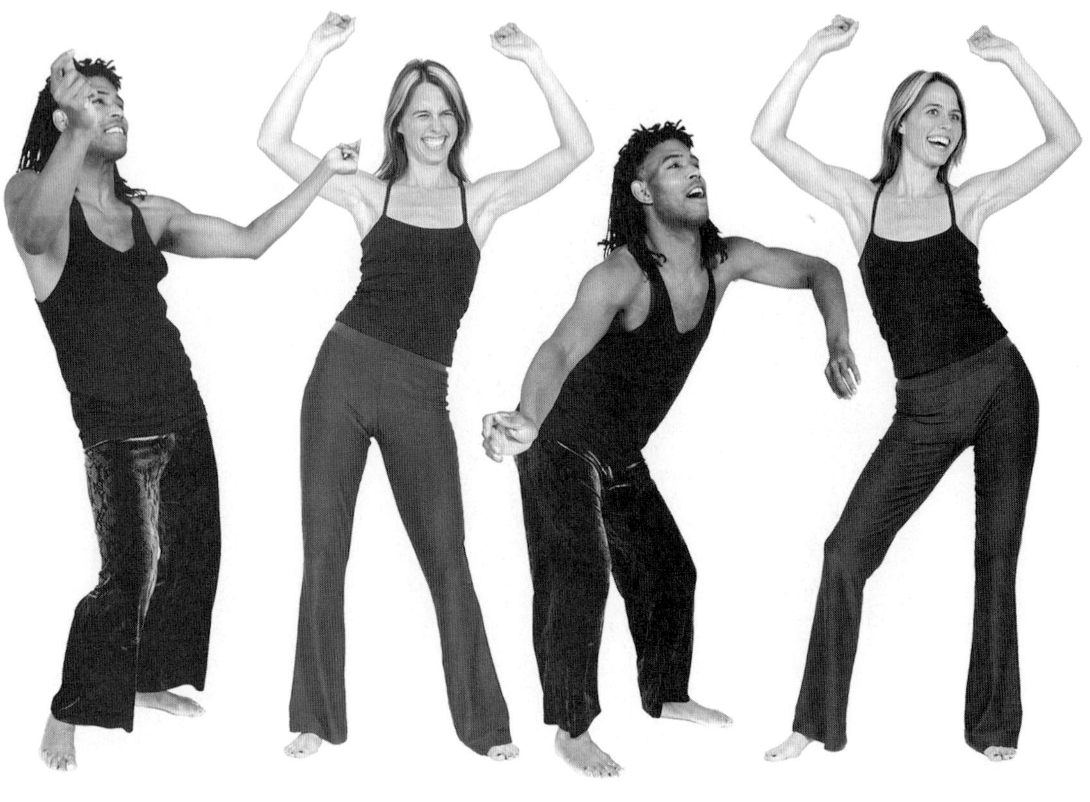

Bump front | Bump right | Bump back | Bump left

BENEFITS: Practicing Hip Bumps keeps your upper body agile and connected to your lower body. This move will tone your Core, define your waist, and increase mobility along your spine.

Bump your hips in varying directions, front, back, and each side, as if you were bumping someone out of the way. Sound *ooo.* Focus on rhythmic precision, and stop the bump before it tugs uncomfortably. Alternate directions.

CHEST ISOLATIONS

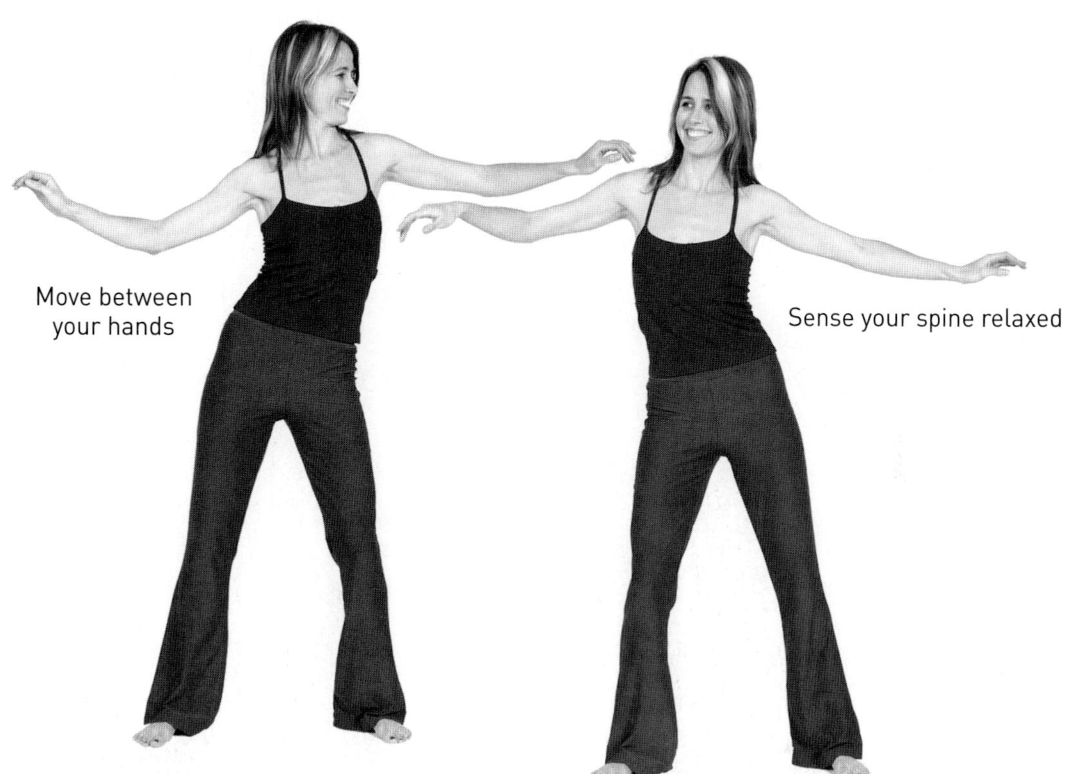

BENEFITS: Practicing Chest Isolations keeps your spine flexible and mobile.

Gently move your rib cage in all directions, placing your hands and arms in space so that you isolate and move only the rib cage. Move it to the front, back, and sides. Open it, twist it, extend it, slide it, and circle it. Focus on rhythmic and fluid movements in all directions. Sound *ahhh!* in a very relaxed way. This move will build the muscles of your Core and will help you improve your posture.

SHIMMY

Move from the
inside out
Hands relaxed at
sides of the body

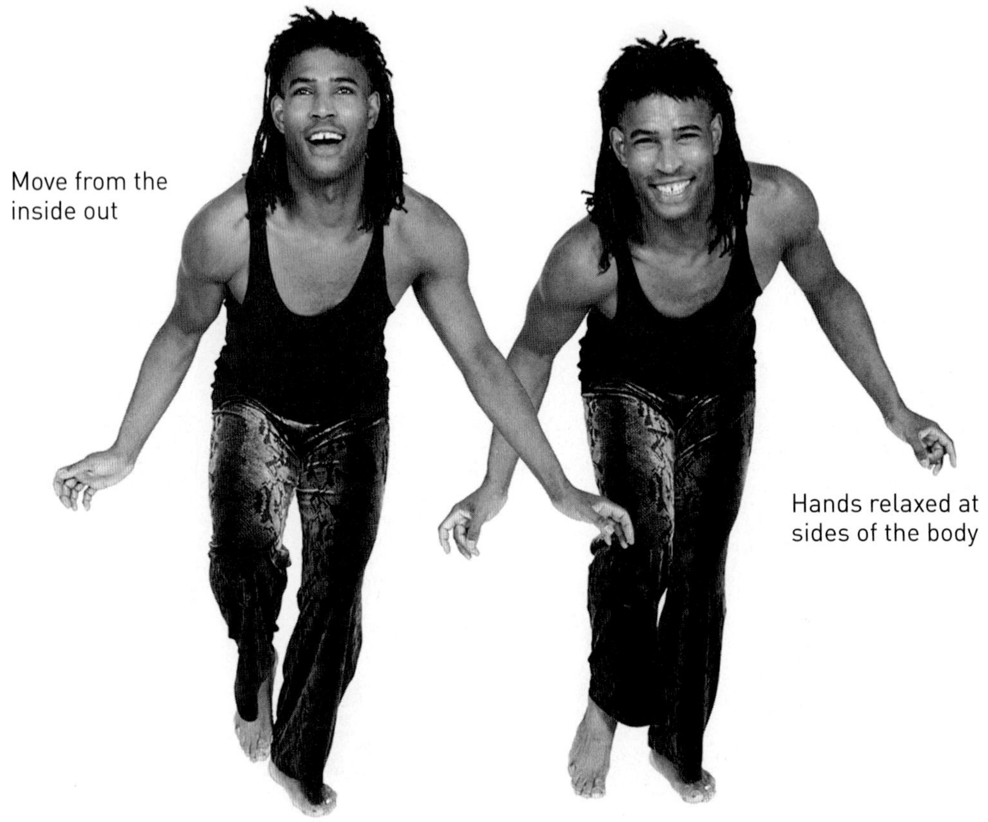

BENEFITS: Practicing Shimmy strengthens your Core and supports your upright posture. This move is great for attaining precision in small movements and building endurance in small muscles.

Vibrate and shake your shoulders, standing upright or moving front and back, as if you are shaking water off. Relaxing your lower jaw, so that the neck and shoulder girdle muscles naturally relax, will allow your arms to hang loosely. Make your movements continuous, instead of jerky. Sound the vowels *a, e, i, o, u* as you shimmy.

UNDULATION

Look up and open the front of your spine
Wave from the top
Look down to open the back of the spine
Wave from the bottom
Sit back to undulate the low back
Feet hip width apart

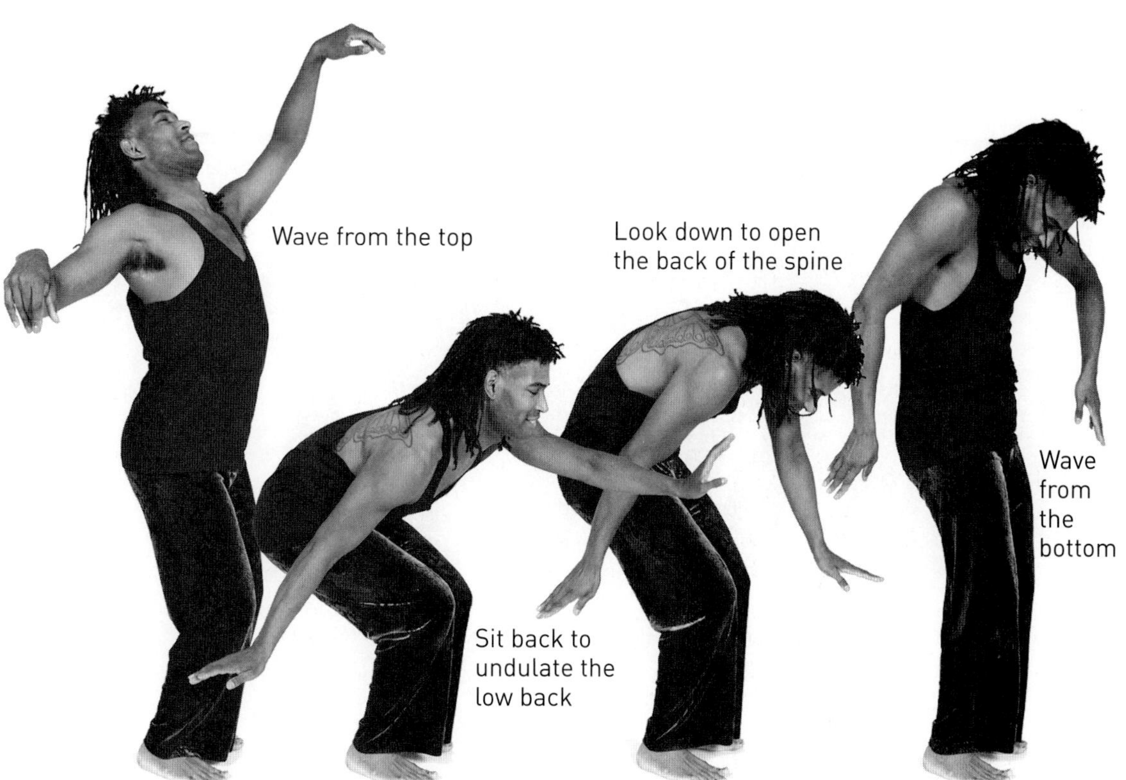

BENEFITS: Practicing Undulation keeps energy flowing along, and through, your entire spine. This move is perfect for releasing tension in the back and bringing power to the Core.

Standing in Open Stance, undulate, or wave, your spine—from top to bottom and then bottom to top. Imagine that your spine is a third arm. As you do the move, sense the spaces between your vertebrae. This mental focus will help release neuromuscular energy and chi that may be blocked in the spine. To help make your movements smooth, sound the word *yessss.* Practice in all stances.

SPINAL ROLL

Inhale and look up to open and lengthen
Look down as you unfold into a full rise
Slide down
Exhale to round up
Relax in "A" Stance
Sink into a strong Base
Push away to rise

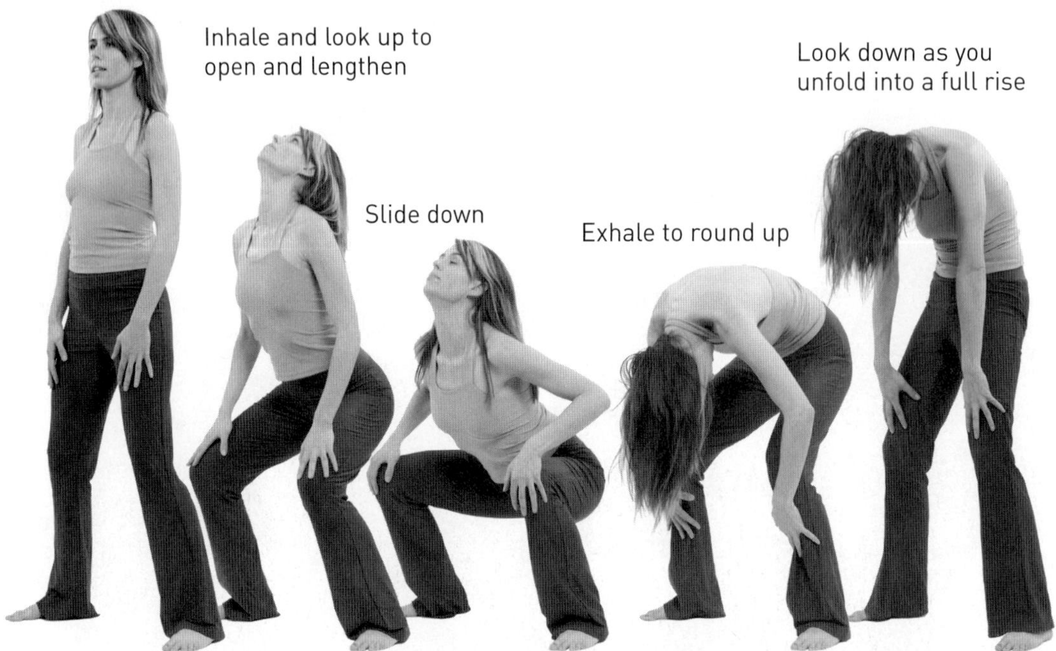

BENEFITS: Practicing Spinal Roll keeps your spine strong and flexible. It's terrific for self-healing the spine and back.

Standing in "A" Stance, inhale deeply and look up and sense the front of your body lengthening and opening. Use your hands for support and slide them down your legs, sinking to a point at which your body says, "Enough, I can't go farther." As if you were a rag doll falling asleep, exhale and look toward the earth; then round up, pushing your feet into the floor, while sliding your hands back up your legs to return to a standing posture. Do the whole movement smoothly, and coordinate your leg and spine mobility. Imagine your spine waving like seaweed in the ocean. Sound the word *hummm* quietly, as you round up, feeling the vibration in your jaw and skull. Focus mentally on energy leaving you as you go downward, and then filling you again as you rise.

HEAD AND EYE MOVEMENTS

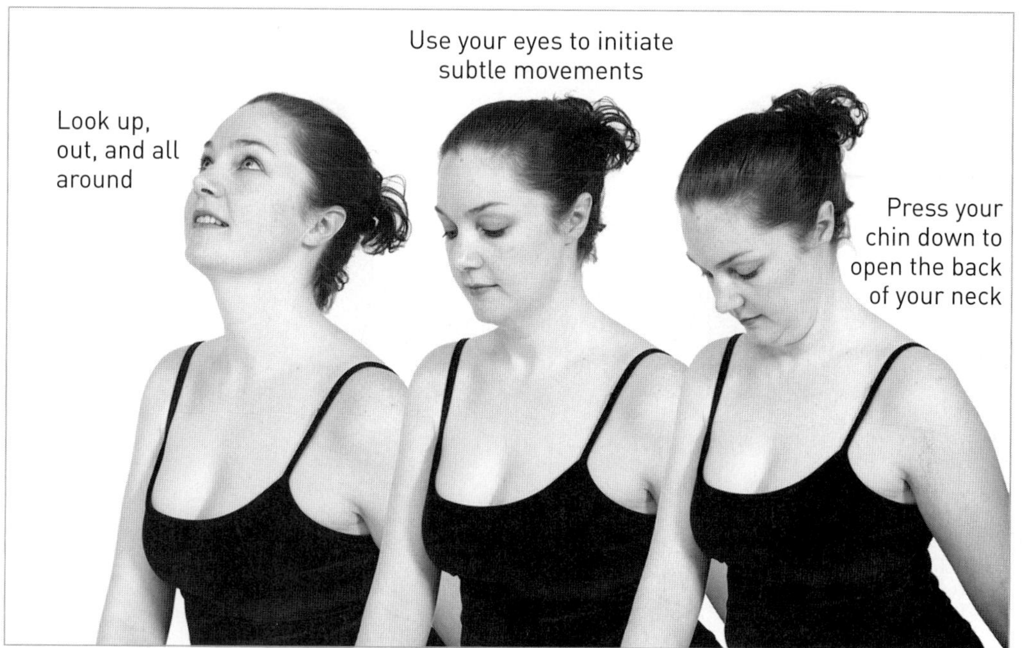

BENEFITS: Practicing Head and Eye Movements teaches you to look wherever you go.

Look in any direction with your eyes, as if you were following a butterfly, and then follow that direction with a move of your head. Use your eyes to "seduce" your head, through natural curiosity, into moving. Look, and then move, in all directions. Next, follow a body part, such as your hand, with your eyes. To enhance relaxation, keep your lower jaw slightly open, and let the tip of your tongue press lightly into the roof of your mouth. Now, nod your head, shake it, and roll it. Your head is the heaviest of your body weights, and this move helps you find the proper balance for it, eradicating the tension that comes from holding it upright all day long. As you do the moves, sound *yes, no,* and *maybe* exuberantly, tying them to the body language gestures of nodding and shaking your head.

BLOCKS

Palm away
Forearm pulls up to protect your forehead
Ready Position, elbows back, palms up
Elbow pulls back

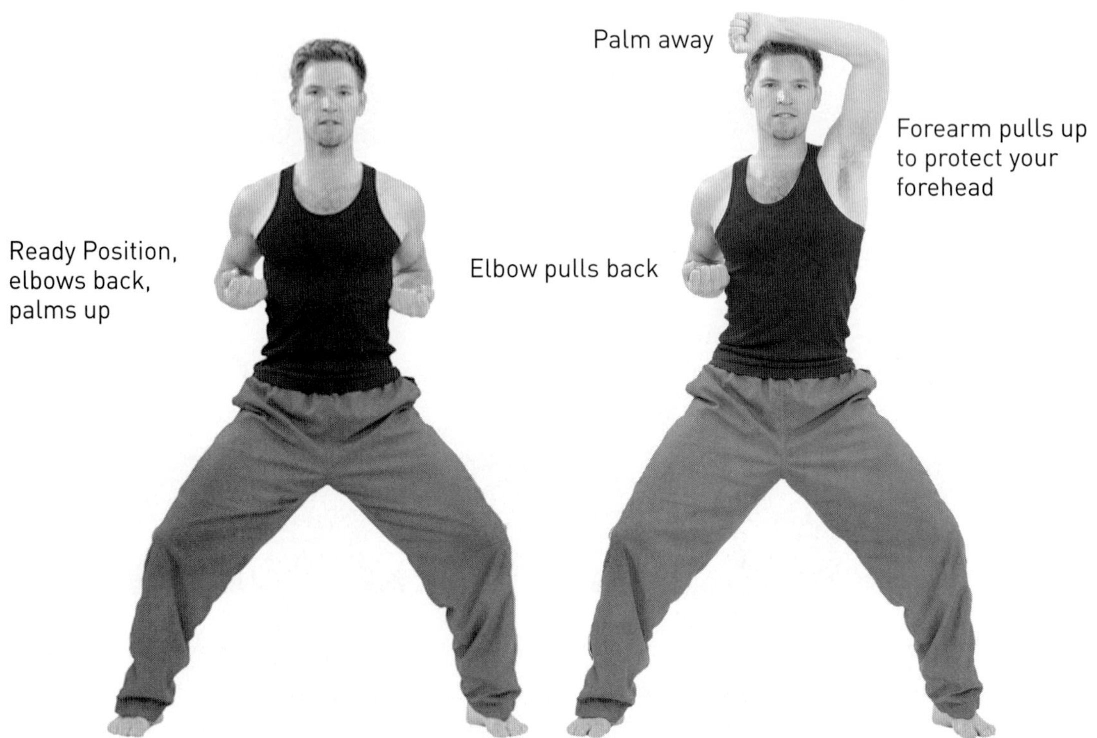

UPWARD BLOCK: Grounded into a strong and stable Sumo Stance

BENEFITS: Practicing Blocks improves your ability to start and stop, creating dynamic upper body coordination. These blocks will build your arm strength and speed and will naturally endow you with added physical confidence.

There are four basic blocks: Upward, Downward, Inward, and Outward. Practice all of them in Riding (Sumo) Stance, and use your forearm and hand as if to shield yourself from any oncoming object. Begin and end each block in Ready Position. Ready Position is palms up, elbows in and pulled back down, with the forearms hugging the sides of the body. Powerful blocks come from moving out of and returning back to Ready Position.

As you do the blocks, the alignment of your forearms stays within an imaginary picture frame. After each block, return to Ready Position, keeping your elbows drawn back and your palms facing up. Keep your lower jaw relaxed and slightly open. As you do each block, exhale and sound *up!, down!, in!,* or *out!* Alternate sides.

To do the Upward Block, start in Ready Position, and simultaneously bring one elbow and forearm up, blocking the area in front of your face and forehead, while the other elbow and forearm draws back to maintain vertical alignment.

To do the Downward Block, start in Ready Position, and simultaneously bring one fist and forearm across, down, and out, blocking the area in front of your groin, while the other elbow and forearm draws back to maintain vertical alignment.

Three body weights aligned
Ready Position,
elbows back,
palms up
Forearm pulls
down to protect
your groin

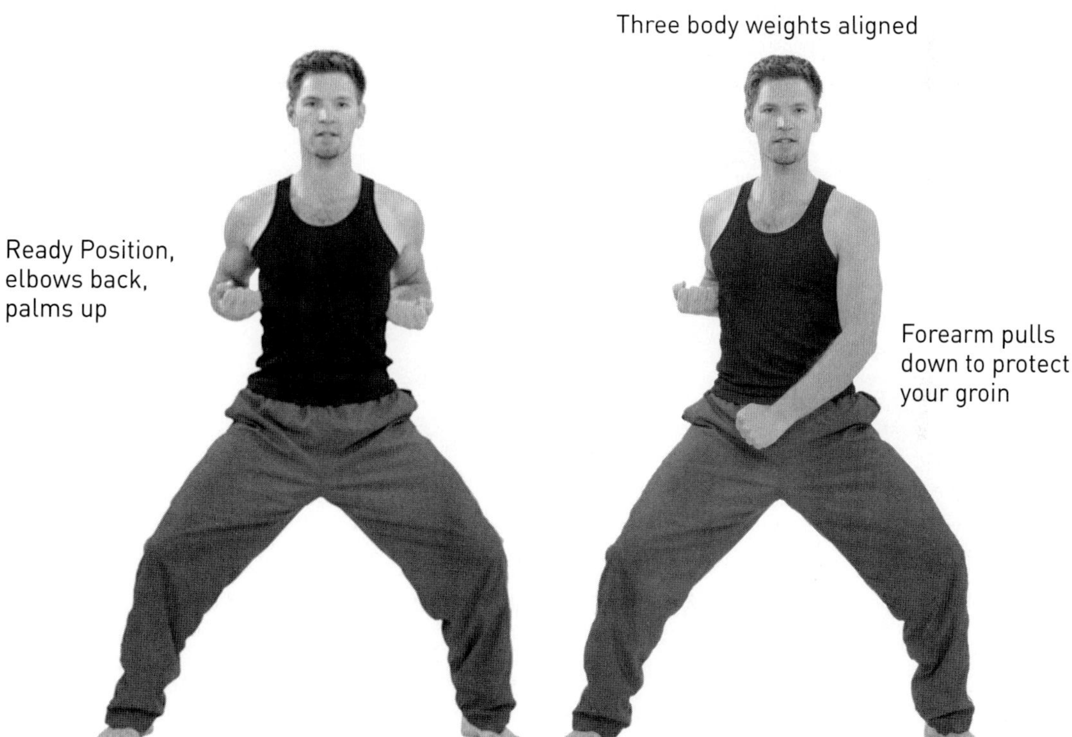

DOWNWARD BLOCK: Keep your ankle, knee, and hip joints agile

To do the Inward Block, start in Ready Position, and simultaneously bring one fist and forearm diagonally across, up, and in, blocking the opposite side of your face, while the other elbow and forearm draws back to maintain vertical alignment.

Ready Position,
elbows back,
palms up
Forearm pulls in to
protect the opposite
side of your face
Hips face front

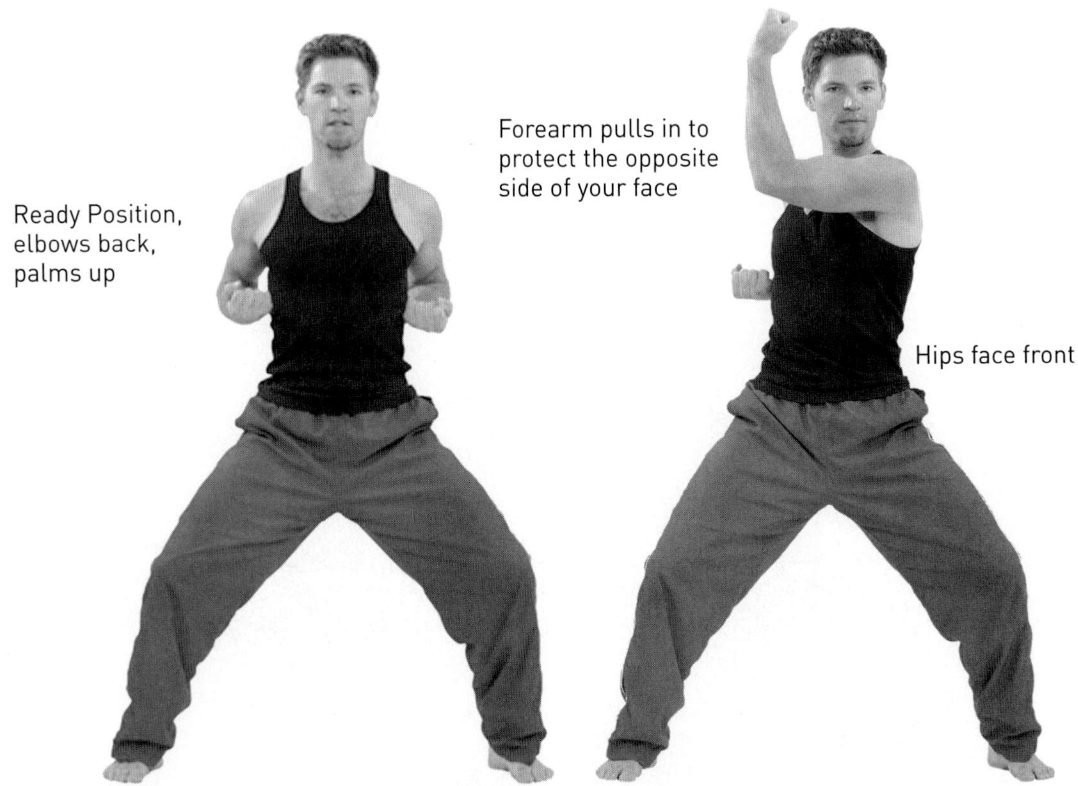

INWARD BLOCK: Sense power from the ground up

To do the Outward Block, start in Ready Position, and simultaneously bring one fist and forearm across, up, and out, blocking the side of your face, while the other elbow and forearm draws back to maintain vertical alignment.

Ready Position, elbows back, palms up
Forearm pulls out to protect the side of your face
Engage the Core

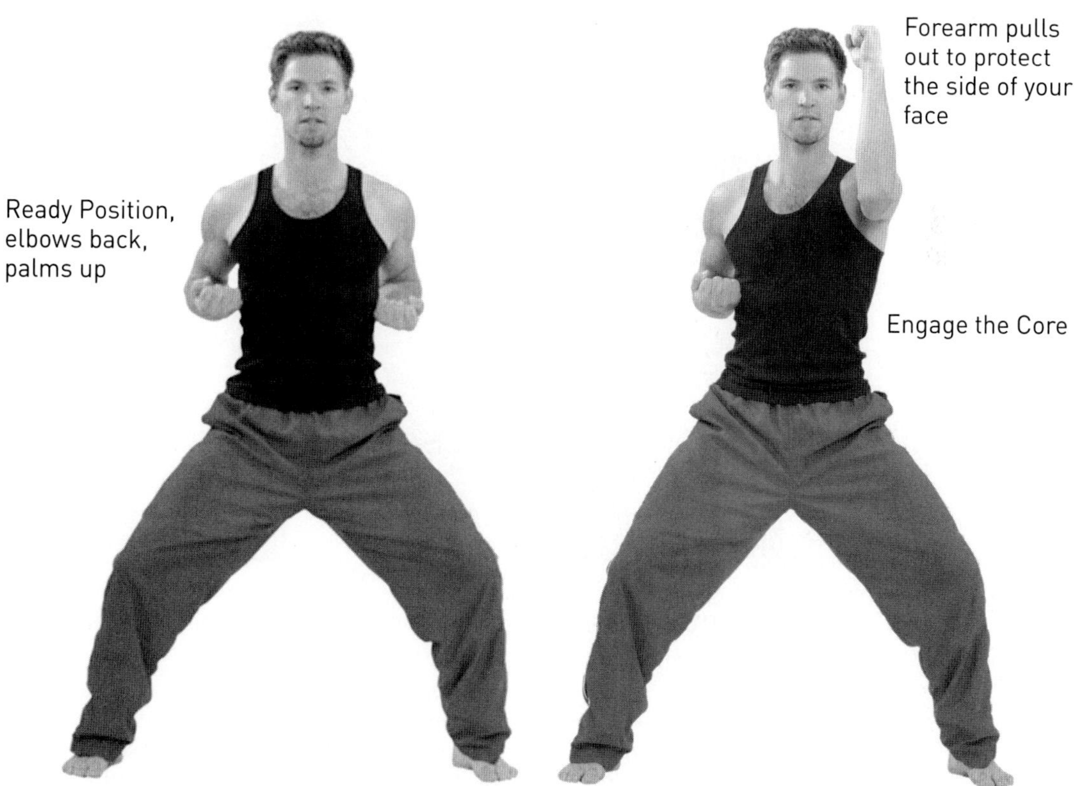

OUTWARD BLOCK: Use your feet for stability

PUNCHES

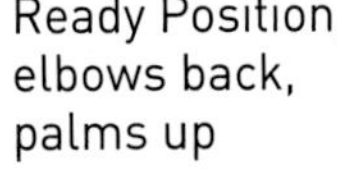

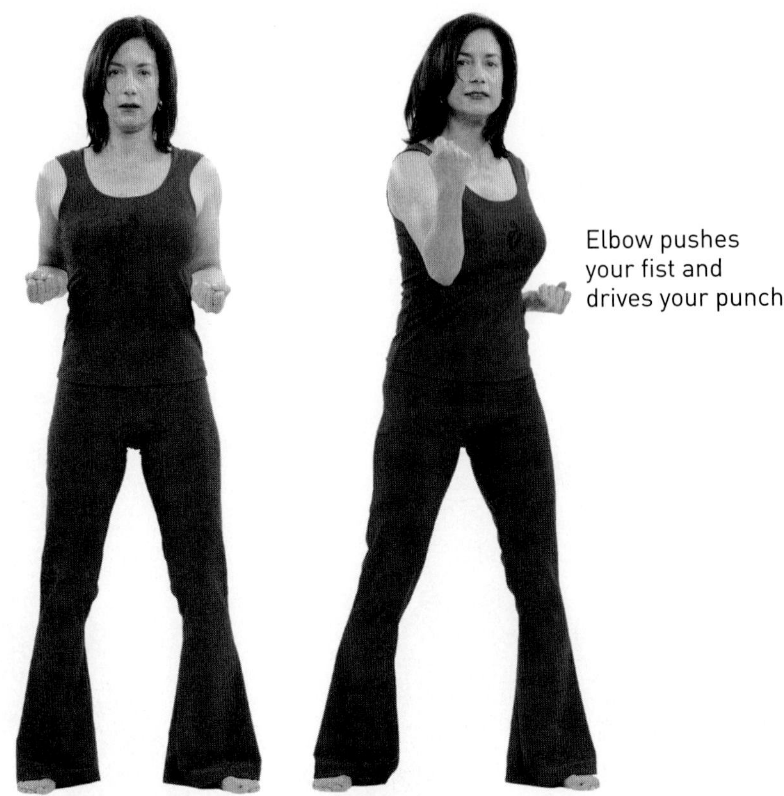

UPWARD PUNCH: Settle into "A" Stance with relaxed knees and hips

> BENEFITS: Practicing Punches is excellent training for moving quickly and rhythmically. These moves strenghten your Core as well as your arms, and will enhance your sense of personal power.

There are four basic punches: Upward, Outward, Across, and Downward. Practice all of them in "A" or Riding (Sumo) Stance, and use your fist as if hitting a punching bag. Begin and end each punch in Ready Position. Powerful punches come from spiraling the forearm bones, which comes from starting with palms up and ending with palms down, as if turning a screw.

As you do the punches, push with your feet, stay agile, and engage the Core of your body. After each punch, return to Ready Position, keeping your elbows drawn back and your palms facing up. Keep your lower jaw relaxed and your mouth slightly open. As you do each punch, exhale and sound *up!*, *out!*, *across!*, or *down!* Alternate sides.

To do the Upward Punch, start in Ready Position, and simultaneously use your elbow to power the punching fist up in front of your face, while the other elbow and forearm draws back to maintain vertical alignment.

To do the Outward Punch, start in Ready Position, and simultaneously bring one fist and forearm straight out to the front of the body, while the other elbow and forearm draws back to maintain vertical alignment.

Three body weights aligned

Ready Position, elbows back, palms up
Spiral your forearm to drive your punch out
Elbow draws back
Engage your Core

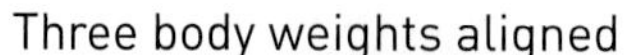

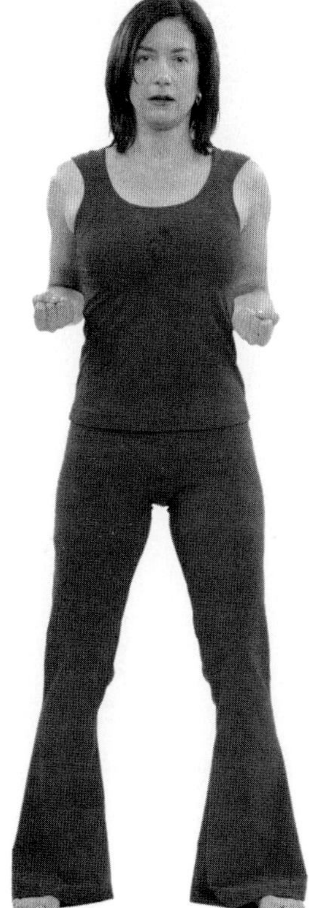

OUTWARD PUNCH: Move from a stable Base

To do the Across Punch, start in Ready Position, and simultaneously bring one fist and forearm across the body, while the other elbow and forearm draws back to maintain vertical alignment.

Ready Position,
elbows back,
palms up
Look where you punch
Spiral out and across,
palm down

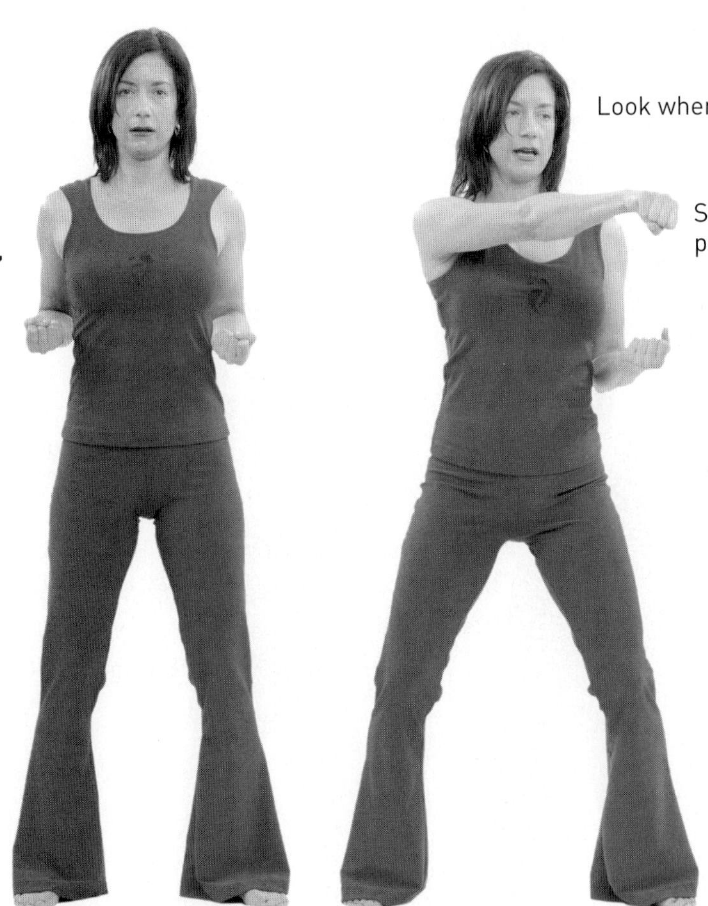

ACROSS PUNCH: Practice in "A" or Sumo Stance

To do the downward punch, start in Ready Position, and simultaneously bring one fist and forearm down in front of the body, while the other elbow and forearm draws back to maintain vertical alignment.

Ready Position,
elbows back,
palms up
Remain vertical as you
punch down

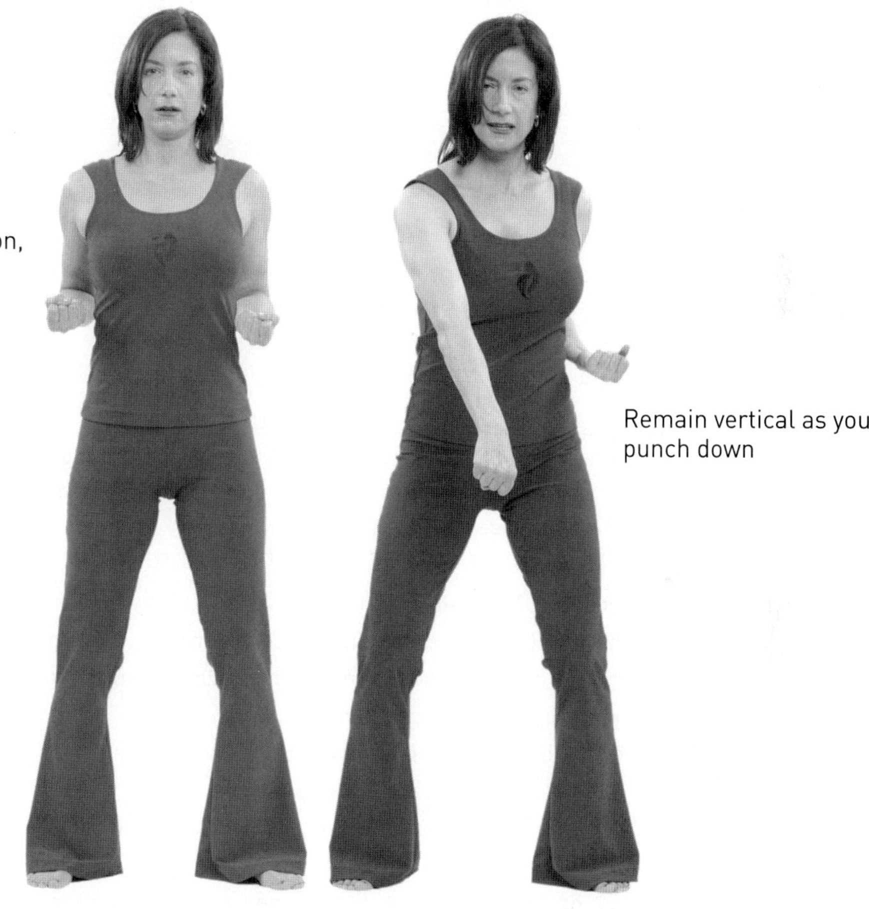

DOWNWARD PUNCH: Parallel feet for knee stability

ELBOW STRIKES

Strike out
Strike down
Strike back
Look where you strike
Ready Position, elbows in and down, palms up
Ground in Sumo Stance
Practice in Bow Stance

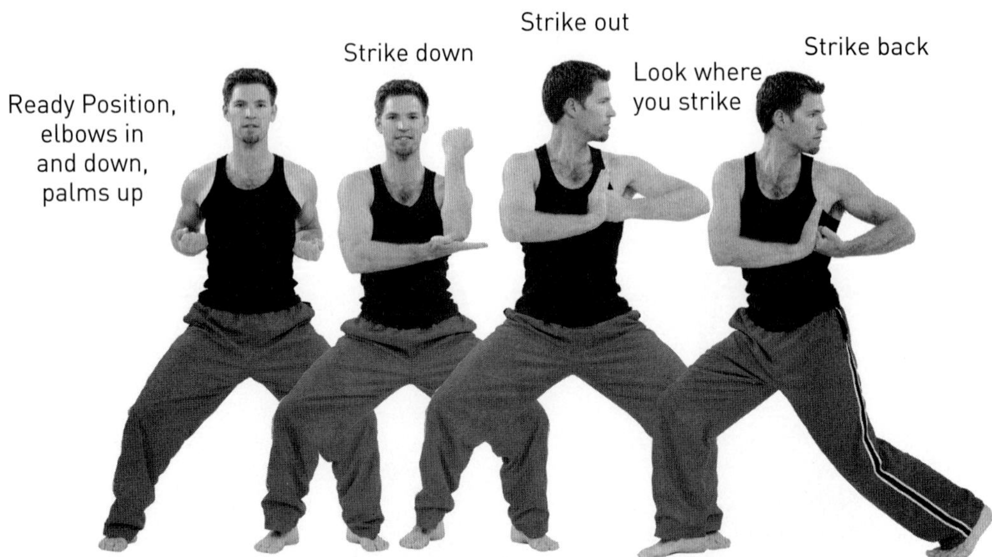

BENEFITS: Practicing Elbow Strikes is excellent for releasing stress and anxiety. These moves will strengthen and define upper chest, back, hands, and arms and will enhance your sense of confident determination.

There are three basic elbow strikes: Downward, Outward, and Backward. Practice all of them in Riding (Sumo) Stance or Bow Stance, and use the opposite hand for support to direct the strike. Powerful strikes come from engaging the whole body. Begin in Ready Position to ground and center.

To do the Downward Elbow Strike, using your opposite hand as a target, strike down abruptly, stopping before hitting.

To do the outward Elbow Strike, use your opposite hand to push and power your fist and elbow out to the side.

To do the Backward Elbow Strike, use your opposite hand to push and power your elbow back behind you.

As you do the Elbow Strikes, push with your feet, stay agile, and engage the Core of your body. Imagine that you are puncturing the space around you. Keep your lower jaw relaxed and mouth slightly open. As you do each strike, exhale and menacingly sound the word *strike.* Alternate sides.

TOUCHING

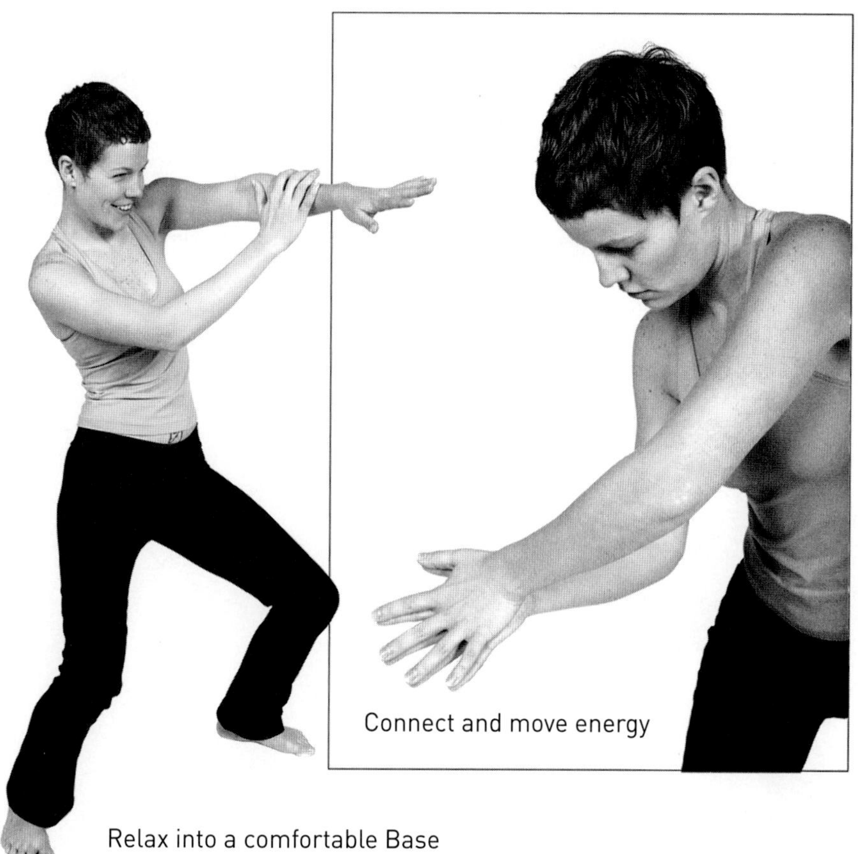

Connect and move energy

Relax into a comfortable Base

BENEFITS: Practicing Touching is excellent training for increasing your Sensory IQ and for improving body awareness. Touch is the act and the art of transmitting non-verbal information and receiving physical information from your environment. It also moves neuromuscular energy and chi into the area you touch and will enhance the grace and mastery you wish to convey in all your movements. It can also help self-heal physical trauma and naturally guide the body into relaxation.

Use your hands simply to touch the things that are around you. Touch your own skin, and the space around you. As you touch, sound the word *chi*. Use both hands.

Practice all hand and finger moves in place, and also while moving freely around the room.

FIST

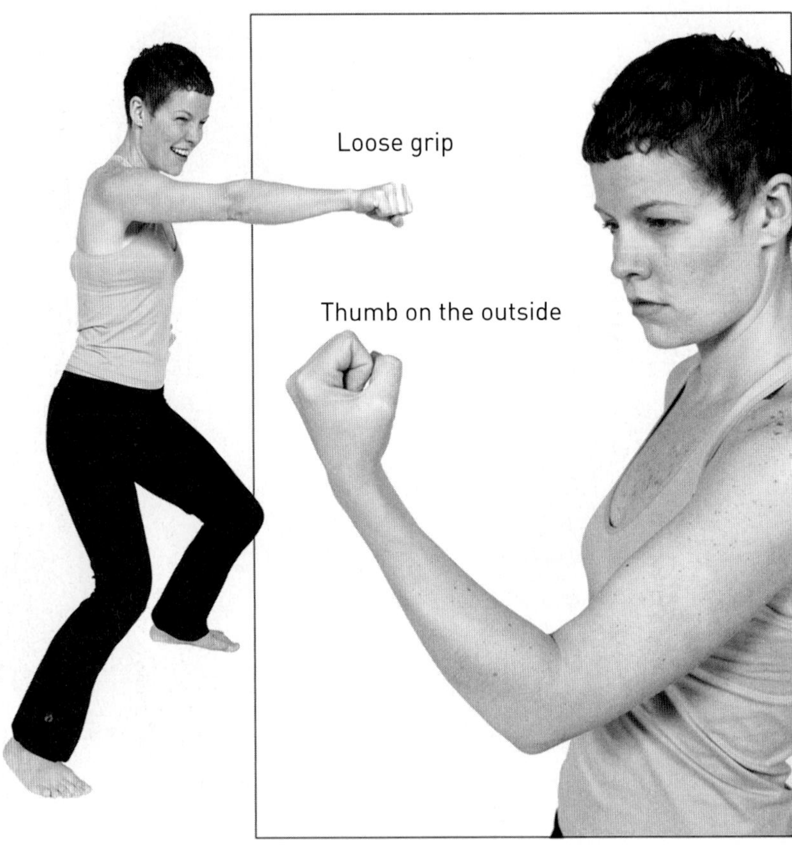

BENEFITS: Practicing the Fist is an excellent energy exercise for drawing energy in. It can also help release negative physical energy and emotions, which tend to build up from daily stress. It's also very effective for bringing strength and tone to the forearms.

Fold all your fingers into the fists of your hands, and shake them emotionally, as if you were in the process of exuberantly winning something, such as an athletic contest. Keep your thumbs on the outsides of your closed fists. As you make your fists, confidently sound the phrase *I made it!* to add to the feeling of joy and victory this move can generate. Use this move for expressing positive emotion—anything from triumph to joy. Use both hands.

PUMPS

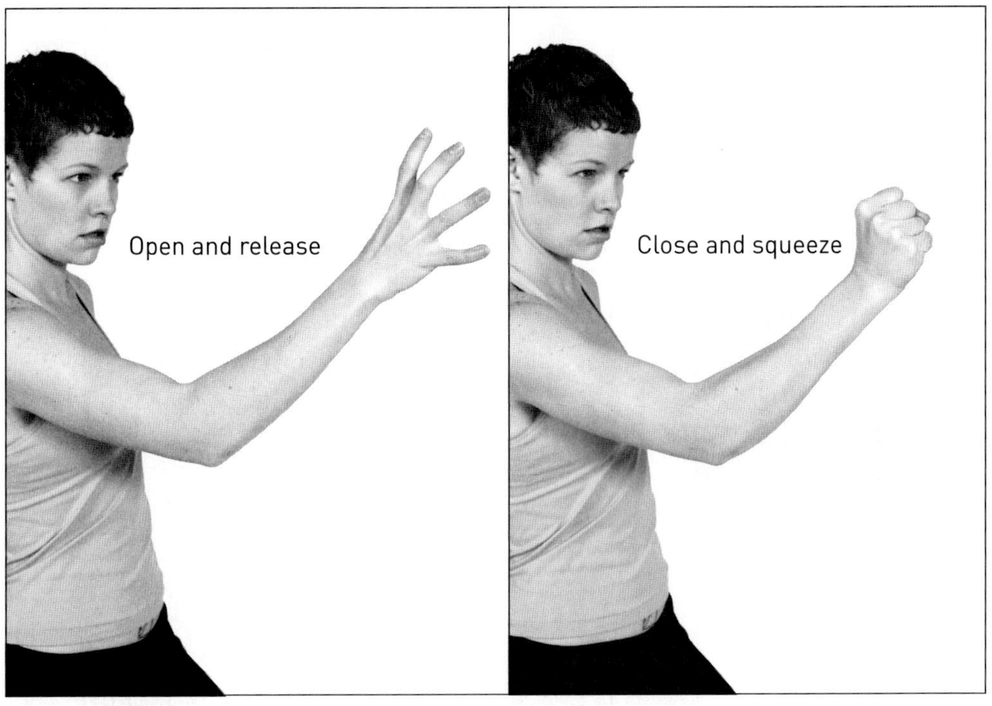

BENEFITS: Practicing Pumps reminds you to keep tension out of your neck and shoulders by keeping your hands active. This move builds power in the forearms, the fingers, and the wrists and can be helpful for people with repetitive use injuries, such as carpal tunnel syndrome.

Squeeze and then relax the palm and fingers of your hand, as if you were milking a cow. Use your thumb forcefully, and periodically change the tension in the squeeze. Sense for an increasing sensation of relaxation in your hands after each pump. Sound *ooooo,* using this sound to stimulate soft, loving contractions in your hands. Use both hands.

STRIKES

Strike out
Pull back
Push through the heel of your hand
Relax into a comfortable Base

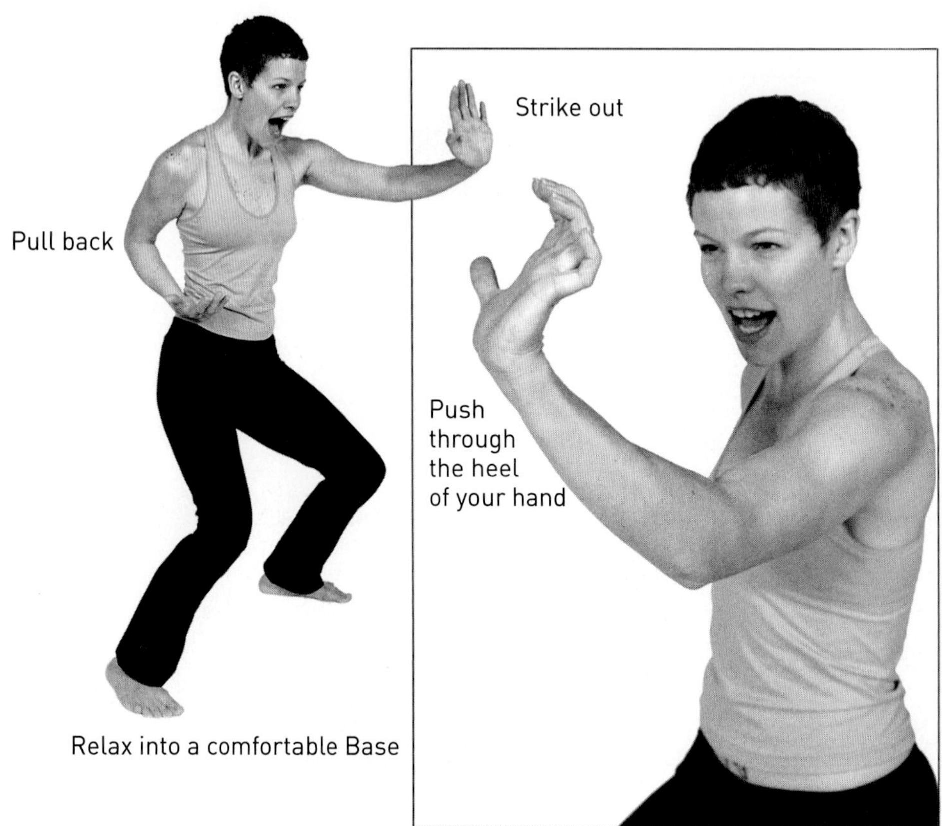

BENEFITS: Practicing Strikes keeps your hands and wrists integrated into whole-body movement. Strikes are perfect for learning to move with precision and for developing quick reactions. They build powerful arms, and heighten self-confidence.

Strike out with the heel of your hand, as if forcefully pushing someone out of the way. Stop suddenly before your arm is fully extended and sense the positive tension in your arms and hands that protects your elbow joint. As you strike, let it all rip, sounding the word *stop!* to release pent-up energy and emotion. Alternate sides.

CHOP CUT

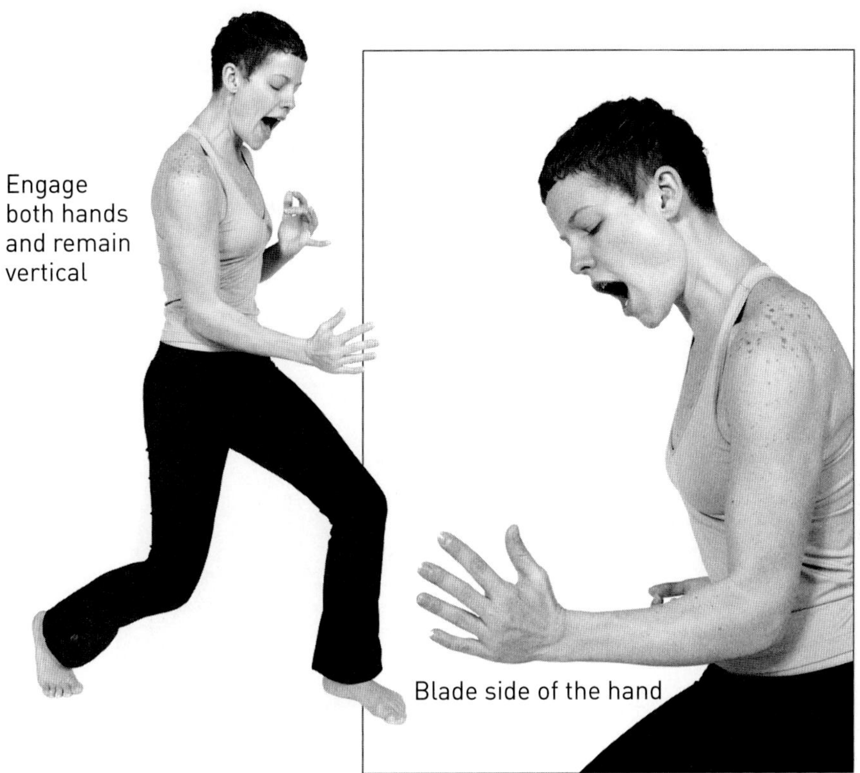

BENEFITS: Practicing Chop Cut is an excellent exercise for affirming your personal power. This move is effective for building strength in the arms and shoulders, and it is superb for releasing stress.

Chop the air with the edge, or "blade side," of your hand, as if you were executing a karate chop. Keep your thumb and fingers extended, and your wrist mobile, to support a powerful chopping action. As you chop downward, imagine that you are vanquishing something that is holding you back from achieving all that you desire and rancorously sound the word *because!* Use emotion and sound to move closer to your dreams. Alternate sides.

WEBBED SPACES

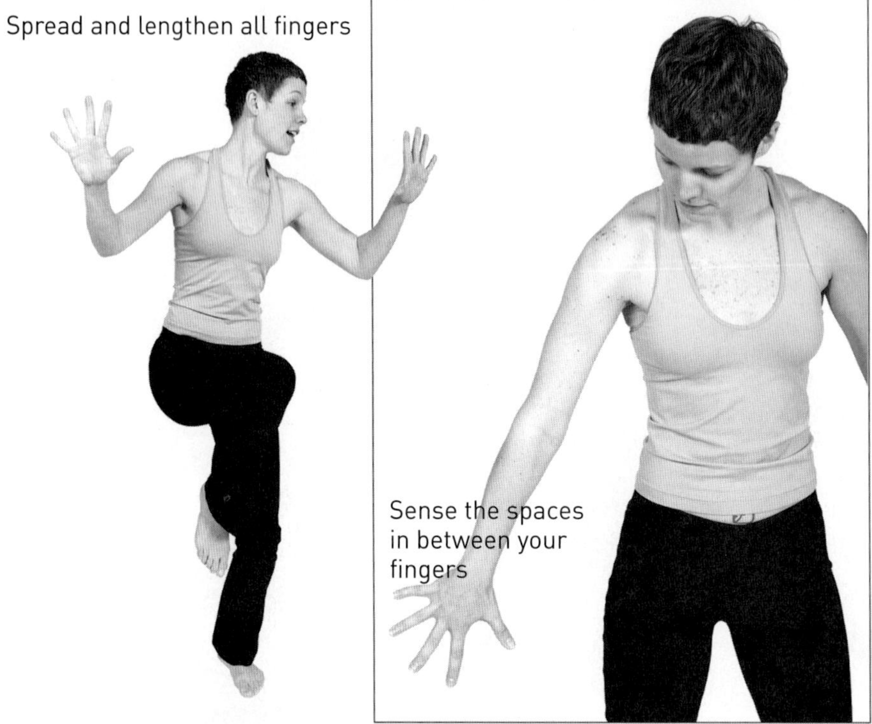

BENEFITS: Practicing Webbed Spaces improves hand agility, coordination, and sensitivity. This move helps you use your hands with greater precision, and it strengthens your hands, wrists, and fingers. It also magnifies your hands' sensitivity to the energy fields that surround them, thus improving your Sensory IQ. Use this move for expressing physical and emotional tension, and for deepening the dramatic expressions of your hand gestures.

Spread your fingers, and open the spaces between them, as if you were yawning with your hands. Sense for the positive tension in your hands and imagine a multi-banded light moving through their webbed spaces. Now, extend each finger, while vigorously separating all of them, making even more space among them. Sense the energy fields surrounding each finger. Move your hands freely and anywhere in space. Imagine your hands as pretty hand fans. As you do the move, sound the word *coool,* as you focus on the sensation of temperature changes in your separated fingers. Use both hands.

PALM DIRECTIONS

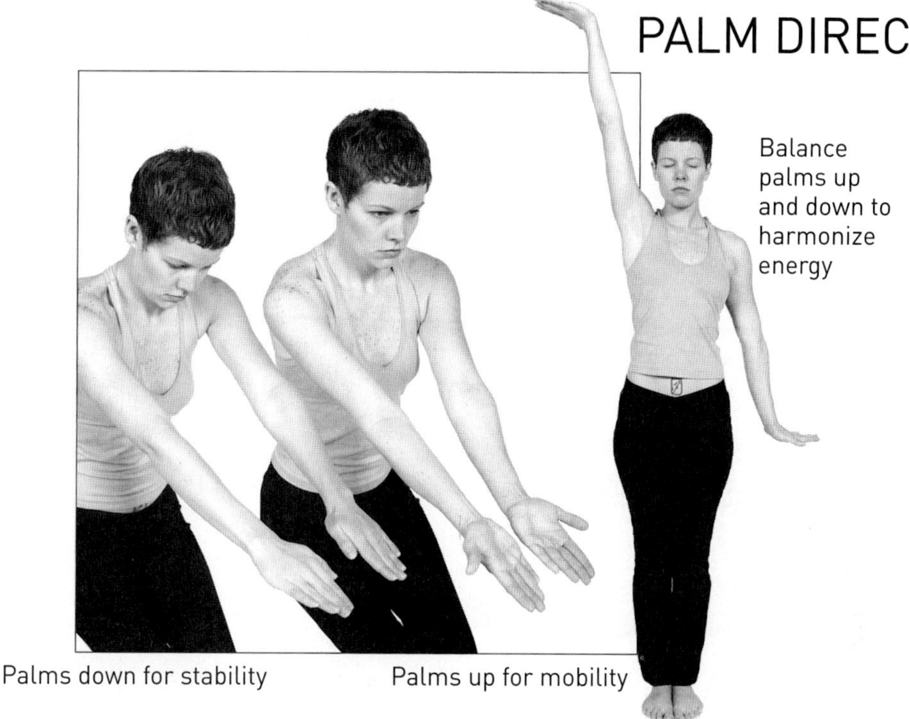

Balance palms up and down to harmonize energy

Palms down for stability

Palms up for mobility

BENEFITS: Practicing Palm Directions keeps your shoulder joint and shoulder girdle open so that you can breathe more fully. Changing Palm Directions allows you to use the Body's Way to get the most power from the arms. Palm Directions also express emotions. Palms up, for example, is a universal body language indicator of openness. This move not only connects you to your emotions but is vitally important for achieving optimal function of the shoulders.

First, with arms lengthened, consciously change the directions of your palms, and notice what Palm Direction feels best in your shoulder joint. Then move your arms freely, bending and extending them, at the same time, change the direction of your palms and seek comfort in your shoulder joints. When your palms face up, it opens the shoulder joint, and makes more room to facilitate lifting your arms above your head. When your palms face down, it closes the shoulder joint, which provides more stability. Keep your lower jaw relaxed and mouth slightly open. As you change Palm Directions, vary your speed and sound the vowels—*a, e, i, o, u*—matching the speed and length of your sounds to your movement. Use both hands and follow the hands with your eyes to safely engage your head.

FINGER EXTENSIONS

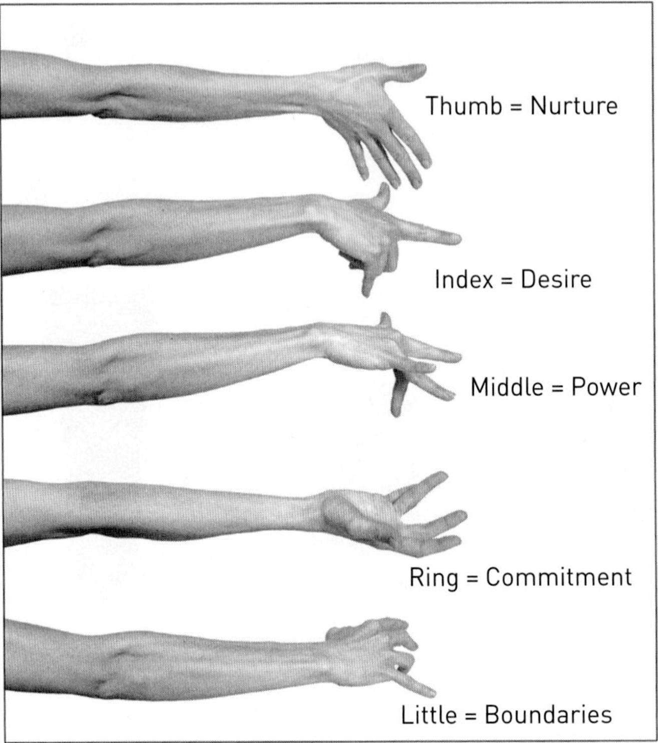

BENEFITS: Practicing Finger Extensions helps move energy in and out of your upper body, and keeps it from getting clogged in your neck and shoulders. Finger Extensions are ideal for learning to move your hands with precision and for strengthening your hands. This move also potentiates your ability for expressing hand and arm gestures that speak powerfully, through the voice of the body, from your heart and soul.

Extend and point your fingers, one at a time, sensing for different qualities of energy. Each finger is associated with a subtly different form of energy, and connects to a different emotion. In Nia, your thumb is your nurturing finger, your index finger is the finger of desire, your middle finger is the power finger, your ring finger is the commitment finger, and your little finger is the finger of boundaries. As you move each finger, sound the word that is associated with it: *nurture, desire, power, commitment,* or *boundaries.* This will help you connect your physical body with your emotional body and your spirit. Use both hands.

FINGER FLICKS

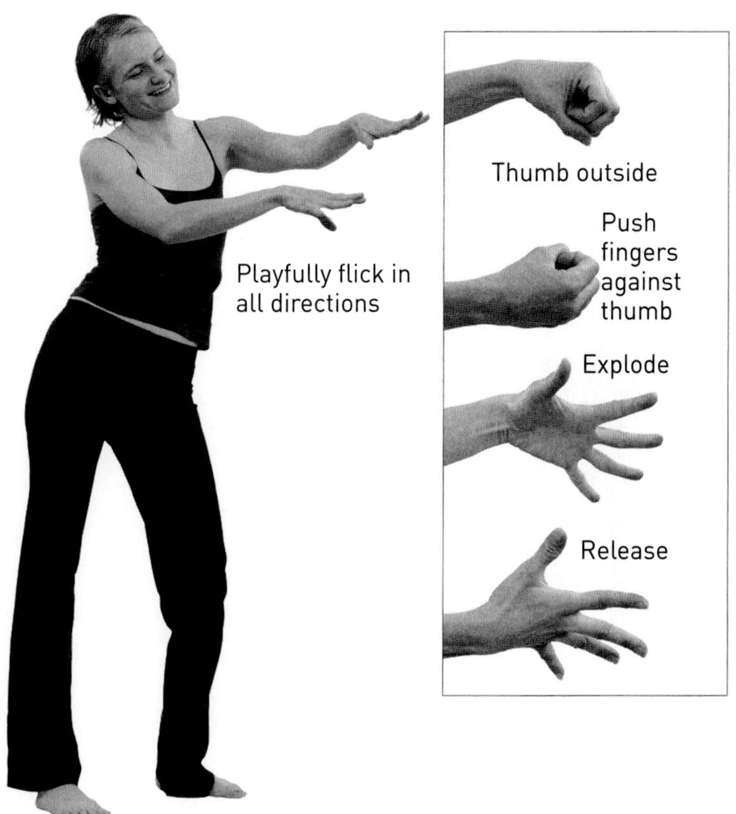

BENEFITS: Practicing Finger Flicks conditions your forearm muscles and hands, keeping energy flowing into and out of the hands and keeping tension out of the neck and shoulders. Finger Flicks strengthen the forearm, the fingers, and the hands. They also rid the hands of tension, which commonly builds up during the day, due to the extraordinary amount of fine-motor movements the hands must continually perform.

Place your thumb over your four fingernails, pushing them against the thumb to create positive tension, and then flick your fingers out, as if you were flicking water off them. Do this with your arms extended and also with them hanging down in neutral. When your arms are extended, keep your hands below your shoulder level, so that the flick uses relaxed power. Change the direction of your palms for movement variety. As you do the move, boldly sound the word *flick*. Use both hands.

CREEPY CRAWLERS

Play with
changing palm
directions
Engage both thumbs
and all fingers

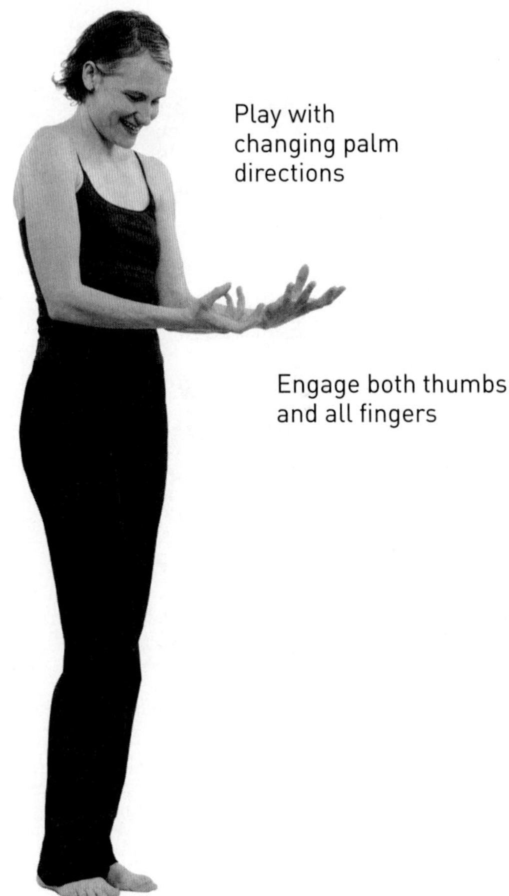

BENEFITS: Practicing Creepy Crawlers helps your fingers, hands, and forearms remain strong, flexible, and agile. This move empowers you to move with precision and keeps the fingers, hands, and wrist joints mobile and dispels tension.

Wiggle all of your fingers, including your thumbs, as if you were tickling someone. Keep your elbows bent, and occasionally change the positions of your palms, to keep your shoulders and neck relaxed. As you do it, be playful and mischievous and make the sound of laughter (which will also help tighten your abdominals). Use both hands.

SPEAR FINGERS

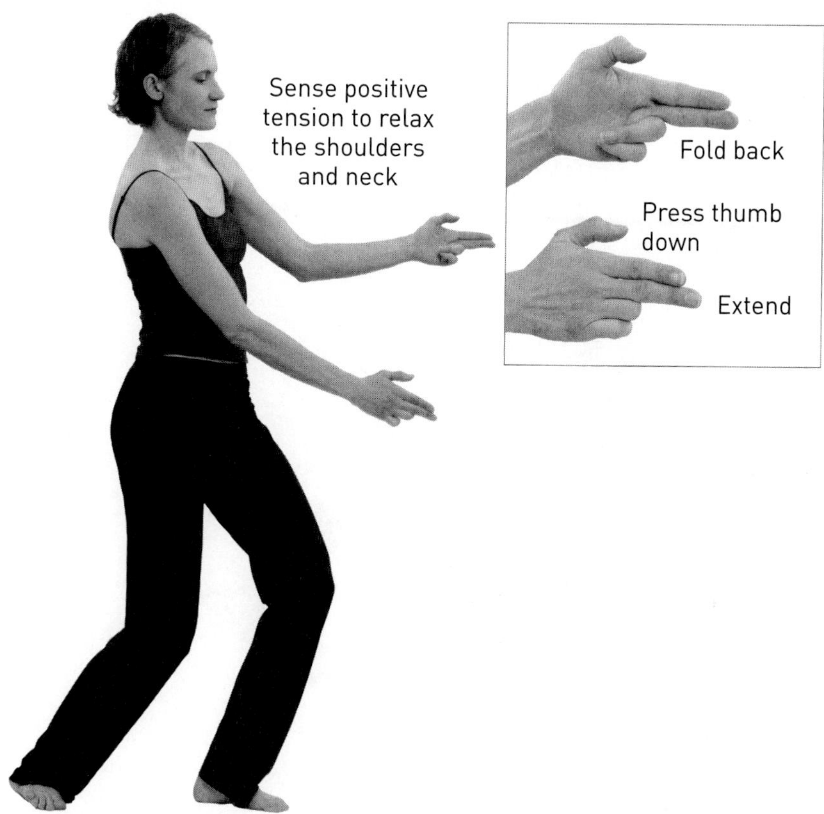

BENEFITS: Practicing Spear Fingers increases body awareness. This very simple move will help eliminate the effects of hyperextension of your elbows and will mediate the tension that tends to build up in your wrists, elbows, shoulders, neck, and jaw. Emotionally, it will trigger a sense of confidence and self-efficacy.

As if saluting with your hand, extend your index and middle fingers, and fold in half your ring finger and little finger. Cock your thumb as if pressing on a water pistol. Move your arms freely through space, bending and extending them, and sustaining your arm extension, sensing the positive tension this hand technique provides to your arm and hand muscles. As you press your thumb down, sound a sibilant *sssss* in a confident tone. Use both hands and change palm directions to spiral the forearm bones.

CATCHING FLIES

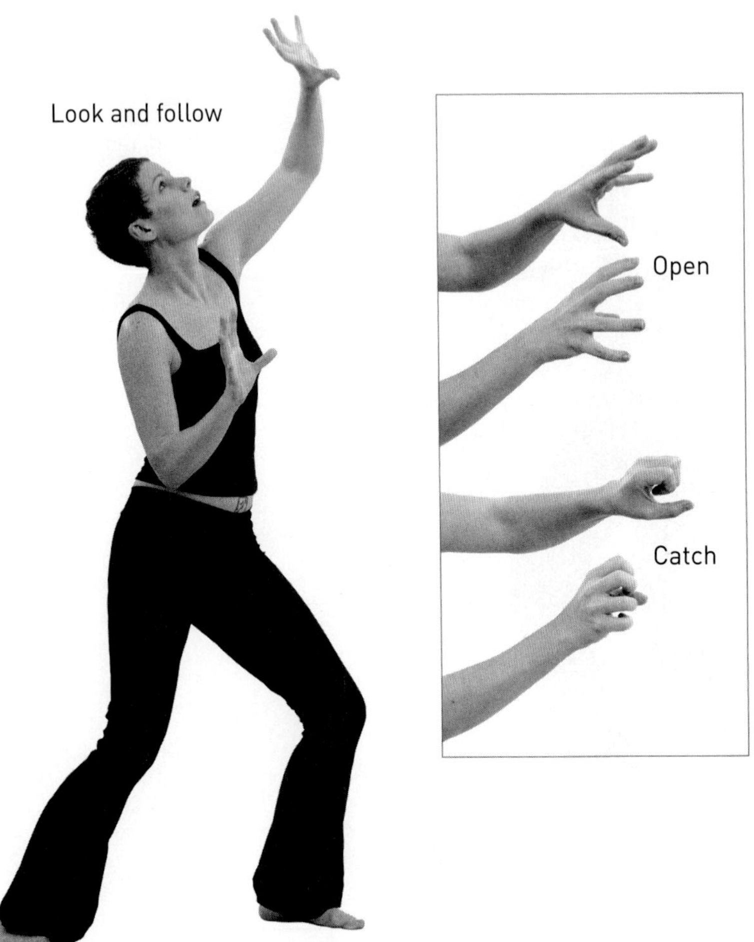

BENEFITS: Practicing Catching Flies increases brain activity. This move neurologically connects your hand, your head, and your eyes and engenders manual dexterity and speed. Emotionally, you can use this move to express aggression, determination, anger, frustration, playfulness, and achievement.

Pretend you are catching flies with your hands as they buzz around the room. Follow them before you catch them. Lead your movements with your eyes, to integrate your hand and your head. As you chase them, sound *buzz!,* and as you catch them, sound *gotcha!* Catch big ones, fast ones, slow ones, slippery ones. Use both hands.

CLAW HAND

Scratch down
Sense positive tension
Practice in all stances and steps

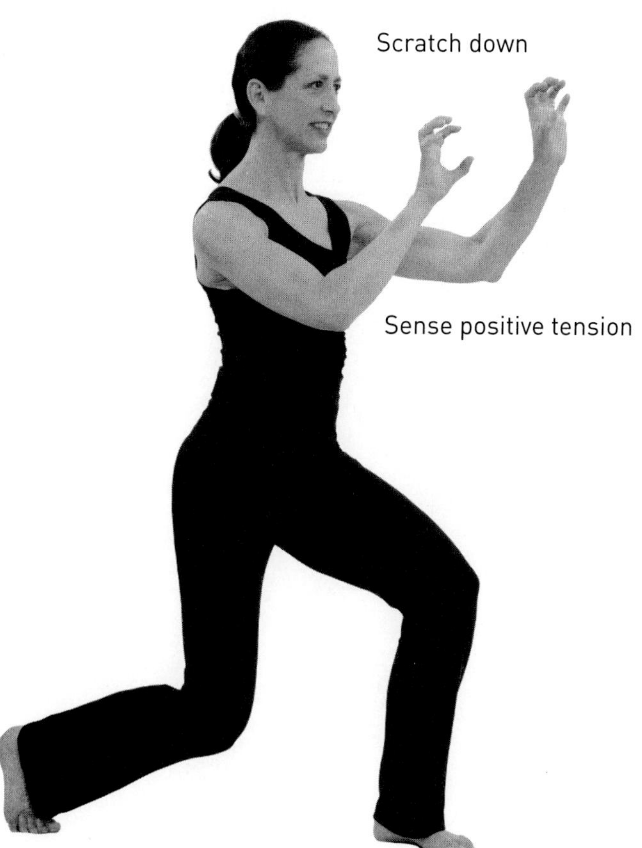

BENEFITS: Practicing Claw Hand strengthens your fingers and hands. This move is great for achieving emotional release, especially when you combine it with sounds. Use it for expressing anger, the survival instinct, animalistic urges, fear, and rage. It will amplify your emotional confidence, and increase your sense of power.

Mimic a claw with your fingers and claw the air, as if you were in a cat fight. Keep your wrists relaxed, and sound a cat's *hissss* as you do the move. Use both hands.

POWER FINGER CROSSOVER

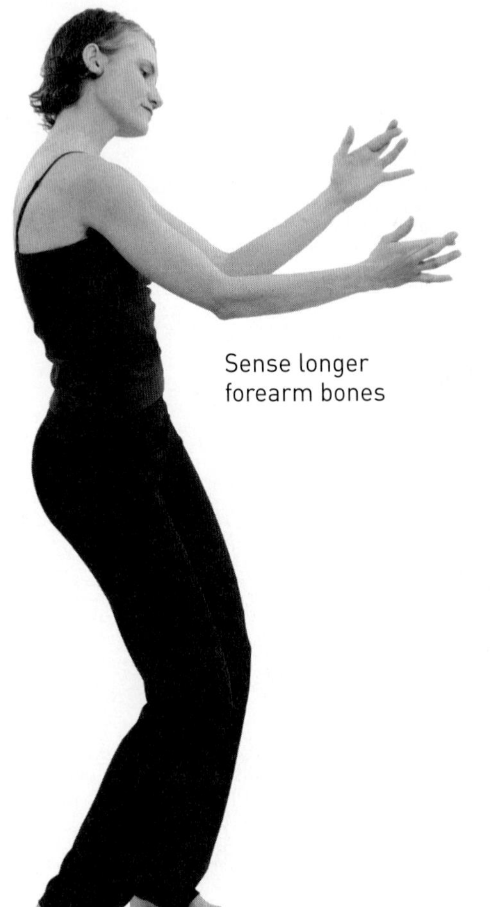

Sense longer forearm bones

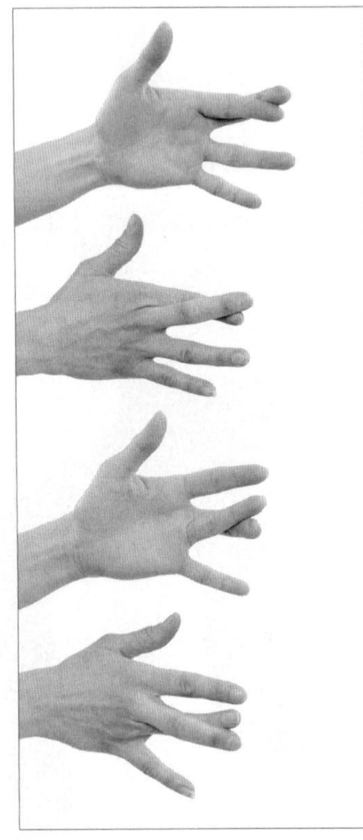

Middle finger crosses index finger

Middle finger crosses ring finger

BENEFITS: Practicing the Power Finger Crossover helps you extend energy along your arm bones and out through your hands, which keeps your neck and shoulders relaxed. It creates positive tension in the hand and adds to awareness of the integration of the hand and arm.

Cross the middle finger (your power finger) over your index finger as if you were crossing your fingers for good luck. Release and then cross your middle finger over your ring finger. Keep your arms long and extended and the cross small. Use both hands. Sound *power* to consciously connect to hand sensation.

BALANCE FINGER

Look around to challenge your balance
Press middle fingers down into earth
Balance on Whole Foot

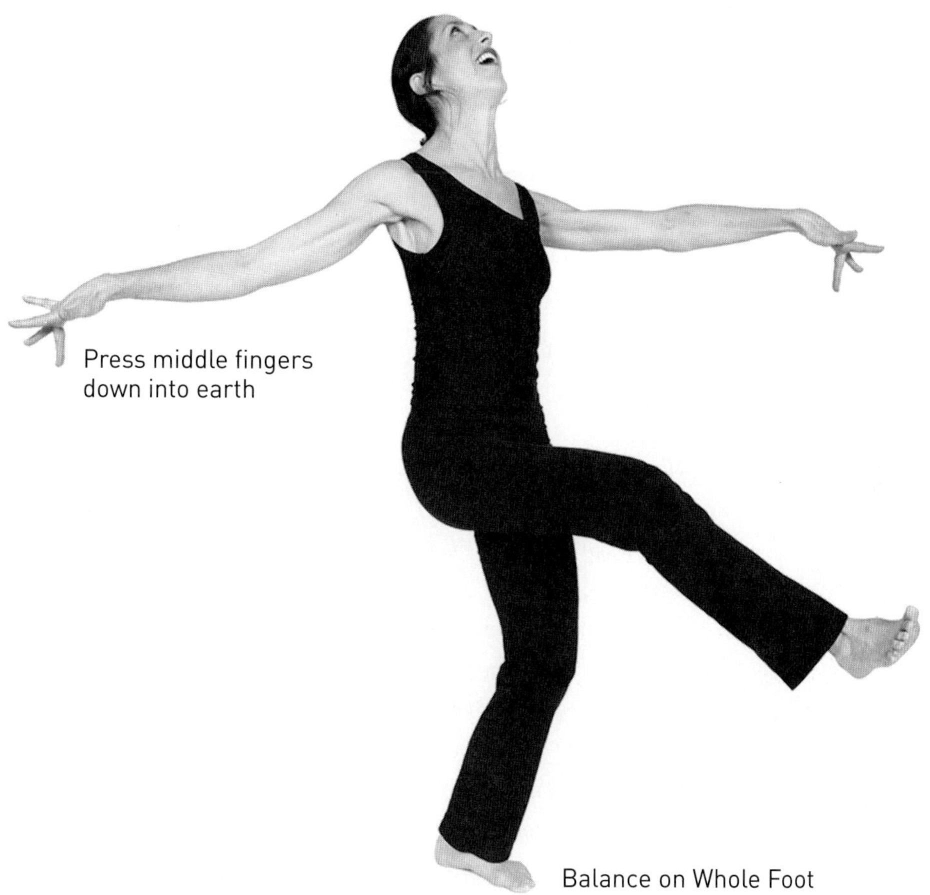

BENEFITS: Practicing the Balance Finger integrates the upper body with the lower body and directs energy through the center of your palm to the center of your body.

Standing on one leg, challenge your balance and use your hands in space for support. With your palms facing down, press your middle finger—the power finger—down into the earth, keeping your other fingers extended straight out. Imagine your middle fingers as powerful magnets. Test your balance by looking up and around and by varying the height of your free leg in space, moving your free leg front, back, and to the sides. Use both hands. Alternate legs. Sound *balance* to release tension.

That's it! All the moves!

In the next chapter, you'll put them all together, and do the Nia workout.

A **Nia** *Story*

BEST SHAPE OF MY LIFE

STUDENT: Karen

CLASS LOCATION: Eugene, Oregon

OCCUPATION: Managerial

Before Nia, Karen was exercising much harder than most people do, but it wasn't having the desired effect. She was walking seven miles two to three times each week, but it wasn't giving her any upper-body exercise. In addition, she'd hoped that her strenuous workout program would help control the chronic headaches that hit her a number of times every month, but it didn't help at all.

Nia had an almost immediate impact. It gave her the upper-body toning she needed, and her headaches diminished dramatically, subsiding to only about one per month. "If I don't do Nia now," Karen says, "I feel sluggish, and when I get that way, I don't feel good about who I am, and I have more headaches!"

Nia is especially effective at helping Karen to control the stress in her life. She manages a large staff, and consults with approximately one hundred clients each day. "If I've had a really frustrating day," she says, "I know I can go to my Nia class and leave feeling relaxed and nurtured." She has even developed the ability to reduce her stress level just by imagining that she is in a Nia class. As she puts it, "I can go to class in my mind."

From Nia, Karen has achieved the highest fitness level of her life. "I'm in the best shape I've ever been in," she says, "and I have a lot of vitality. This has been one of the best life-changing things that I've ever done."

five
The Nia Workout

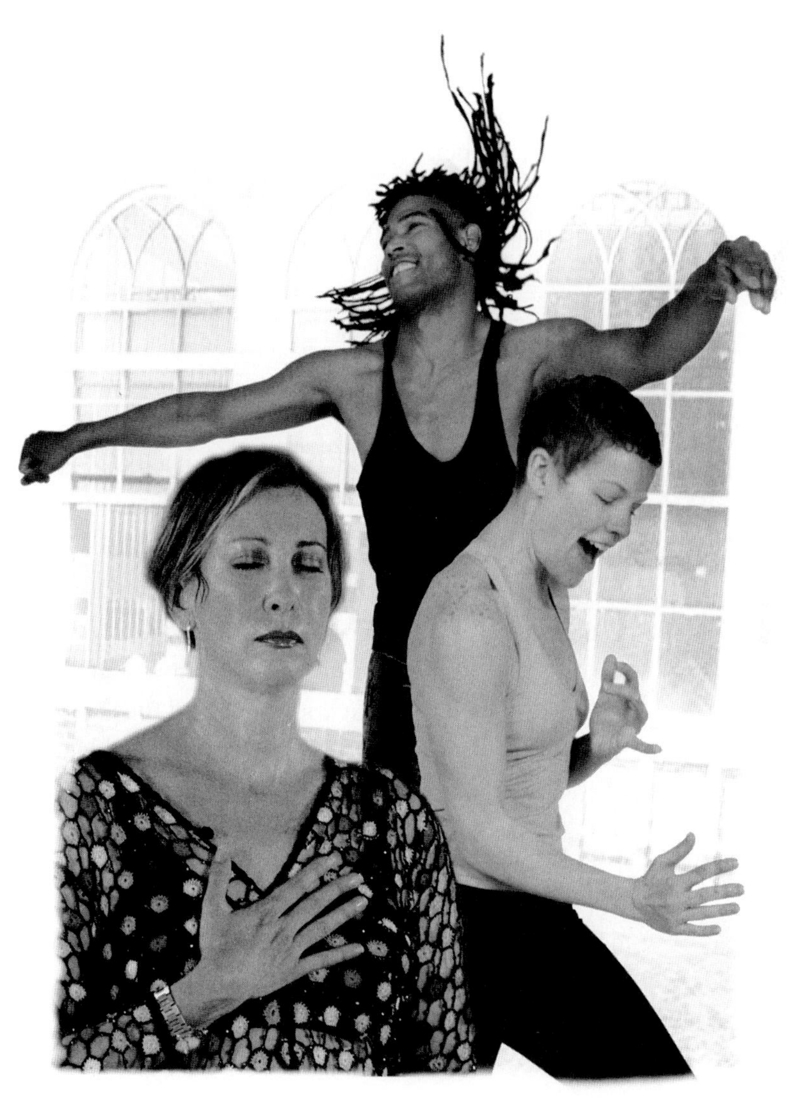

It's time to work out!

This chapter presents two primary Nia workouts—the Classic Nia workout, featuring Debbie, and the Athletic Nia workout, featuring Carlos. They both adhere to Nia's primary Thirteen Principles, but there are distinct differences between them.

You should start with the Classic Nia workout. It is less rigorous than the Athletic workout, even though it delivers a powerful cardiovascular challenge. It may take you some time—several months or even more—to "graduate" to the Athletic workout.

Both workouts use essentially the same movements, but in the Athletic workout, they are performed with more intensity and with a larger range of movement. As you'll see, both variations are presented together, enabling you to progress with each move as you feel ready.

the classic Nia workout

Here are the essential characteristics of the Classic workout:

- Classic Nia is for everyone—from neophyte to dancer to athlete.
- Classic Nia is a learning experience, with an emphasis on gaining new knowledge about your body and the best ways to move.
- In Classic Nia, it is reasonable and acceptable not to expect perfection in your movements.
- Classic Nia is noncompetitive, meaning you grow and change in your own time and in your own way.
- Classic Nia teaches you to play, have fun, and express yourself.
- In Classic Nia, you focus at least as much on your Body's Way as you do on the Body's Way.

the athletic Nia workout

Here are the essential characteristics of the Athletic workout:

- In Athletic Nia, the practice is over and the game has begun. You know your body and can demand more from it.
- In Athletic Nia, you are encouraged to seek perfection in your movements.
- Athletic Nia is more challenging. It builds greater strength, speed, grace, and cardiovascular fitness.
- Athletic Nia stresses more demanding boundaries, challenging your balance, strength, flexibility, and endurance.
- Athletic Nia allows a moderate amount of leaving the floor, with jumps and running.
- Athletic Nia teaches you to merge your Body's Way with the Body's Way.

CUSTOMIZE YOUR WORKOUT

Lighten: To Make It Easier

1. Involve fewer parts of your body in the movements.
2. Keep your movements close to your body.
3. Do fewer repetitions.

Load: To Make It More Challenging

1. Involve more parts of your body in the movements.
2. Make your movements deeper, higher, fuller, and broader.
3. Do more repetitions.

the Nia workout format

The Body's Way reminds us that everything in nature moves in cycles to maintain harmony and balance. The Nia workout moves through seven cycles, each with a unique purpose and each designed to fulfill specific needs and to deliver specific results.

Nia's workout also takes into consideration that you are never the same on any two days, or, for that matter, from moment to moment. While the seven cycles and basic moves remain the same, your experiences, benefits, and results will constantly change based on how you adjust your focus, speed, intensity, and overall intent. Your ability to remain aware and sensitive to your body's ever-changing needs, and to respond to them, will enable you to receive maximum benefit each time you work out. In other words, it's not just the moves that deliver benefits but, more important, it's what you do to personalize them that will deliver ongoing results. Here are the seven cycles:

1. **Set your focus and intent.** Choose a focus and intent from the workout menu. Your focus and intent define what you personally desire to achieve and where you will place your attention in order to achieve it.
2. **Step in.** Prepare physically, mentally, emotionally, and spiritually, by centering and getting ready to work out. Leave behind distractions and activate your body's sensory awareness as a starting point for all action.
3. **Warm up.** Consciously activate the flow of energy in all thirteen joints, increase body heat and respiration, and become aware of how your body is feeling.
4. **Get moving.** Move in space more physically, by combining the five sensations of strength, flexibility, mobility, agility, and stability, to condition your heart and lungs and achieve whole-body conditioning.
5. **Cool down.** Slow down to center, balance, and harmonize the body, mind, emotions, and spirit.

6. **Floorplay.** Use play, gravity, the floor, space, time, and sound to stimulate your body and improve your strength and flexibility. Take advantage of the heat and pliability generated from the previous movement, which now allows you to stretch and open up your joints more fully.
7. **Step out.** Consciously recognize through body sensation the self-healing and fitness benefits you have received. Step out and into your next life experience with renewed health.

A **Nia** *Story*

FINDING POWER

STUDENT: Emily

CLASS LOCATION: Spokane, Washington

OCCUPATION: e-business proprietor

Emily began to do Nia because she was already practicing yoga, but was not achieving an adequate level of benefit from it. Once she had started, she continued to do Nia because, as she puts it, "A Nia class was the only time I felt completely like myself, and completely free. I didn't have to be anything for anyone—it was only for me. It started to heal me."

Before Nia, Emily had experienced chronic anxiety and had difficulty with self-esteem. "I used to hate my body," she says. "I thought that if I were more like everyone else—skinnier, prettier, and wealthier—I would fit in better at school and church. Most of the time I felt that my life was just worthless. I was in a black hole and didn't know how to get out. I was in my mind a lot, daydreaming, in order to escape my feelings and my body. I ate a lot, too. I didn't get obese, but I definitely used food as a way to feel better. Eating helped me feel numb, so I could ignore my body and my emotional pain. But when I would eat, it made me feel even more alienated and worthless."

Nia intervened in Emily's cycle of despair. It created psychological changes even before it inaugurated physical changes. "Nia has helped me relax in every aspect of my life," says Emily. "I'm not so anxious, so stressed to the limit, so repressed and tense. I am slowing down and appreciating every part of my life. Now I know who I am."

The sense of freedom that is very much a part of Nia soon became a part of Emily's own personality. "When Nia came along, I moved my hips, I yelled in class, I threw punches, and I explored my sensuality. I did all this—and found my personal power."

cycle 1 SET YOUR FOCUS AND INTENT

The first cycle is the beginning of every Nia workout. It is the cycle in which you set the focus and intent for your workout. While the moves in this workout will remain the same, you can change your focus and intent for each workout experience and thereby change the workout and its benefits. You'll be choosing your focus from the Nia Workout Menu on p. 263.

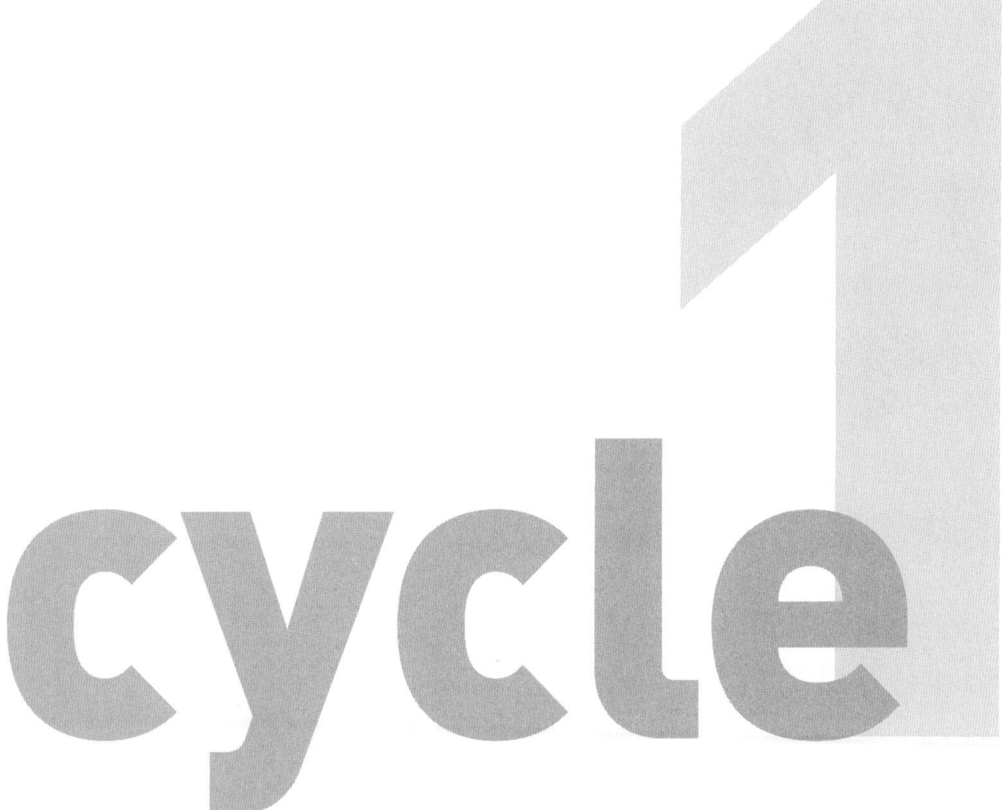

SET YOUR FOCUS AND INTENT

IMAGINE THAT YOU ARE YOUR OWN PERSONAL COACH.

BENEFITS: Focuses your mind, and directs your body, mind, and spirit.

Each time you work out, choose a daily focus from the Nia Workout Menu.

Choose and set your focus and intent

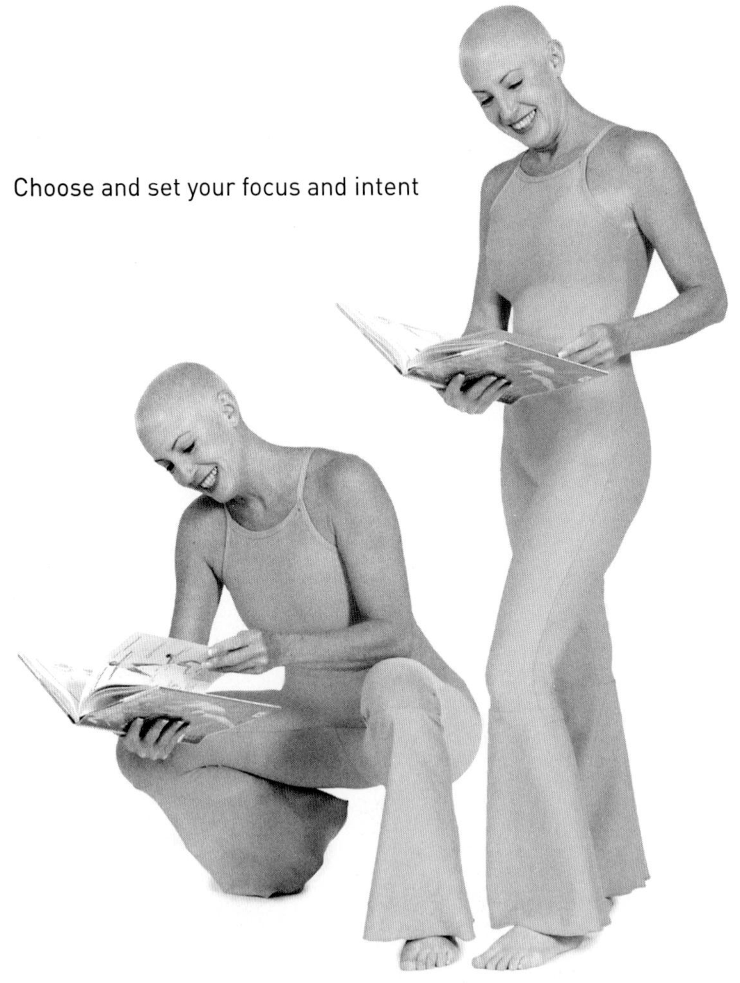

Let what you feel in your body today guide you

cycle 2 STEP IN

The second cycle is the one in which you become body centered and mentally prepare to work out. You center yourself and leave behind all distractions. In this stage, you consciously activate your Sensory IQ and set out to sustain your focus and intent for the entire workout.

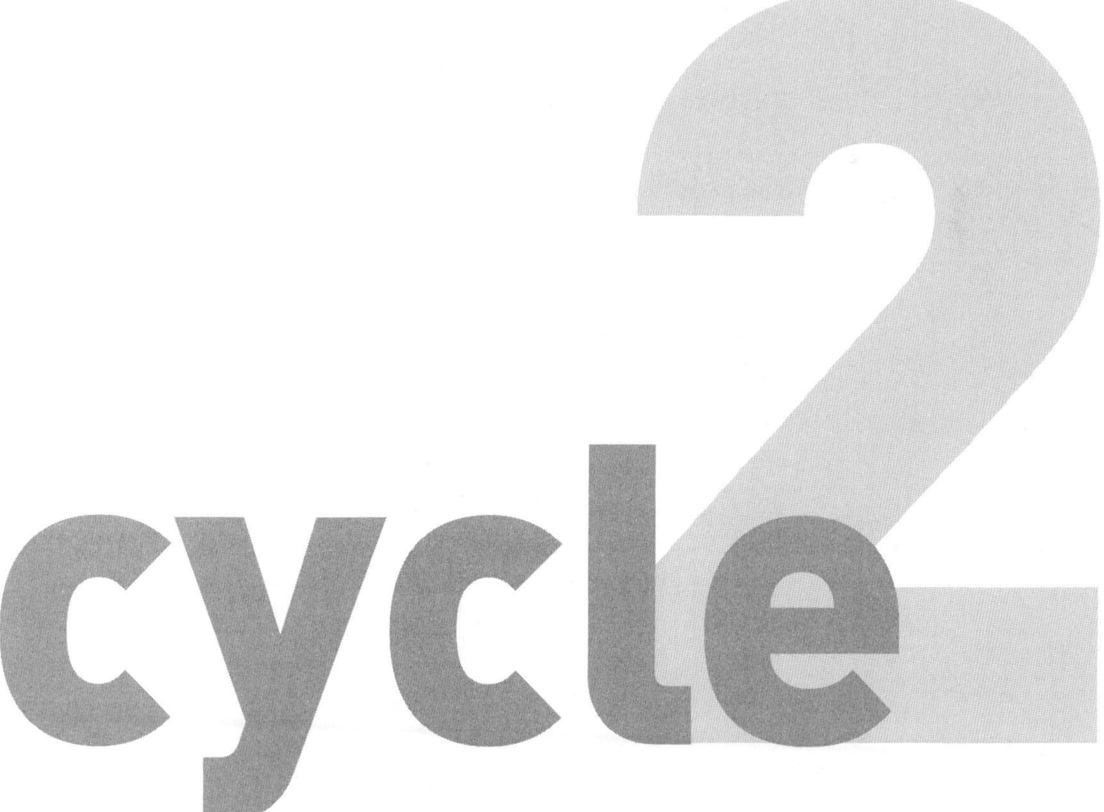

STEP-IN TRIANGLE FOCUS

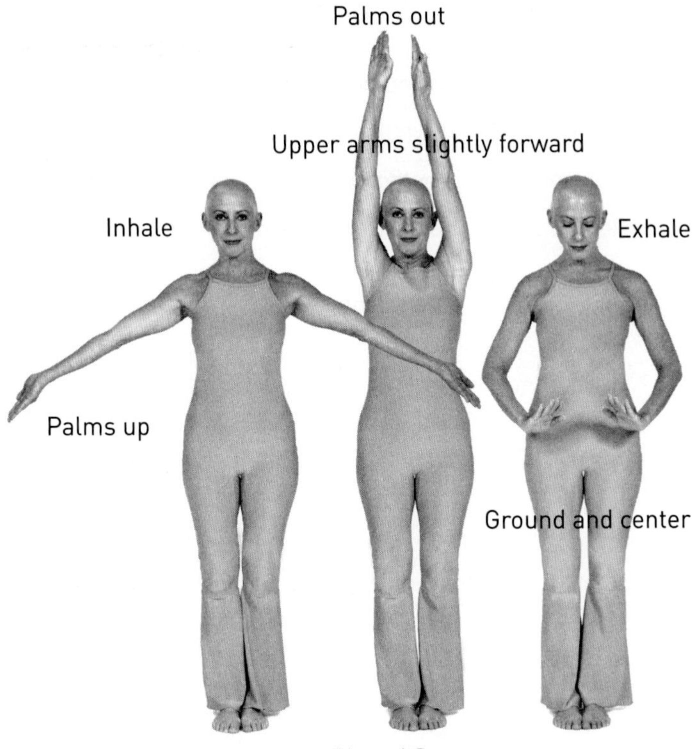

Bringing your focus and intent with you, take two conscious and purposeful steps into the center of an imaginary clock. Turn your palms out, and inhale deeply, as you draw winged arms, slowly and sensually, out from the sides of your body, ending up above your head. Turn your palms out and exhale with the sound *ah,* as you slowly lower your hands and winged arms down to the sides of your body.

With your arms extended, slowly bring your hands up in front of your chest, with your thumbs and index fingers touching to form a triangle. Purposefully look through your triangle and—either silently or out loud—commit to your focus and intent. Inhale deeply and exhale, as you turn your palms in to face each other and slowly draw your hands back toward your chest, your thumbs lightly pressing against your heart. Consciously connect to the feeling of being body centered, and physically, mentally, emotionally, and spiritually prepared. Deeply and purposefully inhale, then exhale. Relax your arms and hands, and bring them back down to the sides of your body.

IGNITE YOUR FOCUS AND INTENT.

BENEFITS: Prepares your body, mind, emotions, and spirit. Consciously tune into what movement forms you will integrate and what you will focus your mind and intention on during today's workout.

CLASSIC: Practice the art of becoming consciously body centered, sensing what it means to be ready to mindfully work out. Turn on your Sensory IQ and tune in to the voices of your body. From this point on, sensation will be your guide, helping you make the right choices and decisions to support personal exploration; growth; and physical, mental, emotional, and spiritual development.

ATHLETIC: Practice is over, and it is time to be your own coach. Use what you have learned from Classic Nia and perform at your very best. All movement choices help you reach goals you set for yourself. Each workout takes you to an edge that you master.

Energetically connect above
Today I will focus on . . .
Now I am ready to work out
Sense stability
Rest on the earth

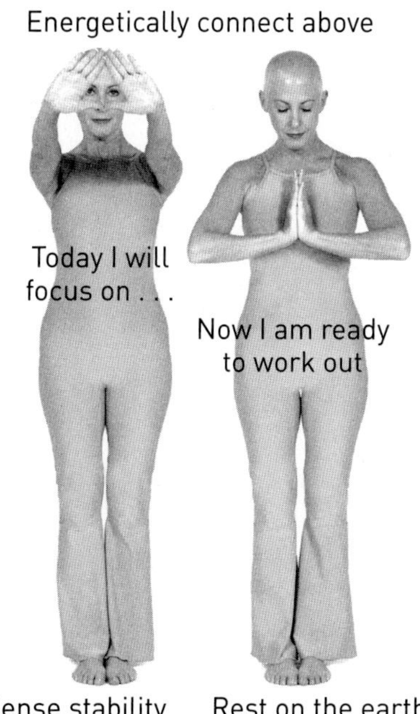

WARM UP

In this cycle, you activate the flow of energy in all of your thirteen primary joints and increase muscle and joint action, body heat, and respiration. You start noticing how your body is feeling today. As you move, you focus on sensations of strength, flexibility, mobility, agility, and stability. You listen to the voices of your body that signal the need for you to either be gentle and lighten the moves or to load and intensify them.

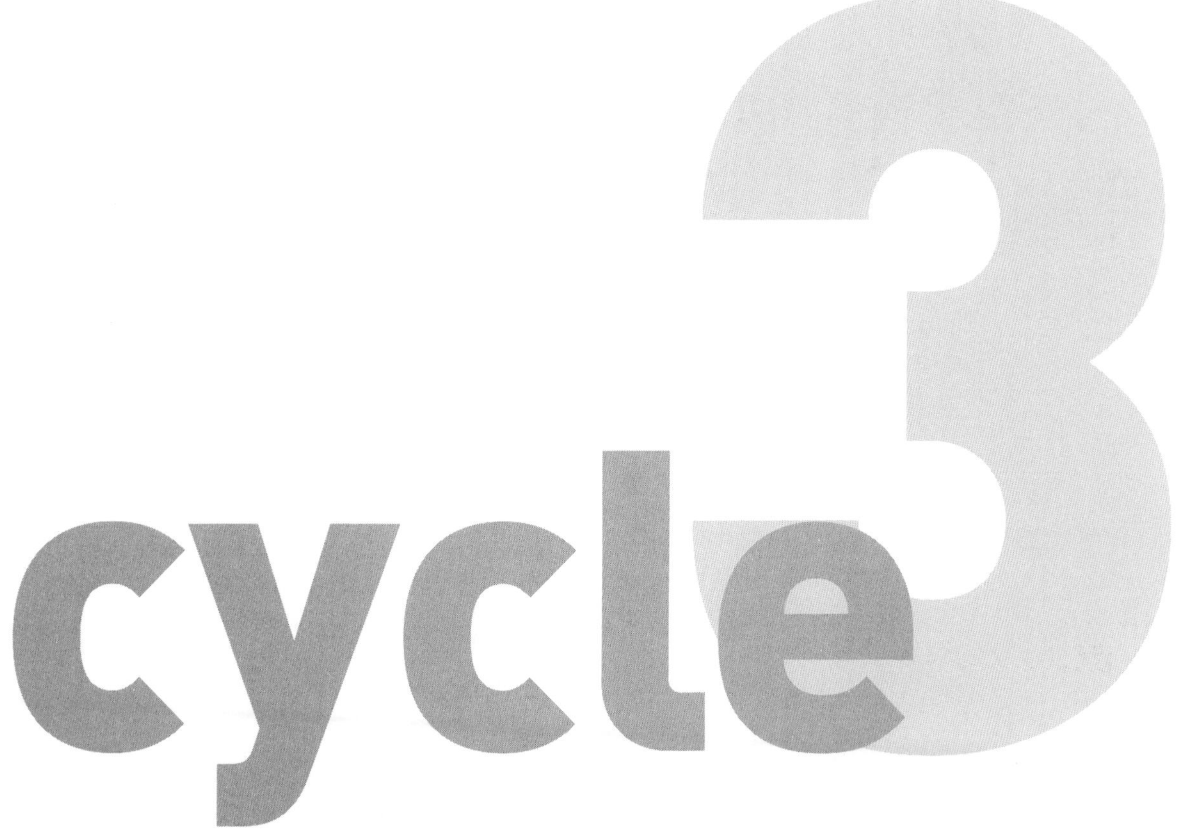

THIRTEEN JOINT STIMULATION

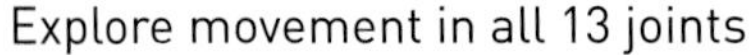

Explore movement in all 13 joints

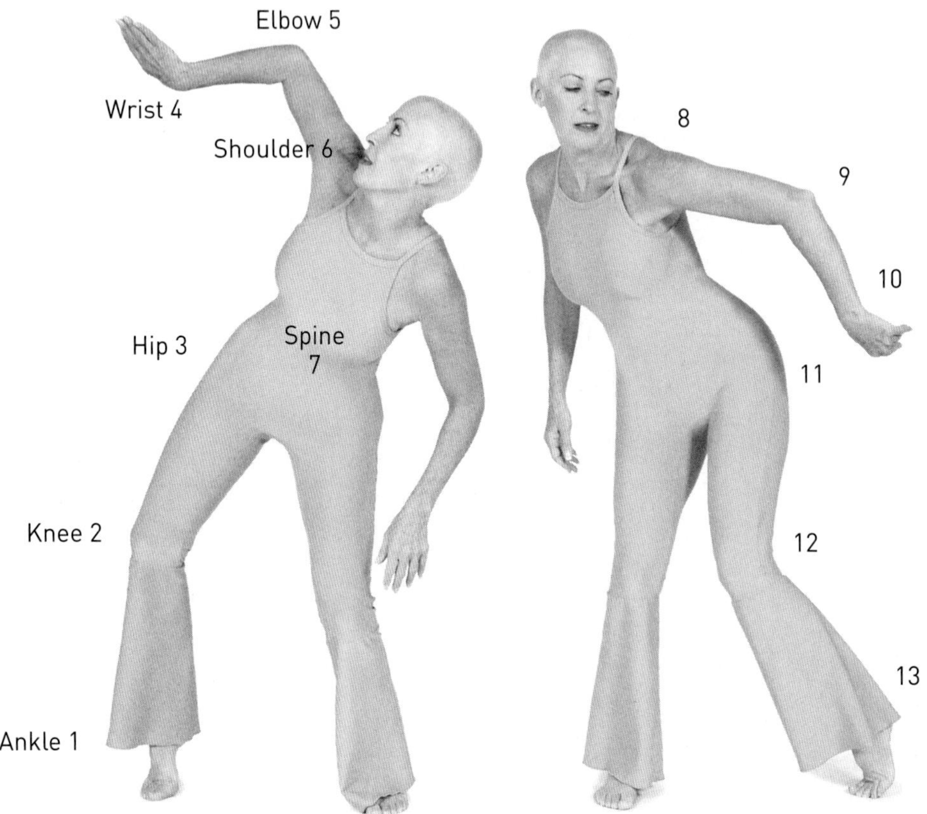

Sense left and right joint mobility

Starting with the left side of the body, stimulate each joint, one at a time. Begin with your left ankle and consecutively move through all the left-side joints. Move your left ankle, left knee, left hip, left wrist, left elbow, left shoulder, and whole spine. As you move each joint, seek pleasure. Now stimulate the right side of your body, one joint at a time, beginning with the right shoulder joint. Move through the rest of your joints (elbow, wrist, hip, knee and ankle). Keep moving each joint until it says, "I'm warm and ready for whole-body movement." Then freely move all of your thirteen main joint systems simultaneously for a couple of minutes. You should now feel sensorily awake and full of energy—alive and ready to move!

IMAGINE THAT YOU ARE A PUPPET BEING MOVED BY THIRTEEN STRINGS.

BENEFITS: Prepares the thirteen main joints and surrounding muscles, ligaments, and tendons for physical movement.

CLASSIC: Practice body–mind integration and consciously guide each joint. Internally explore sensation to learn about how your joints feel today. **Follow Debbie.**

ATHLETIC: Move your joints with more physical intensity and in ranges of motion that will prepare them for supporting you in performing at your mastery level. **Follow Carlos.**

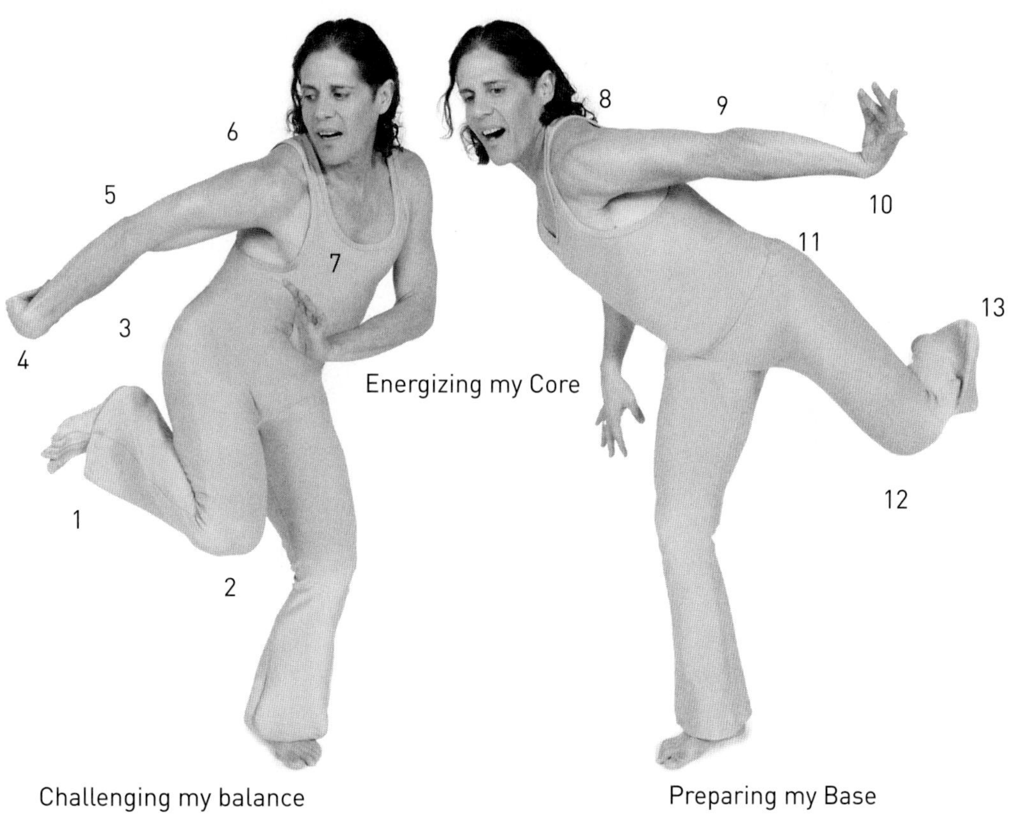

Mastering mobility and agility in all of my main 13 joints

DUCK WALK CREEPY CRAWLERS

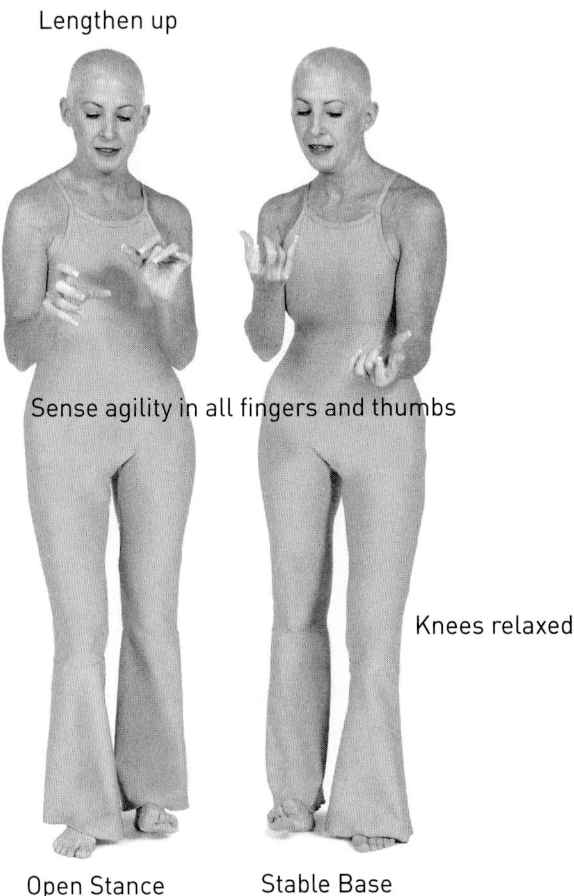

Standing in Open Stance, wiggle all your fingers and thumbs and lift and lower the front of your feet, one foot at a time, alternating sides. Lift as high as possible. Keep your spine vertical, sensing strength in your feet and shin muscles.

Repeat 8 to 16 times—counting each foot as 1 repetition—or until your body says, "My fingers, ankles and feet feel alive, my ankle joints are warm, and my calf muscles are stretched."

IMAGINE YOURSELF WALKING WITH WEBBED FEET LIKE A DUCK WHILE LIMBERING UP YOUR FINGERS TO PLAY THE PIANO.

BENEFITS: Strengthens wrists and hands, defines forearms, stretches and strengthens the lower legs, increases circulation and balance, improves mobility and agility in ankle joints and feet, and helps improve flexibility and strength in calf and shin muscles.

CLASSIC: Practice body awareness and get to know what your feet and ankles can do, sensing their strength, flexibility, and mobility. Explore the natural range of movement in your fingers and thumb and move with the intent to continually seek more and more dexterity.

ATHLETIC: Challenge the strength of your shin muscles and the flexibility in your calf muscles. Speed up your fingers and thumb movement.

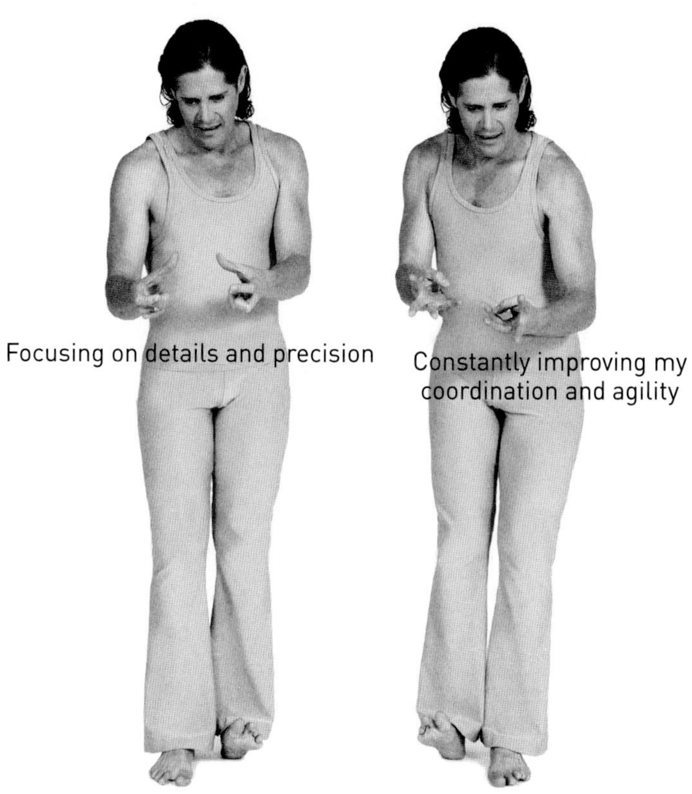

Focusing on details and precision

Constantly improving my coordination and agility

Mastering hand and foot movement

SQUISH WALK SPEAR FINGERS

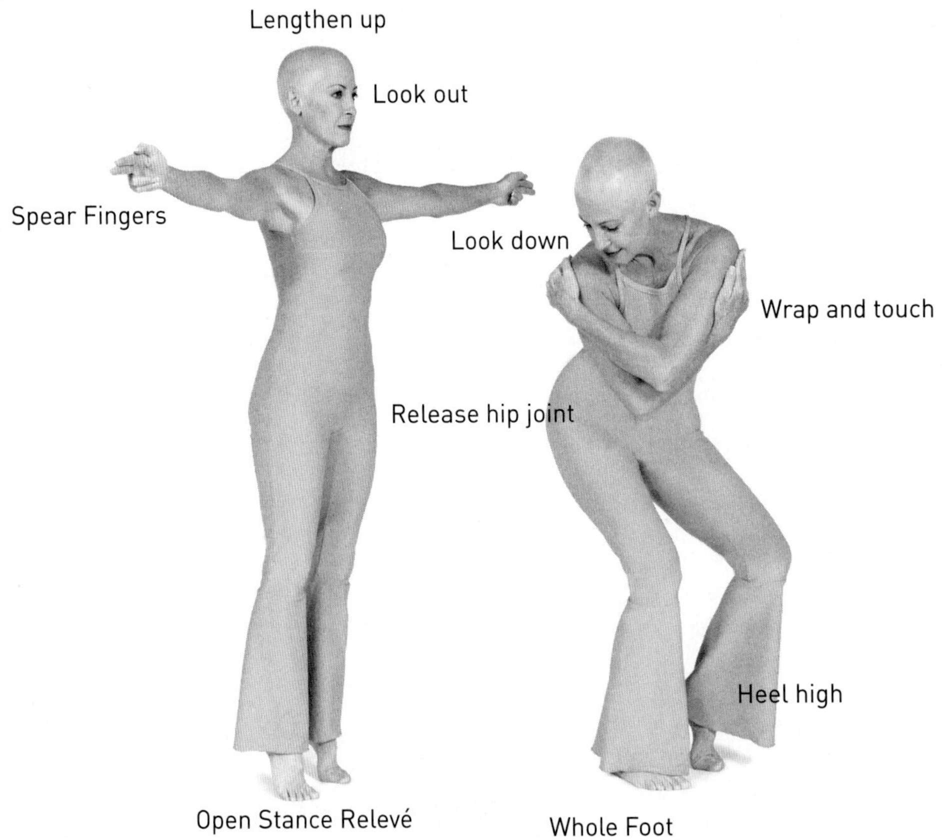

Standing in Open Stance, inhale and rise up, balancing onto the balls of both feet, with Spear Fingers reaching and extending out to the sides of your body slightly below shoulders and in front of your chest. Sense strength in your hands, Core, feet, ankles, and calves. Slowly wrap your arms around you, sinking while sounding *squish* as you bring one heel down and consciously control how you lower your heel, squeezing the juice out of an imaginary orange. Rise back onto the balls of both feet, extending your arms out, and lower your other heel, wrapping your arms around you. Alternate sides.

Repeat 8 to 16 times—counting each foot as 1 repetition—or until your body says, "My ankle joints, calves, and feet feel strong, agile, warm, mobile, and ready to move."

IMAGINE SQUISHING ORANGES WITH YOUR HEELS.

BENEFITS: Strengthens foot and ankle relationship, improves balance, increases flexibility in shoulder joints, strengthens hands, defines arms, increases mobility in your ankle joints and feet, and gives definition and strength to calf muscles.

CLASSIC: Practice turning the feet slightly in to improve balance as you rise into Relevé. Sense the stretch in your feet and ankles and pause before you squish down. As you relevé and squish down, seek the sensation of fluidity by using your Spear Fingers to integrate the upper body with your lower body.

ATHLETIC: Create more precision by extending energy along your bones and sink deeper.

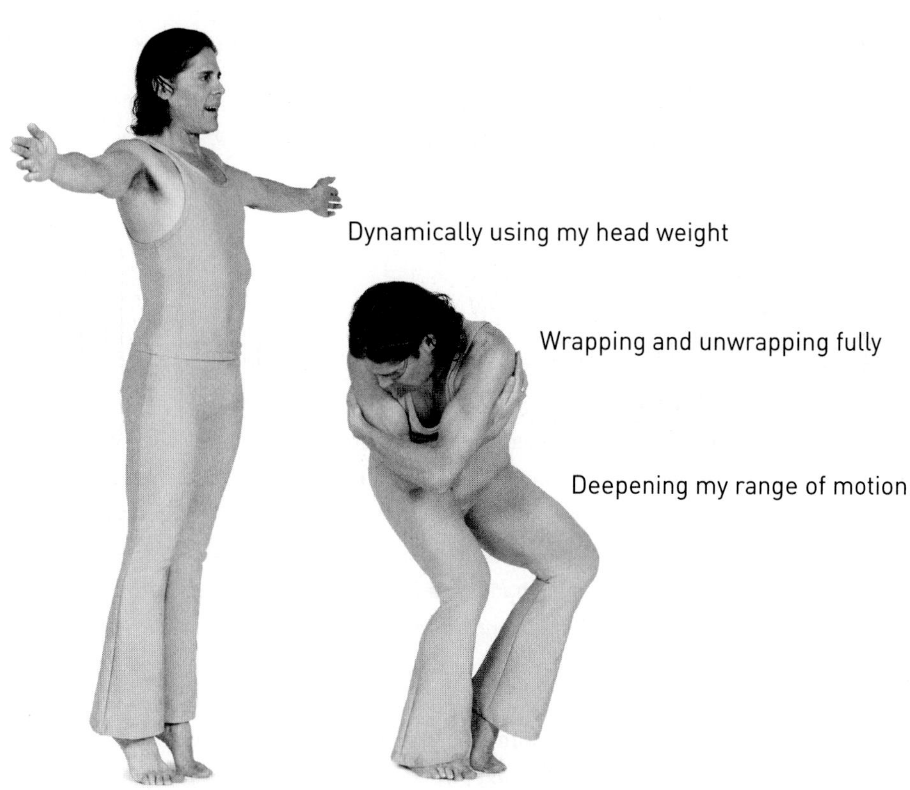

Dynamically using my head weight

Wrapping and unwrapping fully

Deepening my range of motion

Seeking perfection in my balance

Working my feet and ankles

SPINAL MELT

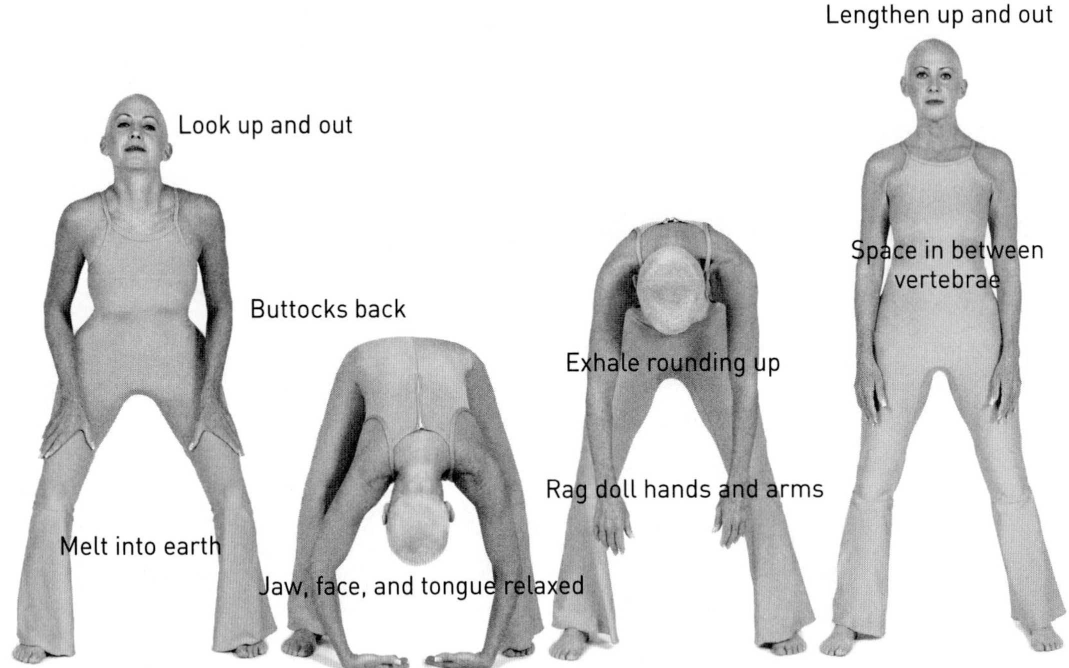

Standing in "A" Stance, look up and inhale, and slowly slide your hands down your thighs as you lower your buttocks back and down, into an imaginary chair, sensing a generous stretch along the front of your Core. Then exhale and melt over your feet and round over your thighs, sensing each space between the vertebrae while keeping your head, hands, and arms loose. Inhale and exhale and push your feet into the earth and rise up slowly, stacking one vertebra at a time.

Repeat a minimum of 8 times—counting rounding down on 4 counts and then rounding up on 4 counts as 1 repetition—or until your body says, "My spine and Core feel flexible, mobile, warm, and ready for more dynamic moves."

IMAGINE YOURSELF AS A SINKING RAG DOLL, FALLING DOWN AND SLOWLY ROUNDING AND RISING UP.

BENEFITS: Increases spine, knee, and hip joint flexibility and strengthens your back and legs.

CLASSIC: Practice moving your buttocks back, away from your knees, and use your hands for support, sliding them down your thighs to maintain alignment and stability. Slowly move in and out of comfortable levels of flexibility, learning about your spine mobility and hip agility.

ATHLETIC: Energetically let go and drop into the earth. Use your feet to generate explosive power from the legs and rise up with energetic precision.

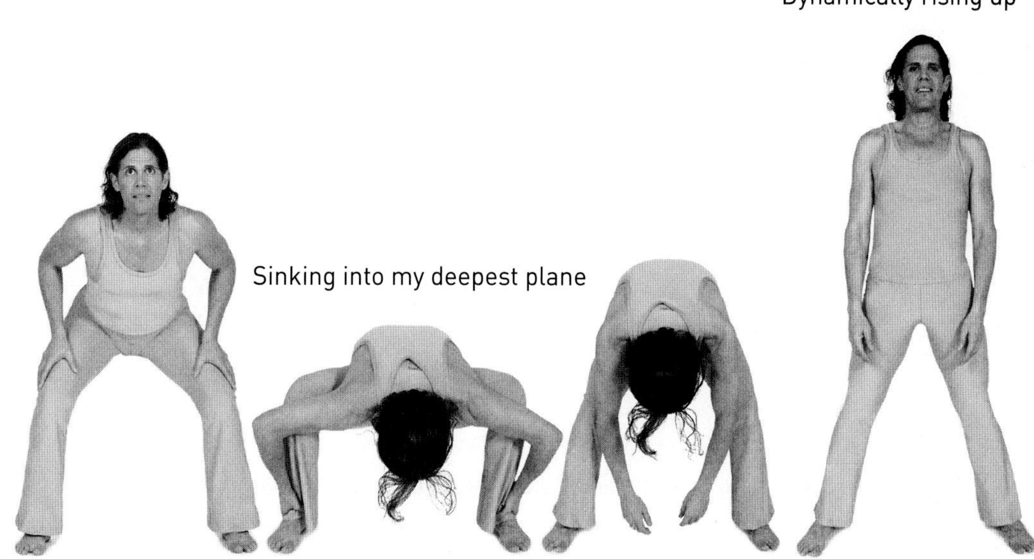

Dynamically rising up

Sinking into my deepest plane

Grounded into my stable Base

Aligned from the ground up

T'AI CHI SWAY

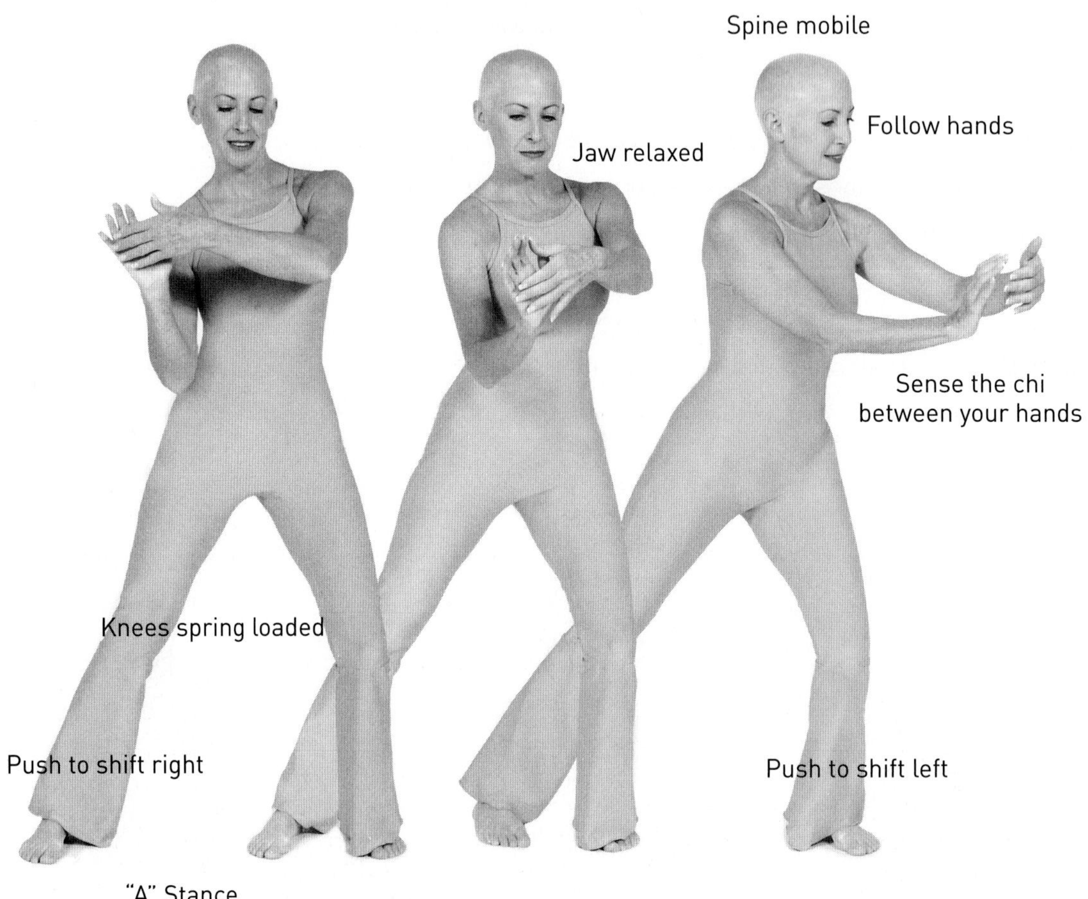

Standing in "A" Stance, fluidly shift your weight to the right, using the power from your left foot to go right, moving your hands in the same direction as you go right. Follow your hands with your eyes. Sense for power in your feet, legs, and hip joints. Exhale to keep your spine agile. Alternate sides.

Repeat 8 to 16 times—counting right-left as 1 repetition or until your body says, "I feel mobile and agile in my legs and stimulated in my spine and upper body. I'm breathing more deeply."

IMAGINE YOURSELF SWAYING LIKE A WILLOW TREE AND YOUR HANDS PUSHING W\ATER.

> BENEFITS: Improves balance, stability, eye–hand coordination, spine and leg strength, and agility.

CLASSIC: Practice following your hands and keeping your feet parallel, to protect your knees. Explore how to fluidly shift weight side to side without stopping at the sides.

ATHLETIC: Challenge your leg strength and Base agility by moving into deeper levels.

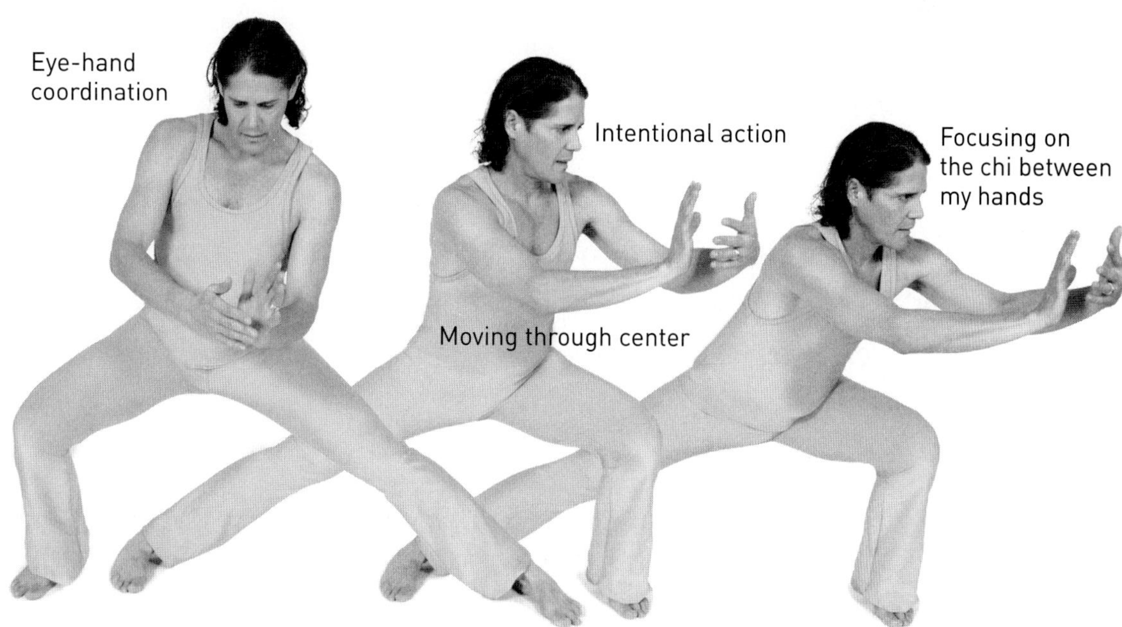

BODY HUG

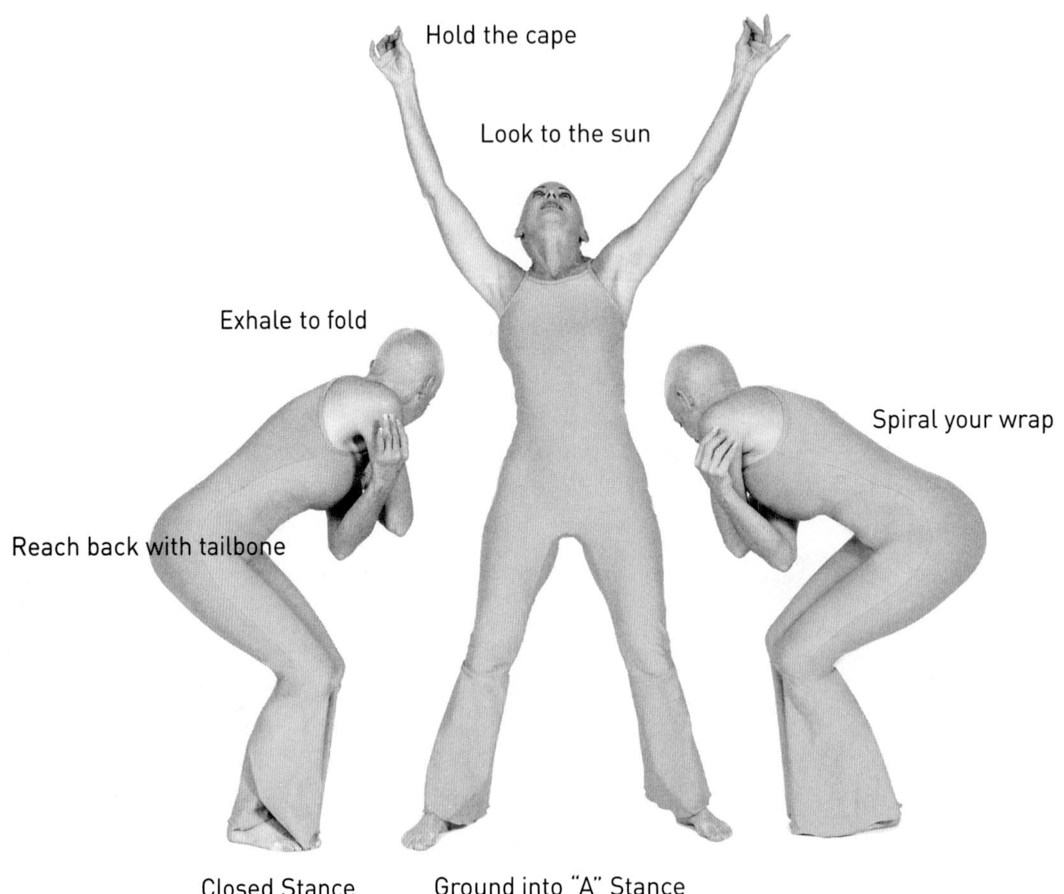

Beginning in "A" Stance, bring your right foot into your left foot and sink into Closed Stance, wrapping your arms and hands around your shoulders, as if wrapping a cape. Now fully rise up, stepping your right foot back out into "A" stance and repeat on the other side. Alternate sides.

Repeat 8 to 16 times—counting each down hug as 1-and, each rise as 2-and—or until your body says, "My legs, hip joints, and spine feel very mobile and agile. I feel connected to the left and right sides of my body, and my breath is accelerated."

IMAGINE YOURSELF WRAPPING AND UNWRAPPING A CAPE.

BENEFITS: Tones and strengthens legs and Core, improves overall agility and flexibility of the entire spine.

CLASSIC: Practice wrapping and unwrapping, shifting weight smoothly, and move in a range of motion that allows you to feel systemic movement.

ATHLETIC: With more speed, challenge your agility, and add more depth and rotation to your Core. Add more length and energy into your Core and arms as you rise up.

With power rising up and along my spine
Challenging my strength and flexibility
Mastering the art of sinking along a vertical line

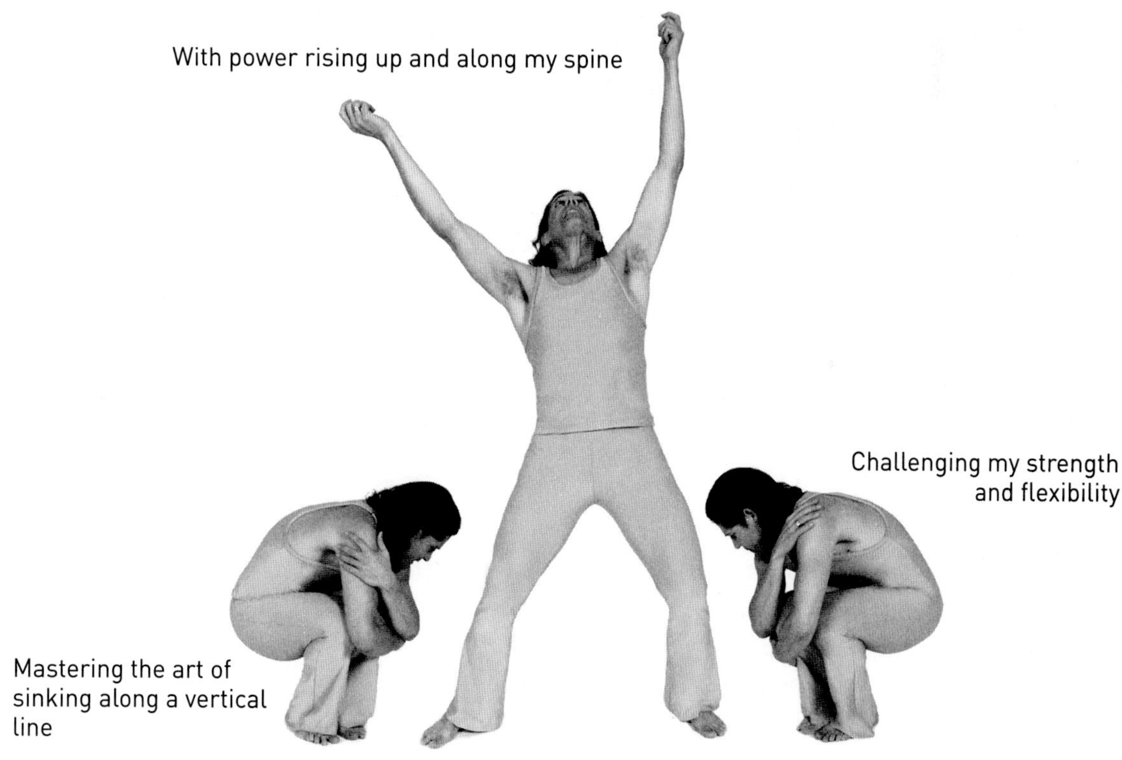

FLAMENCO

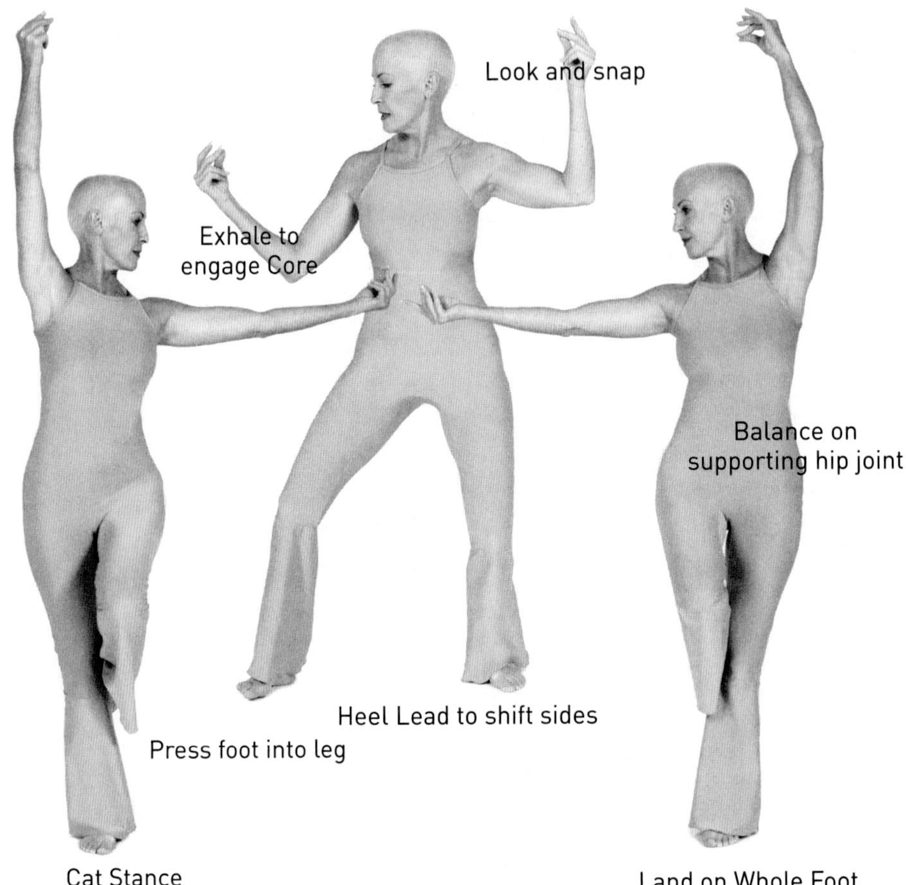

Standing in "A" Stance, shift onto your left foot into Cat Stance as you express grace and power by snapping your fingers, reaching your right hand out and your left hand up. Be theatrical and playful. When you shift body weight and change legs, lead with your heel to use more of the muscles in your feet and legs. Alternate sides.

Repeat a total of 16 times—counting each time you land in Cat Stance as 1 repetition—or until your body says, "My balance is better, I'm breathing deeply, and I'm safely on my way to pleasurable holistic fitness."

IMAGINE YOURSELF AS A GRACEFUL AND POWERFUL FLAMENCO DANCER.

> BENEFITS: Increases balance, leg strength, mobility and stability in the Base and flexibility and tone in the upper body and waist.

CLASSIC: Look to the side you intend to move to, and press your free foot against your supporting leg to help you establish stability and balance in your Base.

ATHLETIC: Swiftly leap from one leg to the other to shift your weight, and draw your knee up higher and with more power.

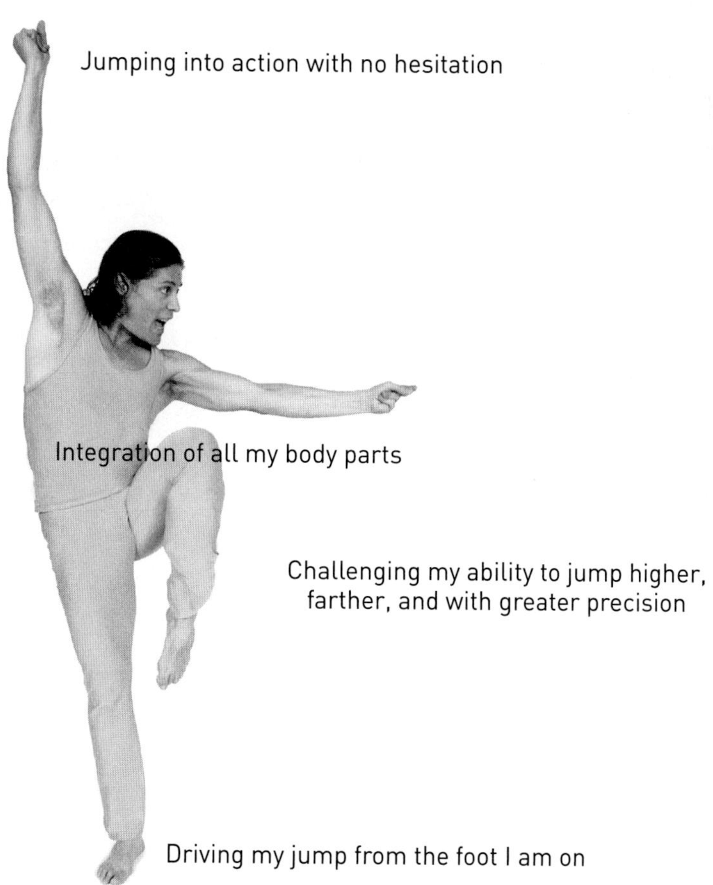

body check

Your entire body should now feel strong and flexible, your muscles warm and agile, and your heart rate safely elevated. Your joints should feel fully mobile and lubricated, and your spirit invigorated. You're ready to move on. If you feel like you've had enough for today, stop. Stretch out and relax. Next time, you can do more. Fitness that lasts is something you build over time.

cycle 4 GET MOVING

In Cycle 4 you condition your heart and lungs. You're going to move through space more vigorously and combine the five sensations of strength, flexibility, mobility, agility, and stability. Nia's cardiovascular cycle integrates the moves of steps, stances, and kicks. You'll be using the martial arts, dance arts, and healing arts to bring variety to the moves.

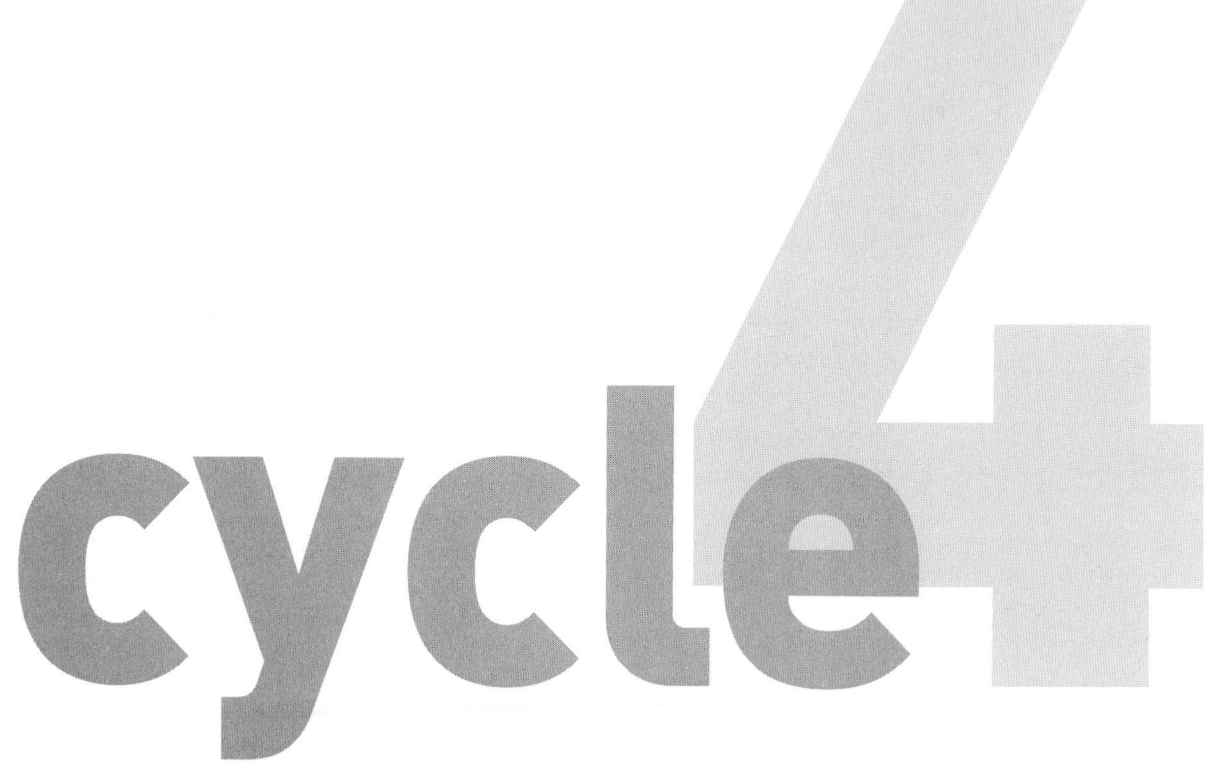

BOW STANCE VEIL DANCE

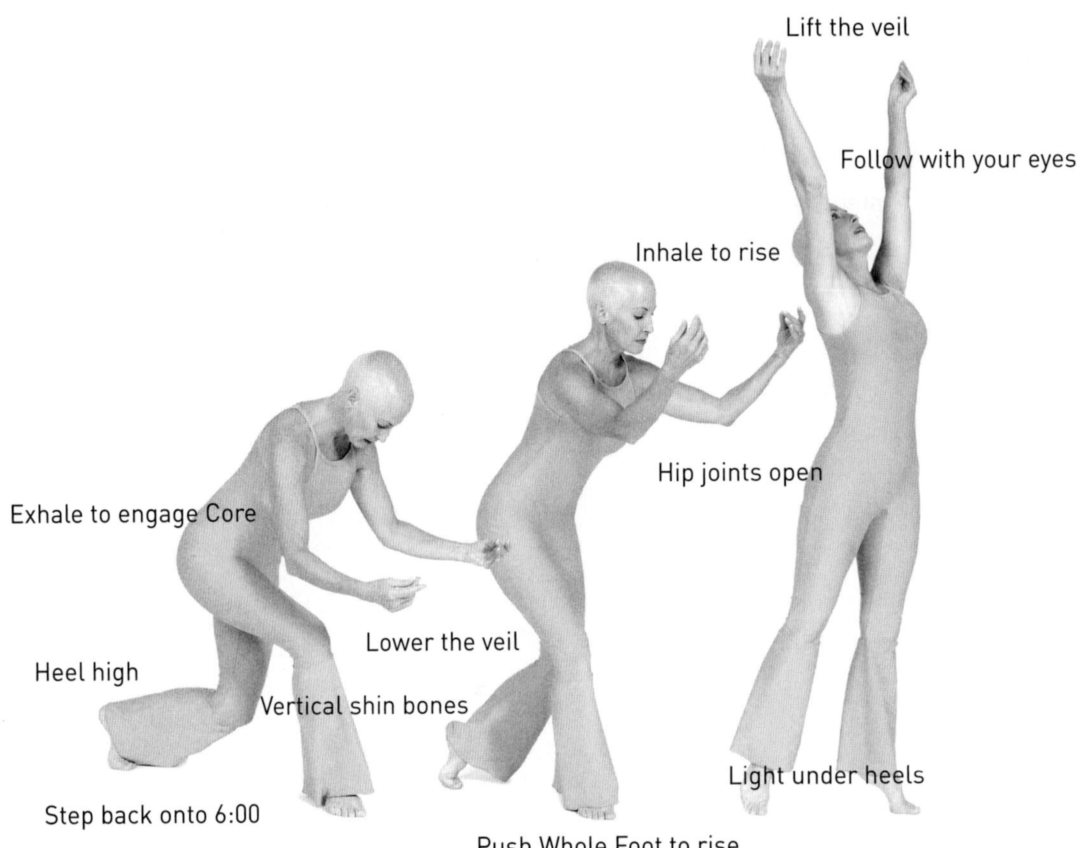

Standing in "A" Stance step back with your right foot into Bow Stance at the 6:00 position; exhale, saying *ho,* as you lower a veil. Then, with the same foot, step (Heel Lead) onto 12:00, and say *hey,* as you lift the veil. Come briefly to a stop in the center of your clock before repeating with the left foot. Arrive at each clock position feeling your whole body—from toes to fingertips—fully charged with energy. Alternate sides.

Repeat a total of 16 times—counting every step at 6:00 as 1 repetition—or until your body says, "That's enough, I'm aerobically ready to move on to my next move."

IMAGINE YOURSELF LIFTING AND LOWERING A LARGE VEIL.

> BENEFITS: Increases aerobic conditioning, coordination, agility, strength, flexibility, and mobility between the upper and lower body and stability in the feet and ankles.

CLASSIC: Practice stepping onto two numbers of your clock, moving in a comfortable range of motion so it feels like ballroom dancing. Use your hands and arms to stimulate deep and full breathing and to invigorate your heart.

ATHLETIC: Move in a bigger range of motion and, with precision, hit the numbers of your clock. As you step back, sink into a deep Bow Stance. Add more hand, arm, and Core power by releasing and throwing the veil.

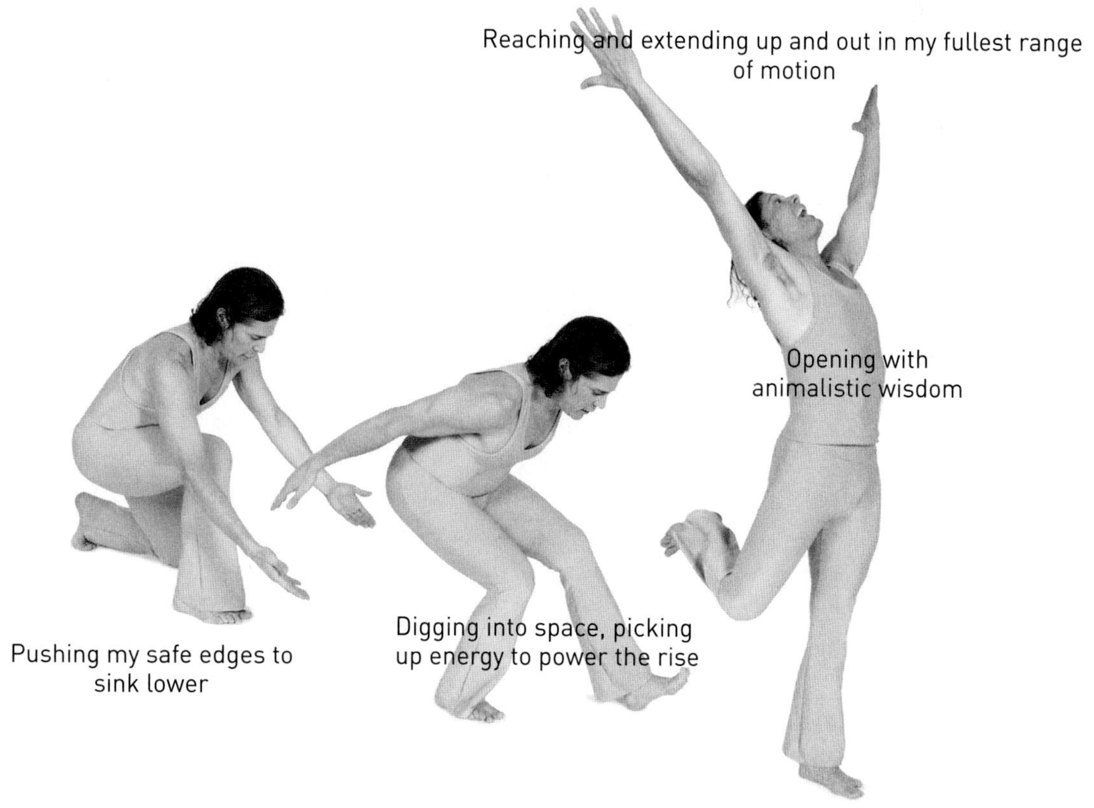

SUMO PALM DIRECTIONS

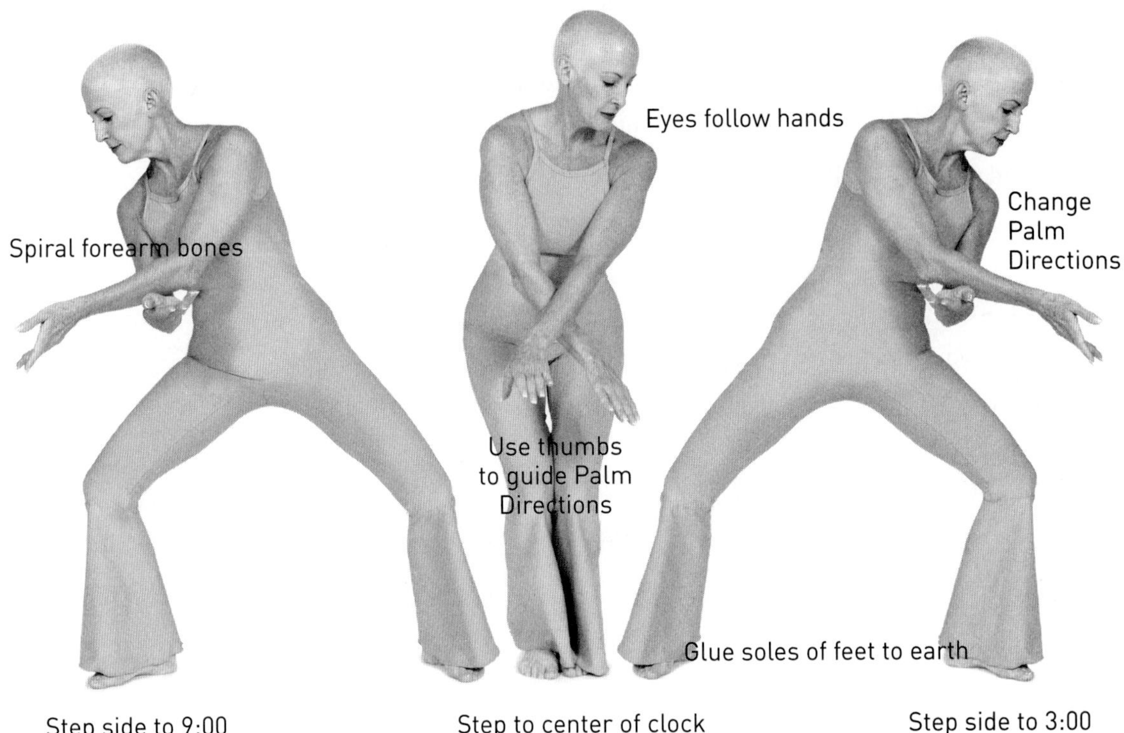

Starting in the center of your Slow Clock, step out with your left foot into Riding (Sumo) Stance onto 9:00 as your hands and arms open (palms up) and close (palms down) crossing and uncrossing them in front of your chest. Step back to the center of your clock and continue opening (palms up) and closing (palms down) your arms in front of your chest. Sense your chest and back muscles getting stronger. Now step out with your right foot into Riding (Sumo) Stance onto 3:00, continuing opening and closing, changing Palm Directions.

Repeat a total of 32 times—counting 1-and [Riding (Sumo) Stance], 2-and [center], 3-and [Riding (Sumo) Stance], 4-and [center] . . . —or until your body says, "This is just what my legs and arms need and I'm breathing deeper and feel balanced."

IMAGINE MAKING WAVES WITH YOUR HANDS.

BENEFITS: Trims and tones arms, legs, and hips. Improves shoulder and hip joint agility, inner and outer leg definition and strength, Core and spine stability. Tones waist, back, and chest.

CLASSIC: Practice moving along the Smile Line, shifting your body weight rather than dropping it. Step out into a range of motion in which you can easily maintain the action of Heel Lead. Use your thumbs to guide palm direction, and keep your elbows close to your body to engage your spine, using it as if it were a third arm.

ATHLETIC: Challenge your energetic coordination by maintaining fluidity in your arm motion while being explosive in your leg motions. Move through three levels with precision, more power, and speed.

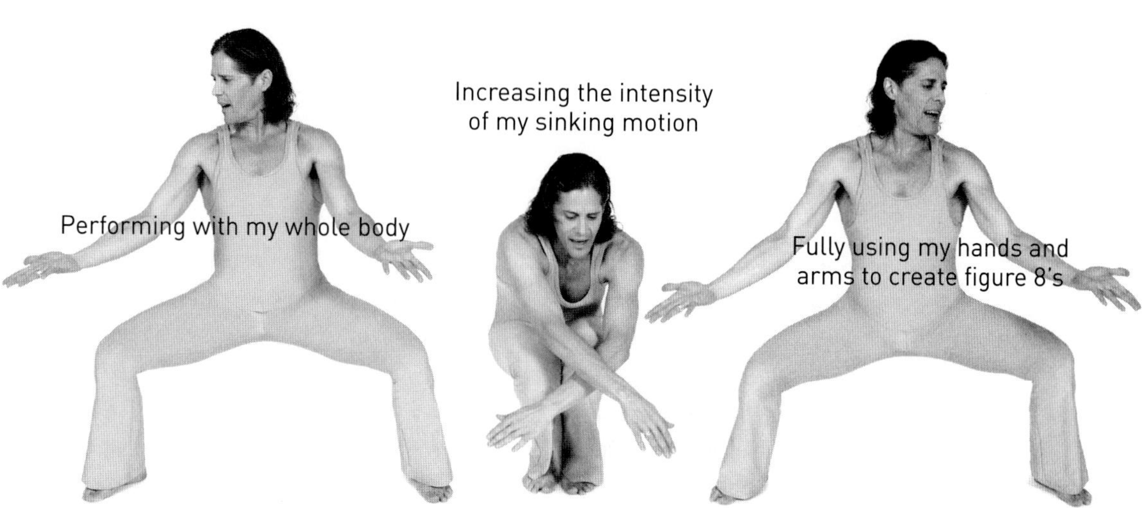

TRAVELING PREPARE KICK

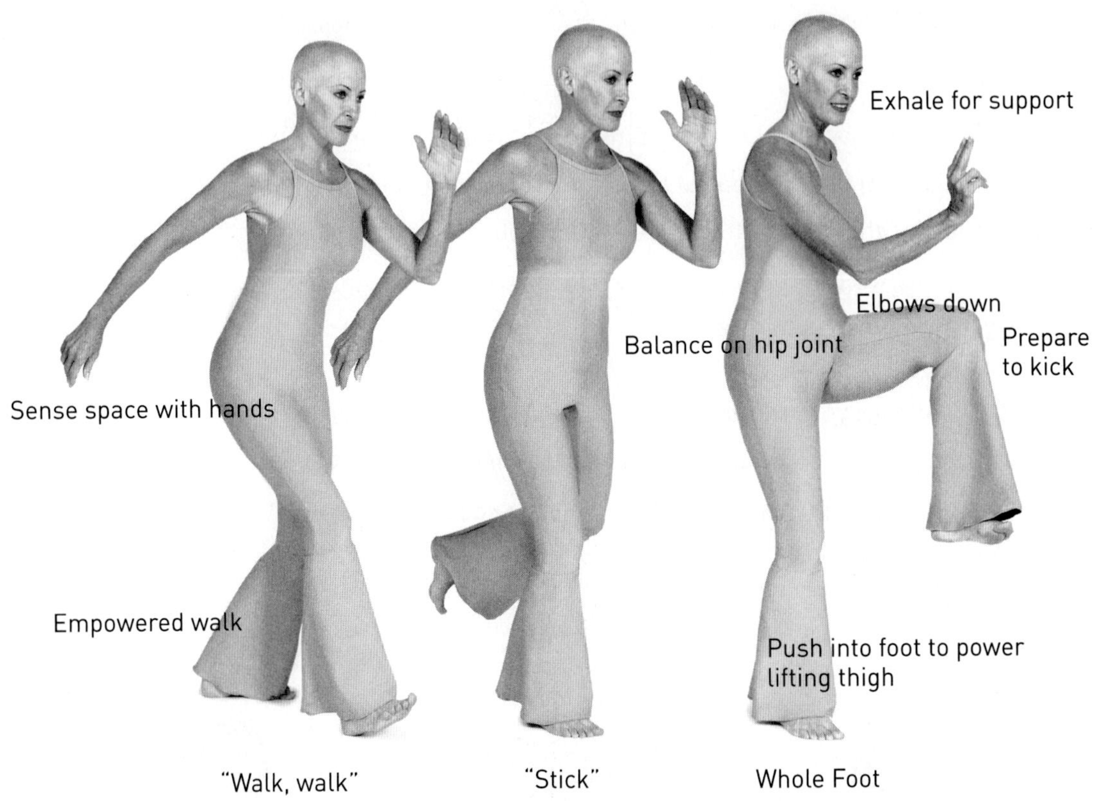

Starting with your left foot, walk forward to a count of four and backward to a count of four. Say *walk, walk, stick, prepare* to find your rhythmic pace. Continue speaking and on *prepare* (count four) bring your thigh up into Prepare Position and use your hands in Spear Fingers to help stabilize your upper body. Sense for balance and precision throughout your whole body. On *walk, walk, stick,* use one or both hands directly in front of you. Repeat on the other side, starting with your right foot. Sense stability and agility in your Base. Alternate sides.

Repeat 8 times—traveling 4 counts forward and 4 counts backward for 1 repetition—or until your body says, "I feel powerful, strong, agile in my whole body, and I'm ready for the action of kicking."

IMAGINE YOU'RE GETTING READY TO KICK BALLOONS UP INTO THE AIR.

BENEFITS: Tones and trims buttocks and thighs, strengthens abdominal and leg muscles. Improves balance, agility, and stability.

CLASSIC: Practice walking and moving your arms naturally. In preparation for learning how to safely kick out, firmly stick your supporting foot on the floor, and smoothly—without losing balance—draw your thigh up. As your thigh comes up, use your hands and arms for stability.

ATHLETIC: Infuse your walk with leg power by crouching as you step down, then fully rise up as you prepare to kick. Move front and back while, at the same time, using your palms vigorously in front of your body, as if attempting to confuse an opponent. With speed and precision, draw your thigh up high keeping your heel in (to spring load the anticipated kick) and use Spear Fingers for stability.

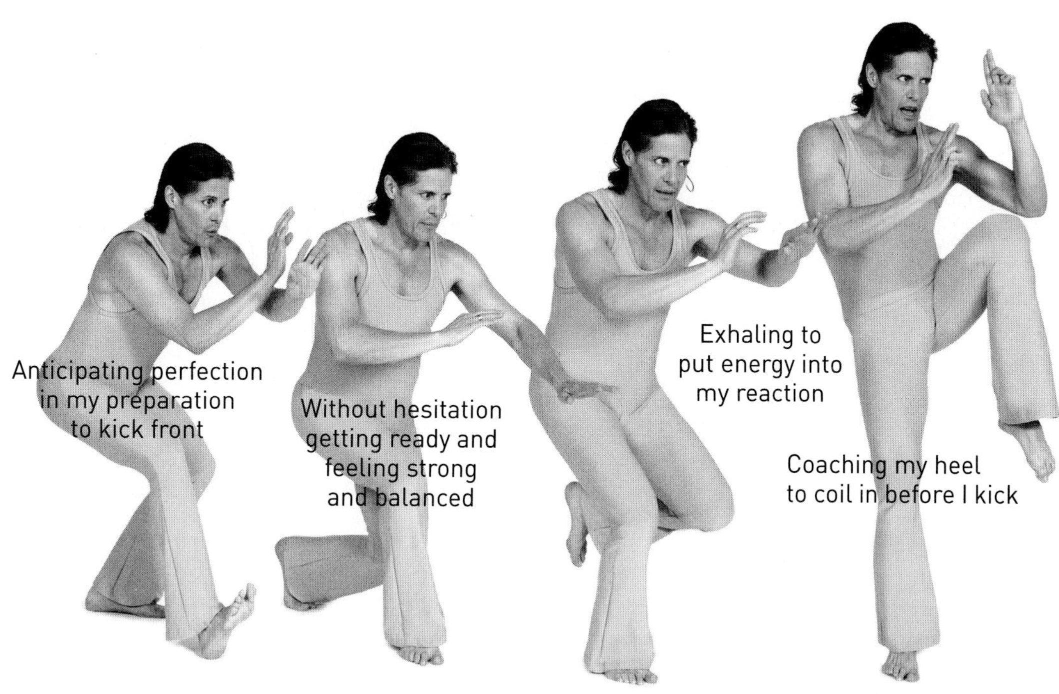

TRAVELING FRONT KICK

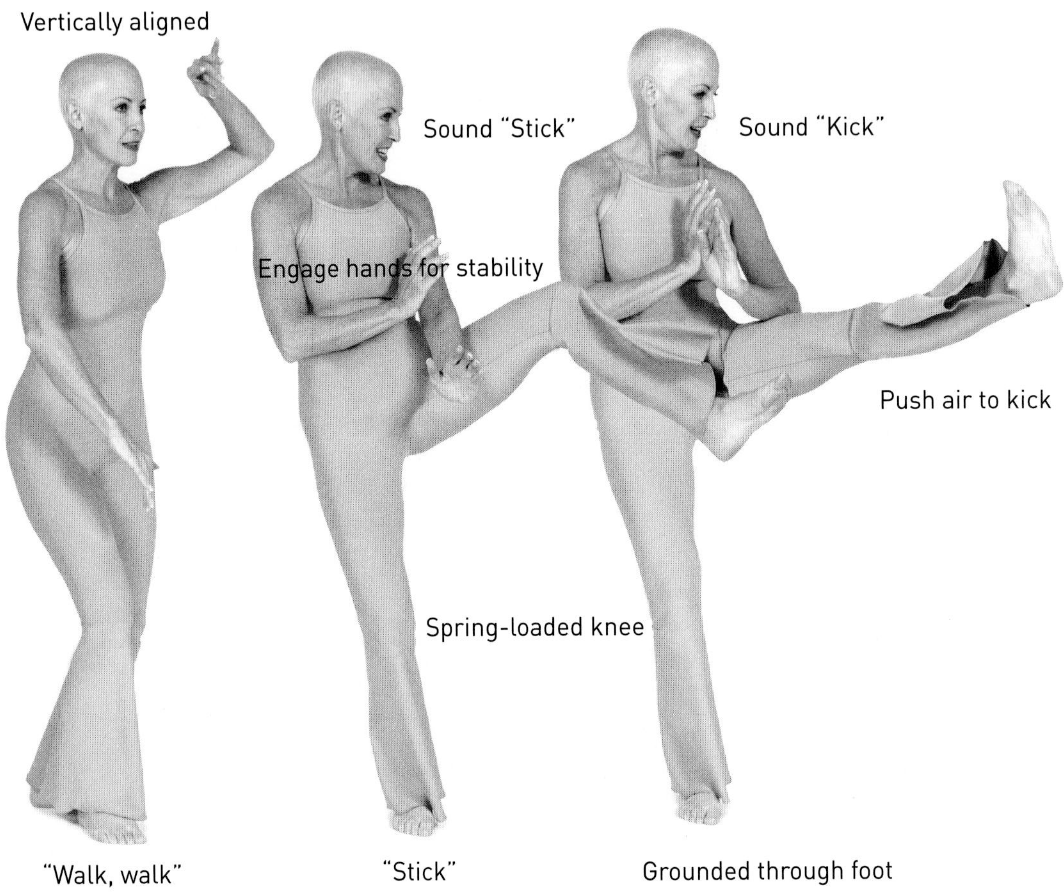

Starting with your left foot and traveling forward and backward to the count of four, kick to the front on four. Say *walk, walk, stick, kick,* and use your hands naturally in front of you for balance and stability. Say a loud *kick,* to engage your abdominal muscles. Sense strength building in the front of your thigh. Alternate kicking legs.

IMAGINE YOU'RE KICKING BALLOONS UP INTO THE AIR.

BENEFITS: Tones and trims buttocks and thighs and strengthens abdominal and leg muscles. Improves balance, agility, and stability and defines frontal thighs.

CLASSIC: Practice coordinating your Base, Core, and Upper Extremities. Kick to a comfortable height, in which you feel strong in your Base and relaxed in your whole body.

ATHLETIC: Reach a new endurance edge by traveling front and back in a crouching position, moving your hands and arms in space faster and with more chaos. Kick higher and with more speed and precision, directing the height of each kick to a target. Challenge your balance, strength, and flexibility by momentarily freezing your kicking leg out in space before you set it down to walk.

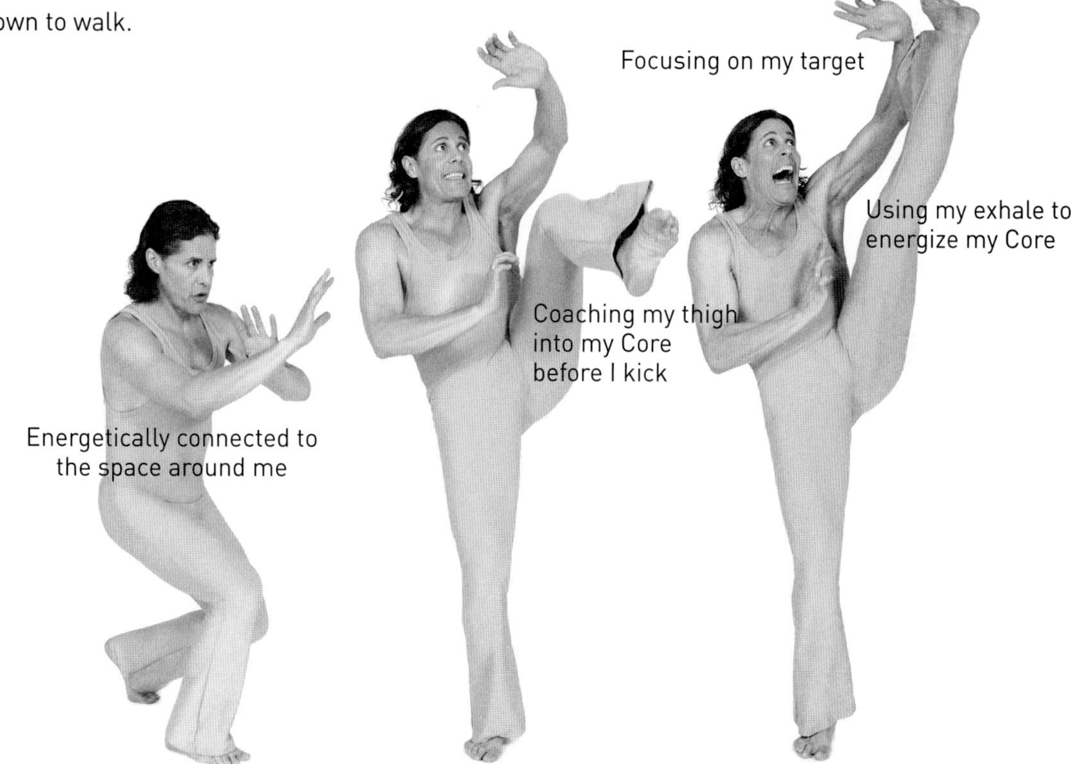

Directing my movement with precision from the ground up

TRAVELING SIDE KICK

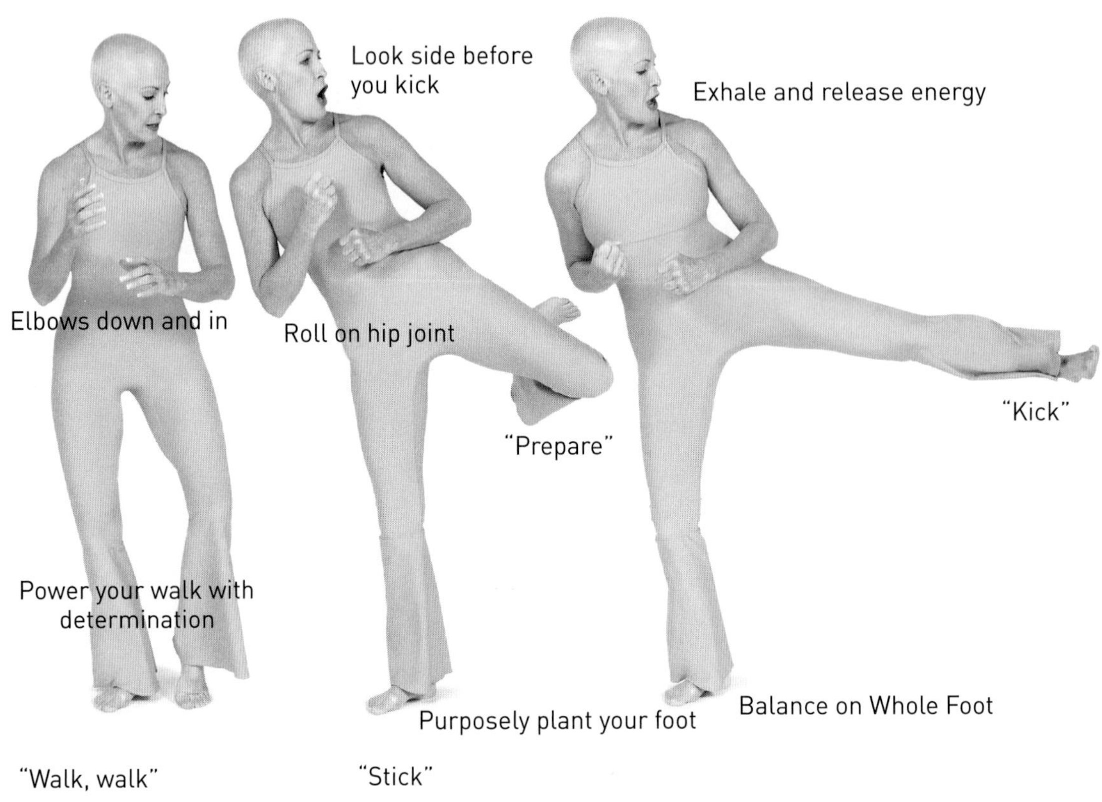

Starting with your left foot, and traveling forward and backward to the count of four, kick to the side on 4. Sound *walk, walk, stick, kick,* and as you kick to the side, make fists with your hands for stability. Sense strength along your outer thigh as you kick side. Alternate kicking legs. For greater balance, look to the side before you kick and kick at a height your Base can support.

Repeat 8 times, alternating sides—walk, walk, stick, kick to the right plus walk, walk, stick, kick to the left equals 1 repetition—or until your body says, "The sides of my thighs are awake and feel powerful."

IMAGINE PUSHING A HEAVY BOULDER AWAY WITH YOUR FOOT.

BENEFITS: Tones and trims buttocks and thighs and strengthens abdominal, Core, and leg muscles. Improves balance, agility, and stability and defines inner and outer thigh muscles.

CLASSIC: Practice pointing your tailbone in the direction you will kick. This naturally tilts the body and balances it over the supporting foot. Sense mobility (a rolling sensation in your hip joint) to keep your Base powerfully relaxed and to move energy up from your Base, into your Core, and out of your upper body.

ATHLETIC: Tightly tuck the heel of your kicking leg into your buttocks as you practice Prepare Position. Coil the power of your kick before you release it. Release the kick with more power and precision, and briefly hold the extension of your Side Kick before you draw your foot back in and place your foot back down.

Cultivating my ability to kick higher
Focused on technique
Drawing my heel in to generate power
Directing my kick by pointing with my tailbone
Rolling on my hip joint

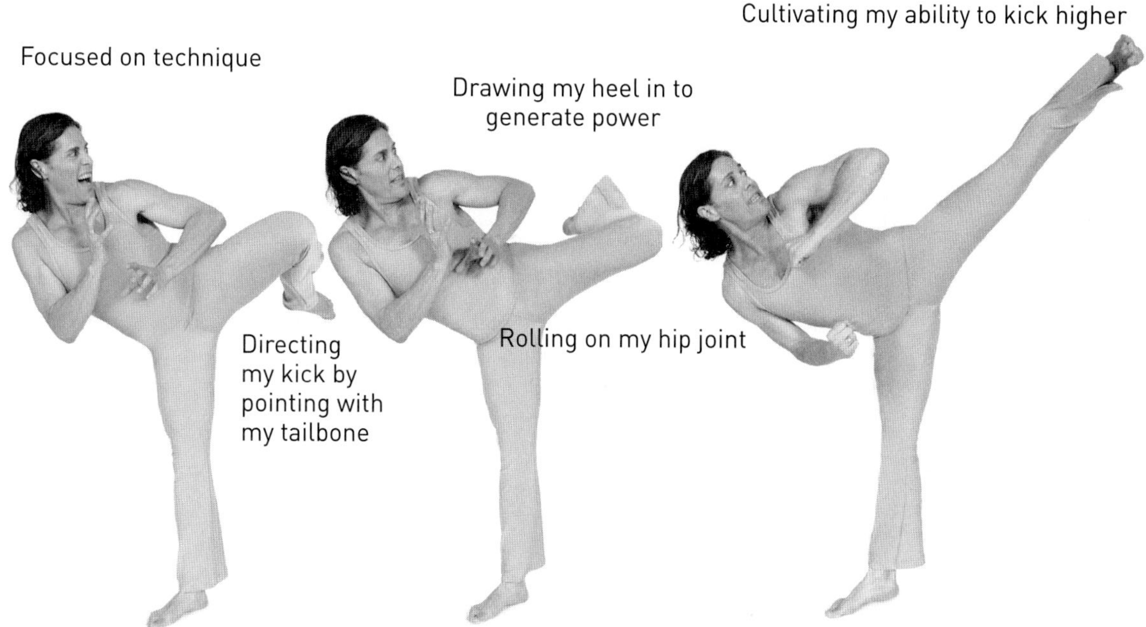

Coaching my body to vertically ground to deliver horizontal power

SINK AND PIVOT TABLE WIPE

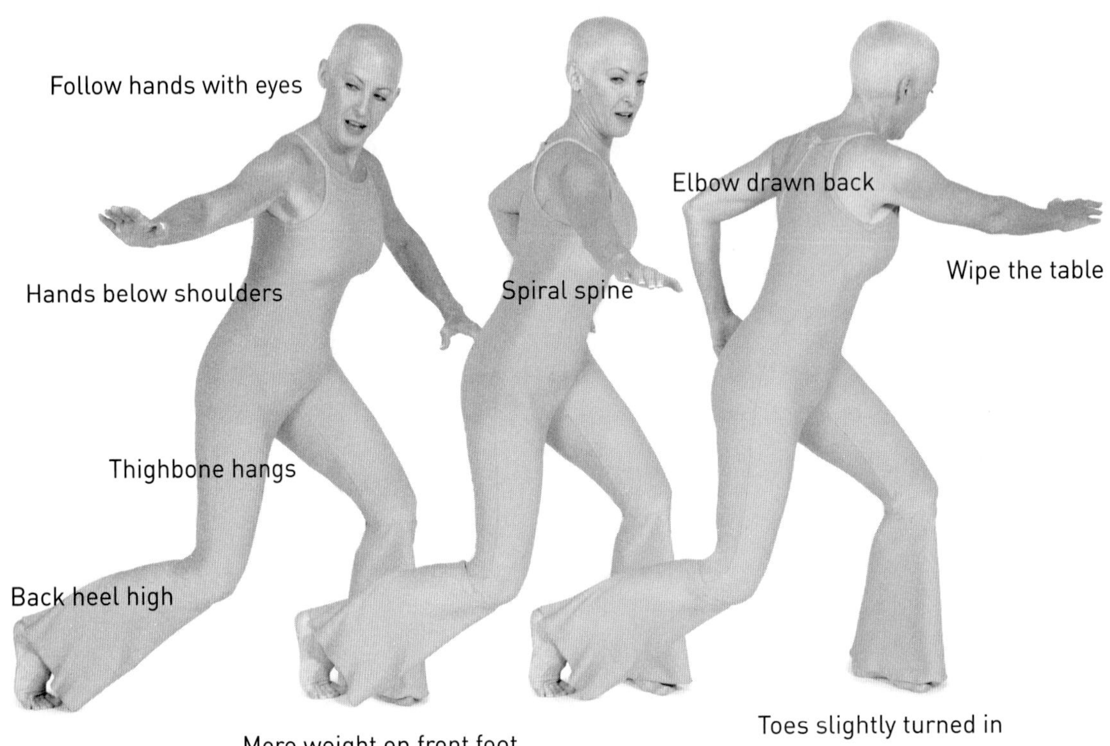

Standing in "A" Stance, sink into a comfortable Bow Stance by shifting your body weight to the right foot and slightly lifting your left foot off the floor, rotating your left thigh to pivot and place the ball of your left foot down as your left hand wipes off a table from back to front. Keeping your back heel high, and your spine elongated, *wipe,* sensing power in your Core as you use your hands to wipe the table. Pivot smoothly from right to left side by picking up and placing your feet with precision. Sense agility in your feet and hip joints as you pivot, and strength and flexibility in your legs as you land. Alternate sides.

Repeat 16 times—each wipe is 1 repetition—alternating sides or until your body says, "I feel coordinated and agile, and in control of my lift, pivot, and place. I feel strong in my legs, and flexible in my upper body."

IMAGINE WIPING OFF A TABLE.

BENEFITS: Tones buttocks and thighs. Defines upper body; improves mobility, agility, and stability in the whole body.

CLASSIC: Practice the sensation of smoothly shifting your body weight and firmly placing the ball of the back foot, as you simultaneously wipe off the table (to integrate your upper and lower body).

ATHLETIC: Master the skill of anticipating the rotation of your back leg by alternating sides with greater agility and speed. Practice moving from right to left while maintaining a low plane as you wipe off the table with more power. Sink into your deepest Bow Stance.

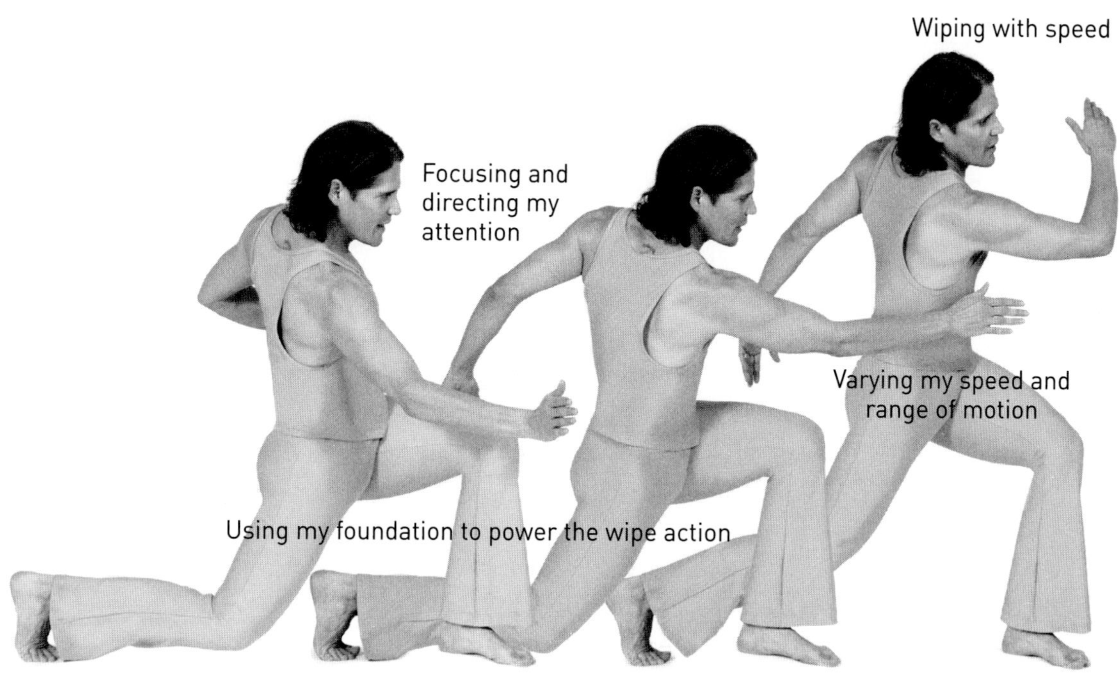

CROSS FRONT CHA-CHA-CHA

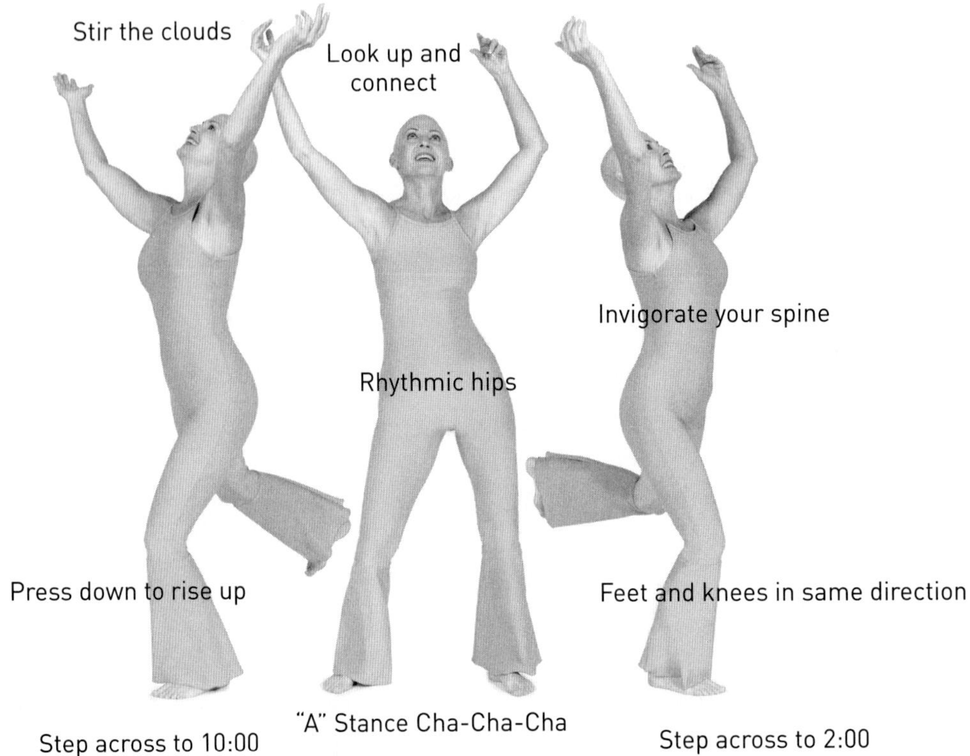

Starting in "A" Stance, Cross Front to the left corner with your right foot (Heel Lead) onto Whole Foot, keeping your left leg relaxed and free. Use your hands freely and "stir the clouds," while saying *oo-ah.* As you Cross Front, follow your hands with your eyes, and sense a long agile and free spine. Come back to center and rhythmically do a Cha-Cha-Cha. Then repeat with Cross Front to the right corner. Sense rhythmic mobility in your hips and spine, as your hands and arms continue to play with the clouds in celebration. Add sound and emotion to invigorate your body, mind, and spirit. Alternate sides.

Repeat 16 times—counting Cross Front Cha-Cha-Cha as 1 repetition—or until your body says, "I am breathing deeply and fully."

IMAGINE YOU'RE CELEBRATING AND PLAYING WITH THE CLOUDS.

BENEFITS: Conditions your whole body. Improves agility and encourages free self-expression.

CLASSIC: Practice using Heel Lead and adapting your Upper Extremity movement to support grounded and agile stepping, mindfully guiding your whole body. Turn and move toward the corners consciously, while also directing your foot, knee, and hips to all face in the same direction you're moving.

ATHLETIC: Burst up and out and into the corners, loading your front foot and leg with more body weight and kicking your back leg up and out. Cover more space and use your hands and arms more aggressively. Cha-Cha-Cha with more of your whole body.

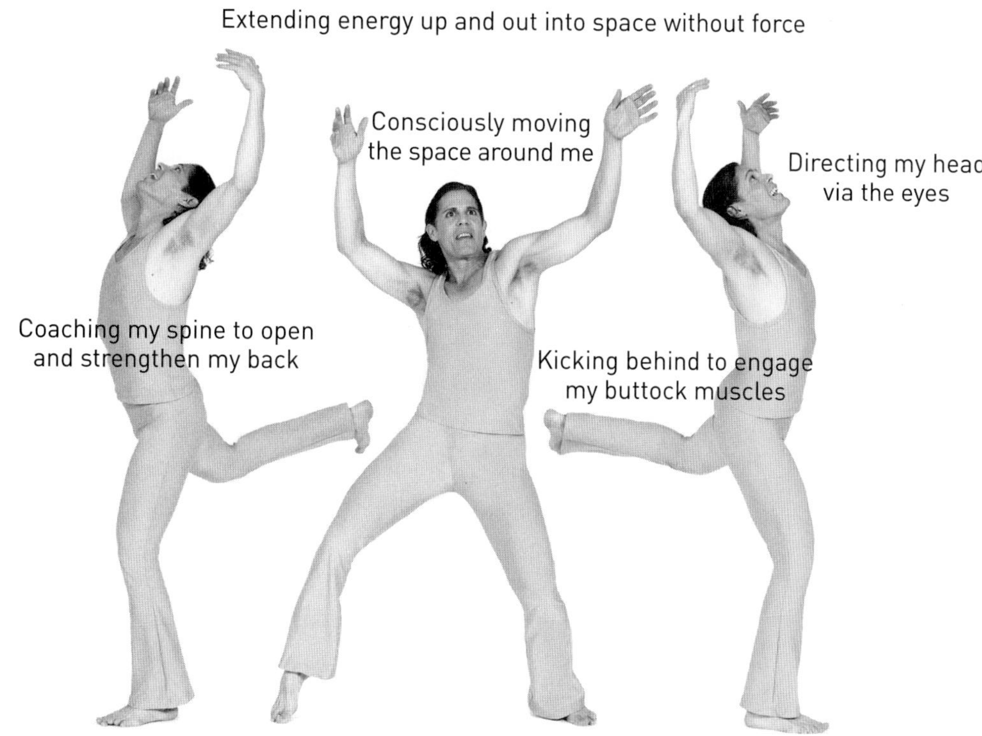

RIDING (SUMO) STANCE PUNCH

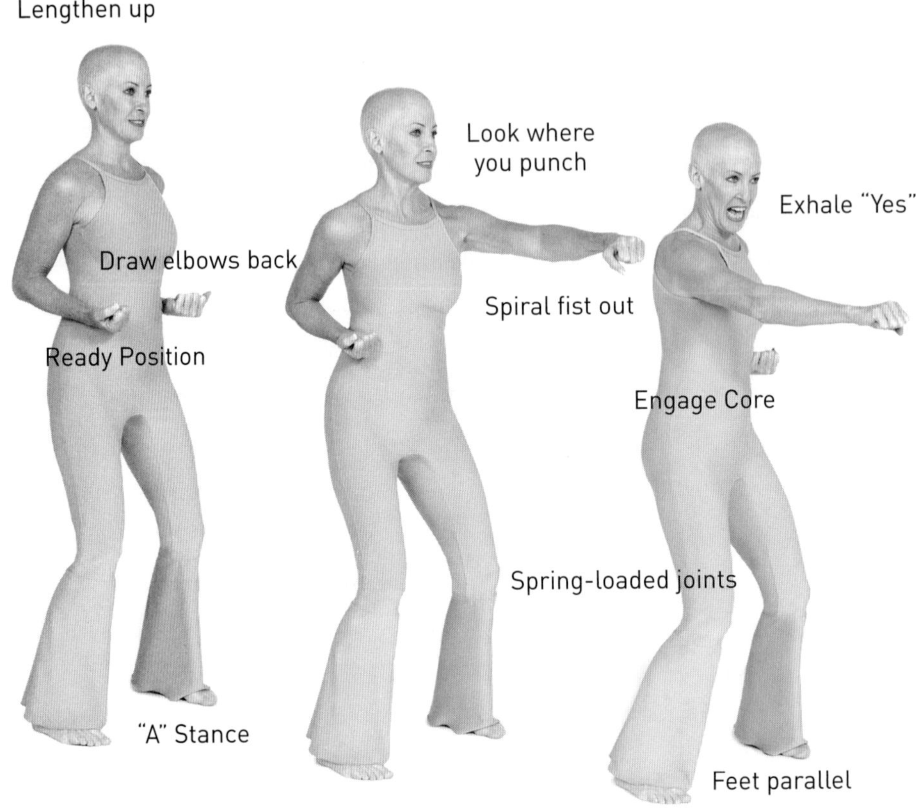

Standing in "A" Stance or Riding (Sumo) Stance in Ready Position, punch out with your right fist as you draw back your left elbow. Stabilize the punch by saying either *no* or *yes* as you punch. Now punch with your left fist, and draw back your right elbow. Always begin your punch in Ready Position, with palms up and fists close to your body, elbows down. Play with doing Upward, Outward, Across, and Downward Punches. Inhale deeply and use vocalizations to gain Core support. Alternate sides.

Repeat 32 times—counting punch right–punch left as 1 repetition—or until your body says, "My arms and upper body are charged and my Core is empowered with breath and dynamic energy."

IMAGINE YOURSELF PUNCHING A BAG.

BENEFITS: Tones and trims the Core and upper body; strengthens the legs, arms, and chest muscles; improves agility in shoulders and elbows; increases mobility and stability of the spine; and improves speed and coordination.

CLASSIC: Practice beginning Punches from Ready Position, palms up. Begin slowly, and learn the art of spiraling the forearm bones to protect your shoulder joints as you punch out. Add speed only after you feel your whole body engaged.

ATHLETIC: Create an agile Base by quickly making minimal (but apparent) weight shifts side to side and punch faster. Visualize targets, varying the height of your punch.

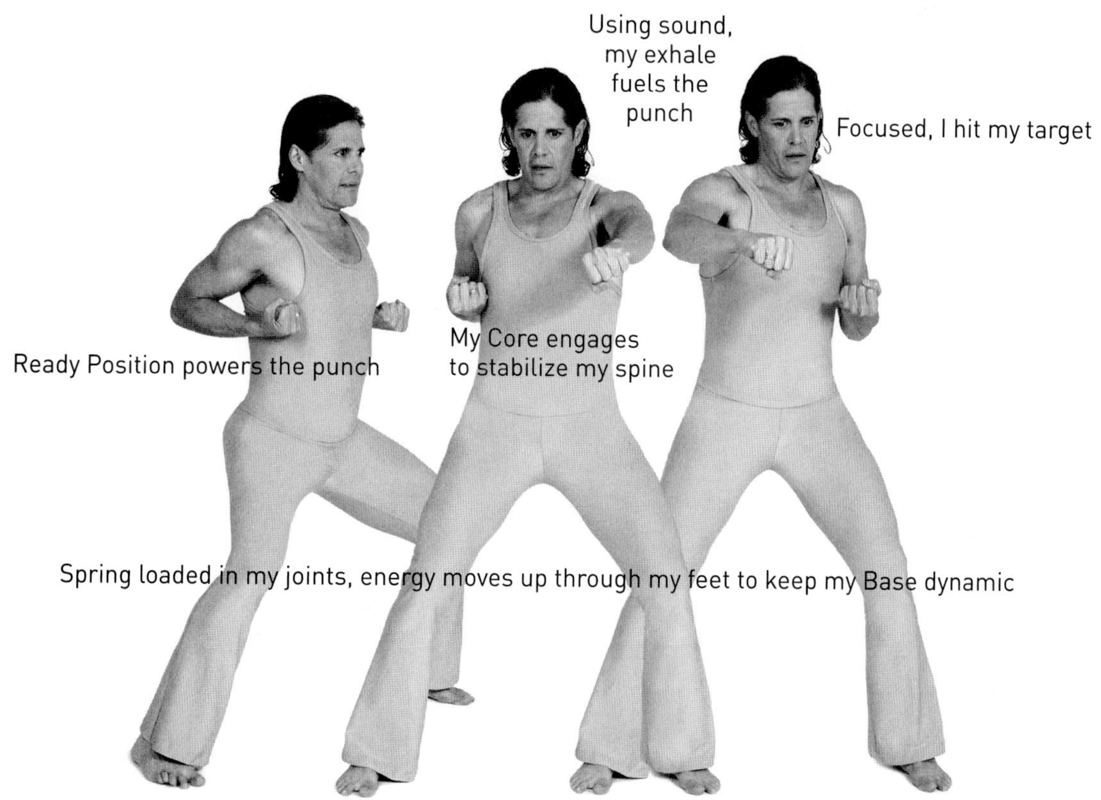

CROSS BEHIND, RELEVÉ, CHA-CHA-CHA

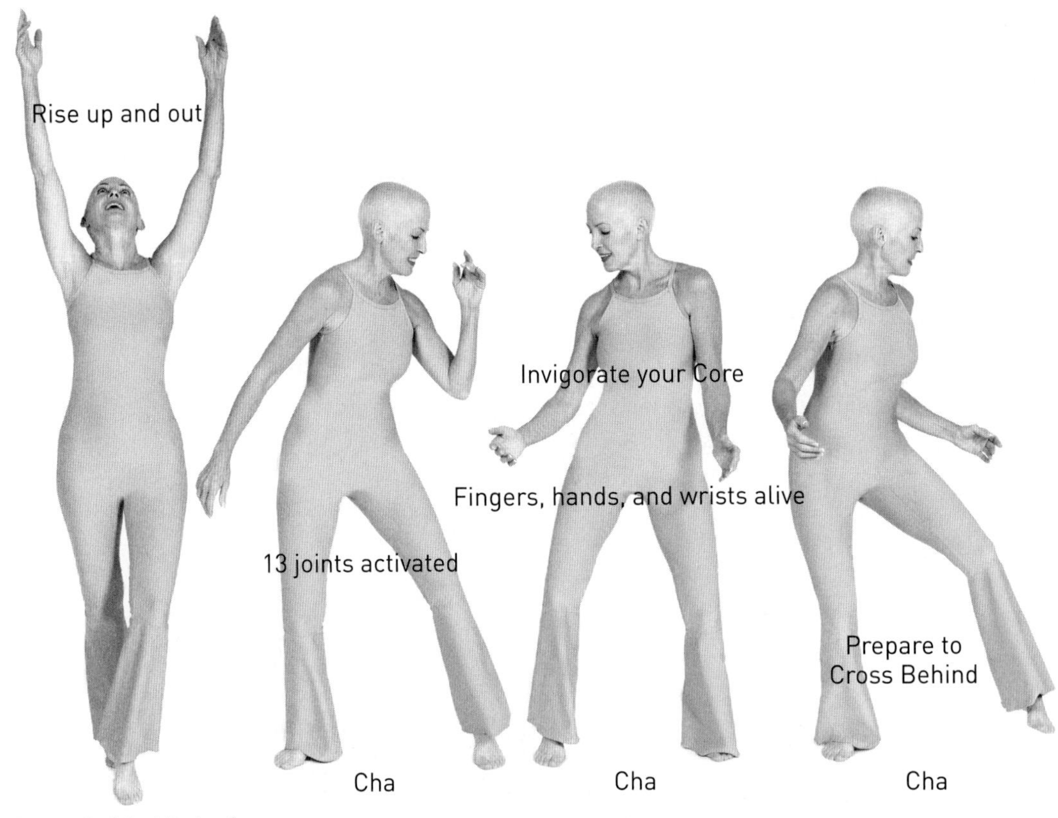

Starting in "A" Stance, Cross Behind with your left foot creating a small "x" with your ankles and rise into Relevé on both feet. Simultaneously look up and reach into the sunlight and sense stability as you rise. Return to "A" Stance and Cha-Cha-Cha with loose and rhythmical arms and hands, hip and spine movements. Now, Cross Behind with the right foot and into Relevé. Use your whole body and hands to engage your chest and back muscles.

Repeat 16 times—counting Cross Behind Cha-Cha-Cha as 1 repetition—or until your body says, "I'm breathing even more deeply and feel fully engaged, agile, and powerful in my whole body."

IMAGINE RISING AND REACHING UP INTO THE SUNLIGHT.

> BENEFITS: Build stability in the feet, strength in the legs, and agility in the ankle, knee, and hip joints. Encourages self-expression.

CLASSIC: Practice using your hands, and sense a harmonious integration between your upper body and lower body as you rise up in Relevé. Learn to bring your ankles close together on the Cross Behind. Learn to rhythmically use your Base in Cha-Cha-Cha.

ATHLETIC: With explosive power, cross your ankles and rise up with more speed. Move more deeply in and out of "A" Stance and Cha-Cha-Cha. Push into the earth to rise and open up the entire front of your body.

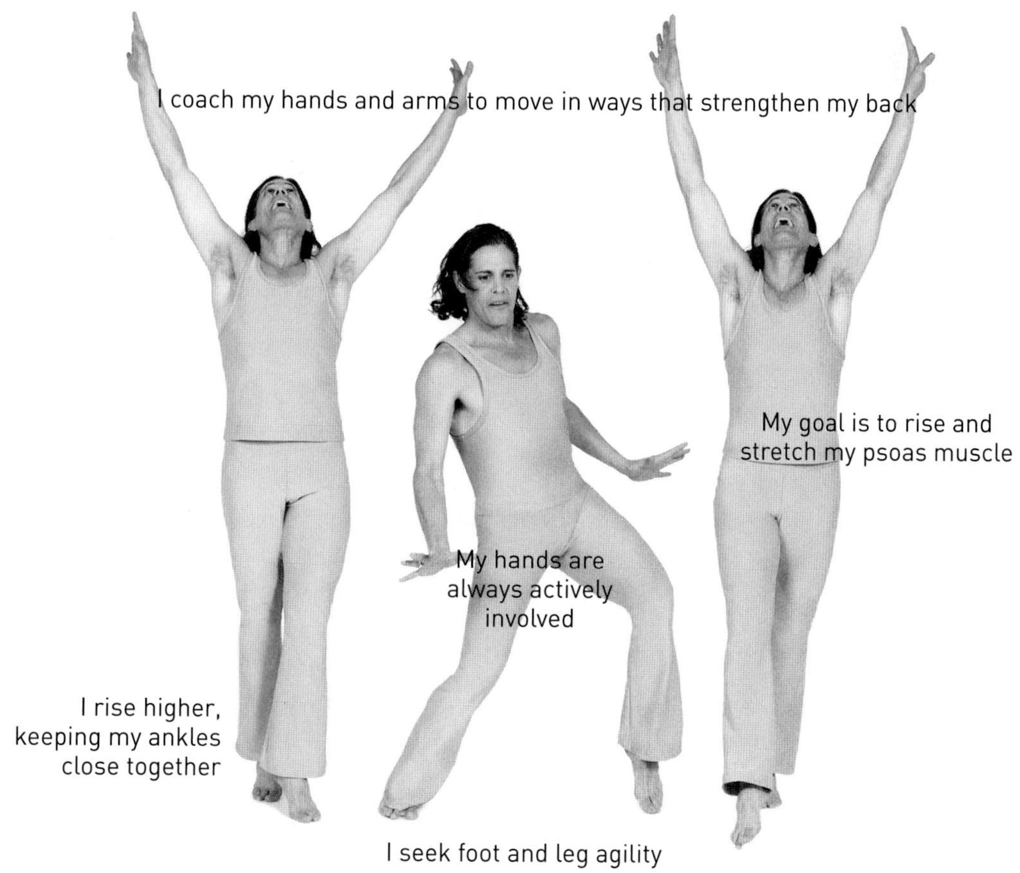

TOUCH FRONT PADDLE

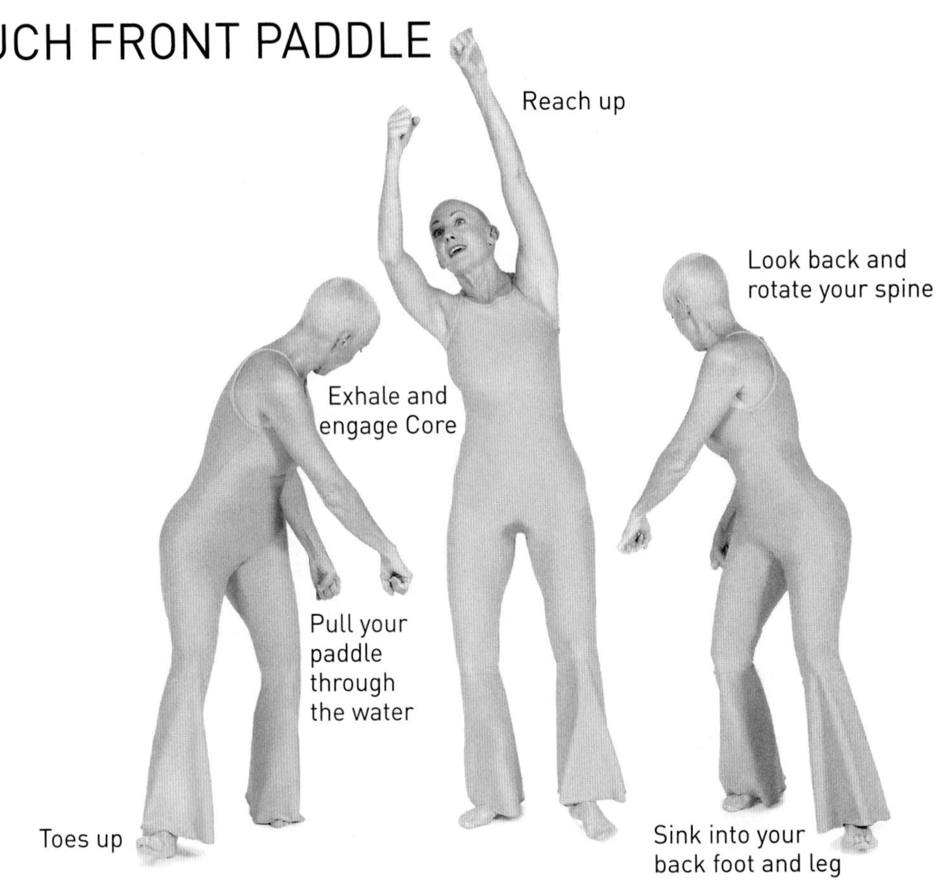

Starting in "A" Stance, shift your body weight to your right foot and touch out to the front with your left heel as you pull your paddle toward your right hip, following it with your eyes. Sense mobility and strength in your Core as you pull the paddle. Now, bring your left foot back to center, lift your paddle above your head, and touch out with your right heel to the front, as you plunge your paddle into the water on your left side. Inhale deeply and exhale as you say the word *pull,* while paddling. Sweep the paddle behind and up as you return to "A" Stance. Create smooth and powerful figure-eight arm motions and maintain momentum. Alternate sides.

Repeat 16 times—counting left then right as 1 repetition—or until your body says, "I'm breathing even more deeply now, and I'm feeling my Base, Core, and Upper Extremities."

IMAGINE YOURSELF PADDLING WITH AN OAR THROUGH ROUGH, CHOPPY WATER.

BENEFITS: Conditions the arms and Core muscles. Tones and trims the waist and increases agility in the spine and between the upper and the lower body. Tones the buttocks and thigh muscles and improves coordination and your ability to shift body weight with precision.

CLASSIC: Practice sinking into your back foot and following the paddle with your eyes. Learn to paddle smoothly.

ATHLETIC: With more intensity, sink deeper and push off, jumping with precision from side to side. Using your full range of motion, paddle high and deep.

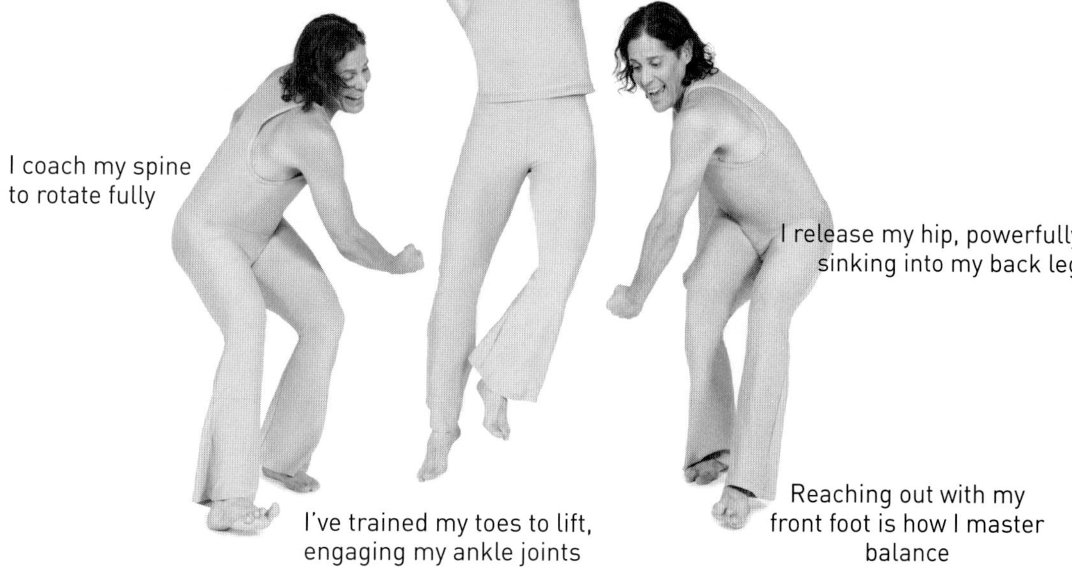

TRAVELING DIRECTIONS KNEE SWEEP

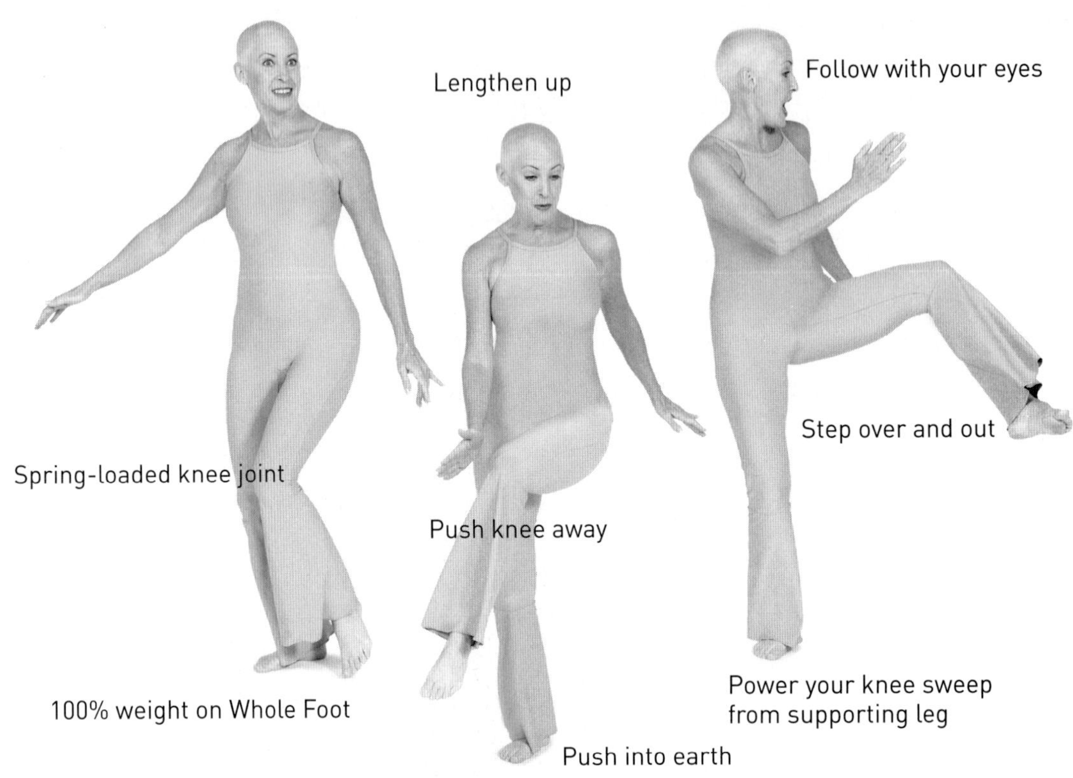

Traveling in directions to the count of 4, beginning with your left foot, walk 1, 2, 3, and on 4 lift your right leg up to the left and sweep it across from left to right. As you bring the sweeping leg up to the left, slap and push the inside of the knee out and away from your body with your left hand. Exhale as you sweep, saying the word *wow,* to synchronize your breath with your body action. Lower your sweeping leg slowly, and plant your foot firmly back down into "A" Stance. Now walk 1, 2, 3, and on 4 Knee Sweep with the left leg. Alternate sides.

Repeat 16 times—counting left then right as 1 repetition—or until your body says, "I've reached my safe edge and can feel my whole body getting stronger and more agile."

IMAGINE YOURSELF STEPPING OVER A BIG BEACH BALL.

BENEFITS: Tones and trims abdominal muscles, strengthens inner and outer thighs, increases Core and hip mobility, and improves balance and overall agility.

CLASSIC: Practice maintaining balance and establish support in the grounded foot. Sweep smoothly and fully from your hip joint while remaining upright and agile in your Core.

ATHLETIC: On the sweep, add more height and leg extension, and slap your ankle.

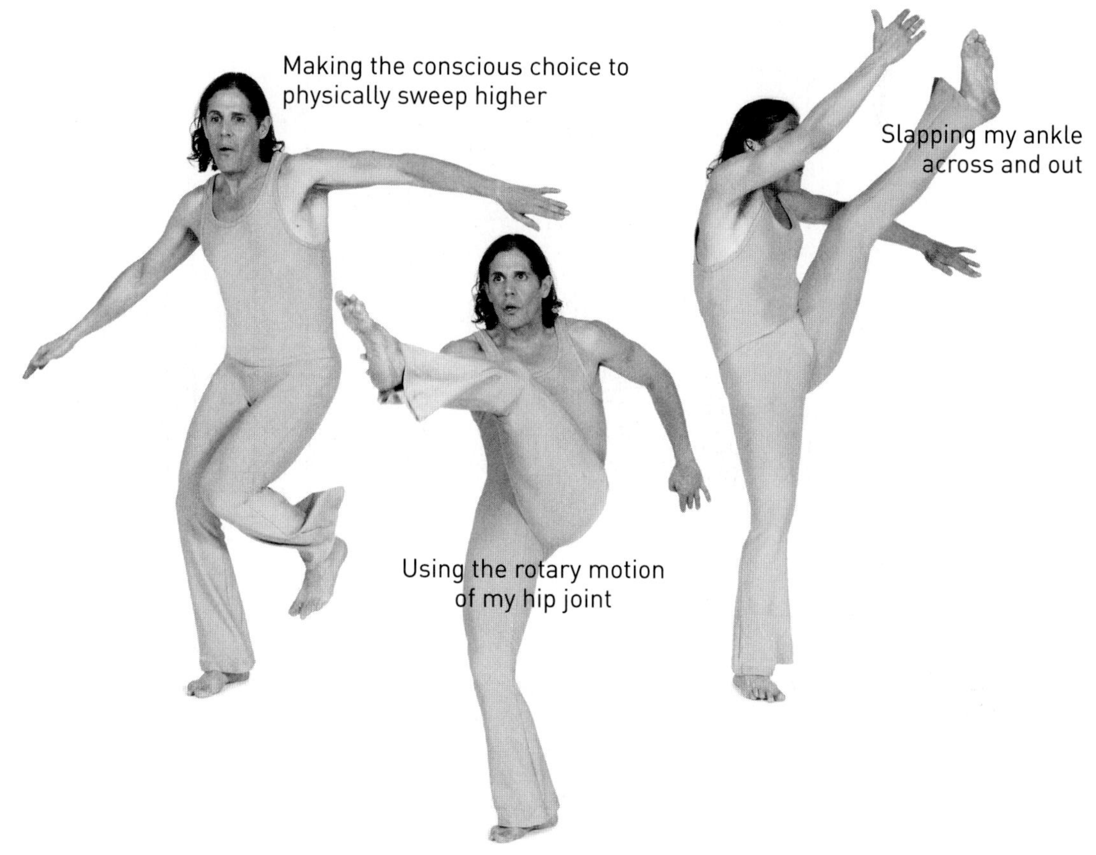

SUMO BLOCKS

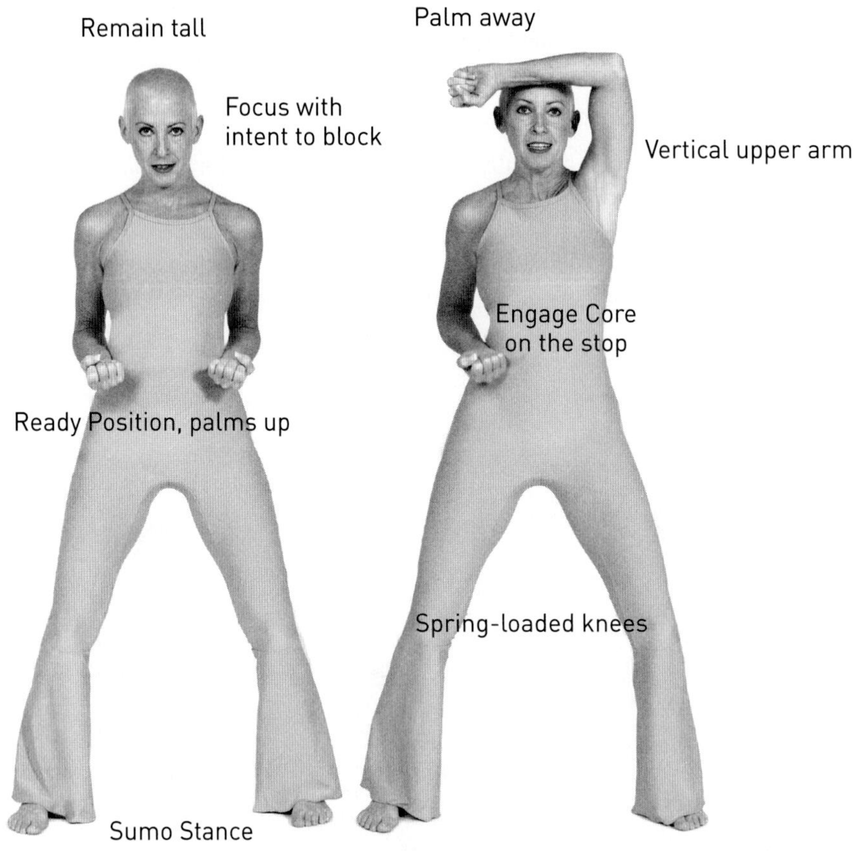

Standing in Riding (Sumo) Stance in Ready Position, lift your right forearm up into an Upward Block with explosive power coming to an abrupt stop in front of your forehead. Exhale, saying *stop!* Sense stability in your Base and Core and agility in your shoulder joints as you come back to Ready Position. Pulling your right elbow down and close to your body, pause briefly before you lift your left forearm up into an Upward Block as you stop your block above your forehead. Alternate sides.

Repeat 32 times—counting each block as 1 repetition—or until your breath, shoulders, and body say, "We've had enough."

IMAGINE YOURSELF BLOCKING YOUR FACE DURING A PILLOW FIGHT.

BENEFITS: Increases lower body stability and strength, Core stability, back strength, and upper body agility. Tones, trims, and defines arms and chest and improves systemic reflex coordination.

CLASSIC: Practice stopping the movement of both arms at the same time, spiraling the forearm bones and turning your palm out when doing Upward Block.

ATHLETIC: Add more speed and challenge your coordination by crossing your forearms in front of your chest in between blocks.

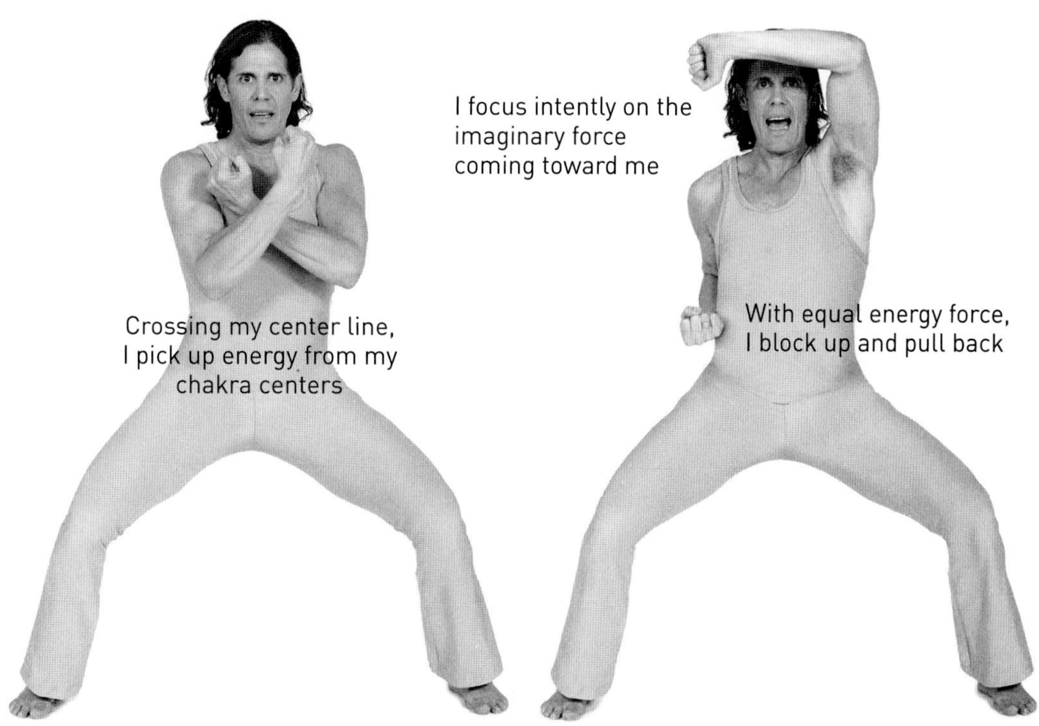

CROSS FRONT, RELEVÉ, CHA-CHA-CHA

Lengthen up
Look up to energize neck and spine
Open heart
Wings back
Squeeze shoulder blades
Loose hip, knee, and ankle joints
Knees spring loaded—no locking!
Strong feet and ankles
Cha-Cha-Cha
Press down to rise
Cross Front Relevé

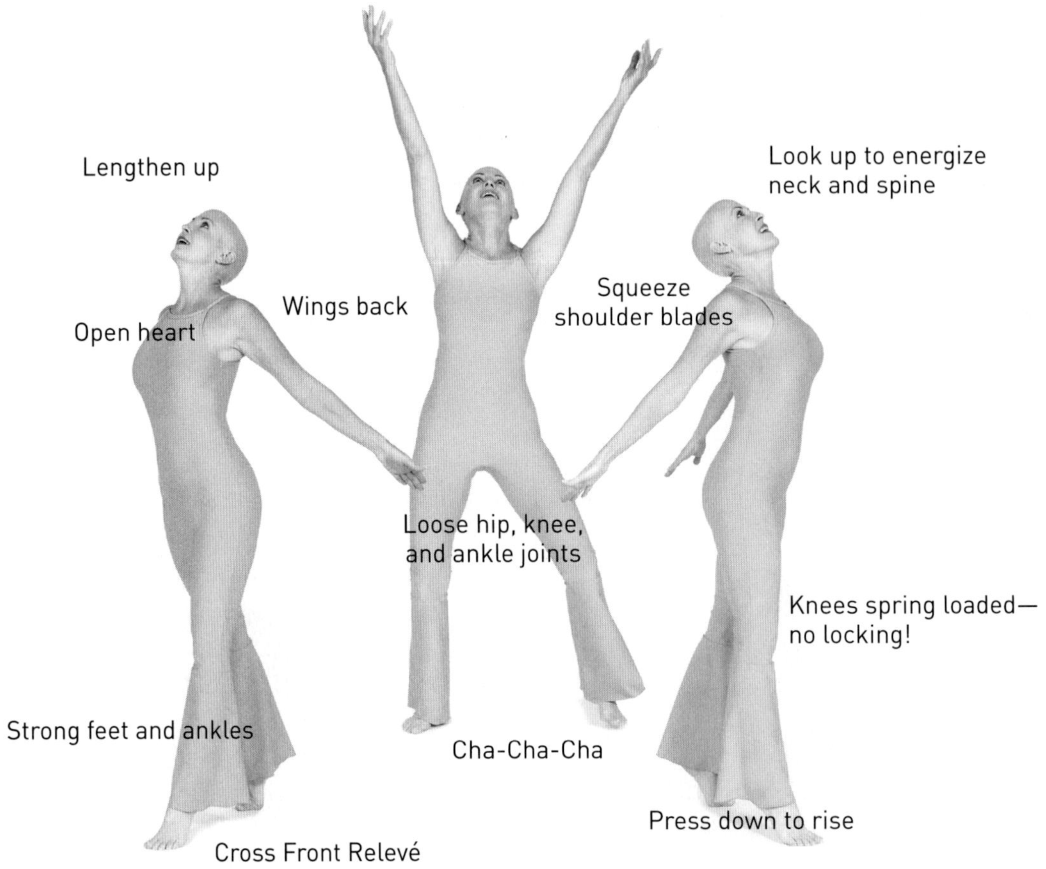

Standing in "A" Stance, Cross Front and rise into Relevé, reaching your hands behind you, palms down, extending energy through all ten fingers. Then step rhythmically back into "A" Stance and Cha-Cha-Cha as you lift your hands and arms like wings while saying *ah.* Repeat on the other side, stepping diagonally onto the ball of your left foot. Look up to fully open your chest, engage your back muscles, and stimulate deep breathing. Sense lightness and grace.

Repeat 32 times—counting each Cross Front Relevé as 1 repetition—or until your breath and body say, "Our spine is longer and stronger, and we're flying high."

IMAGINE YOU'RE A BIRD IN FLIGHT.

BENEFITS: Improves strength in the legs and agility in the ankle, knee, and hip joints. Increases spine flexibility, back strength, and shoulder and arm agility.

CLASSIC: Practice learning how to lengthen systemically and open up the front of your body, using your arms and hands (finger extensions) for balance and stability.

ATHLETIC: With agility and more power, Cross Front and rise into Relevé more swiftly. Reach and extend your wings farther while lifting and extending your back thigh.

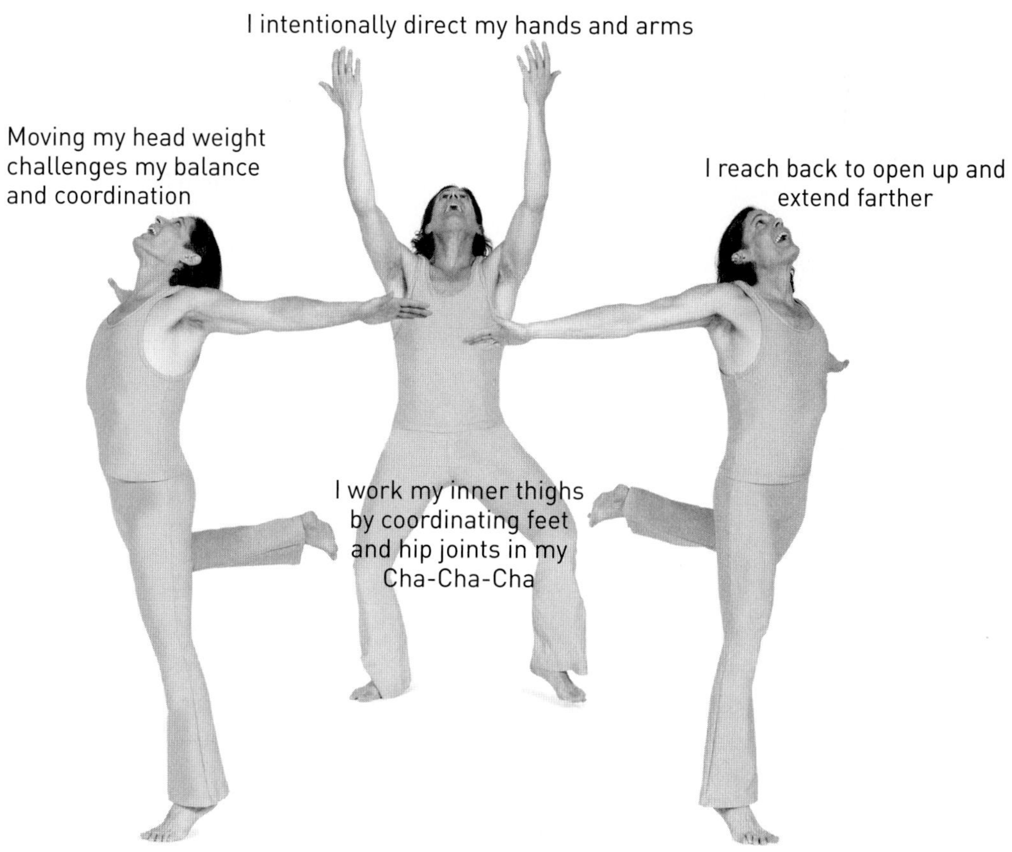

CROSS BEHIND, SINK, CHA-CHA-CHA

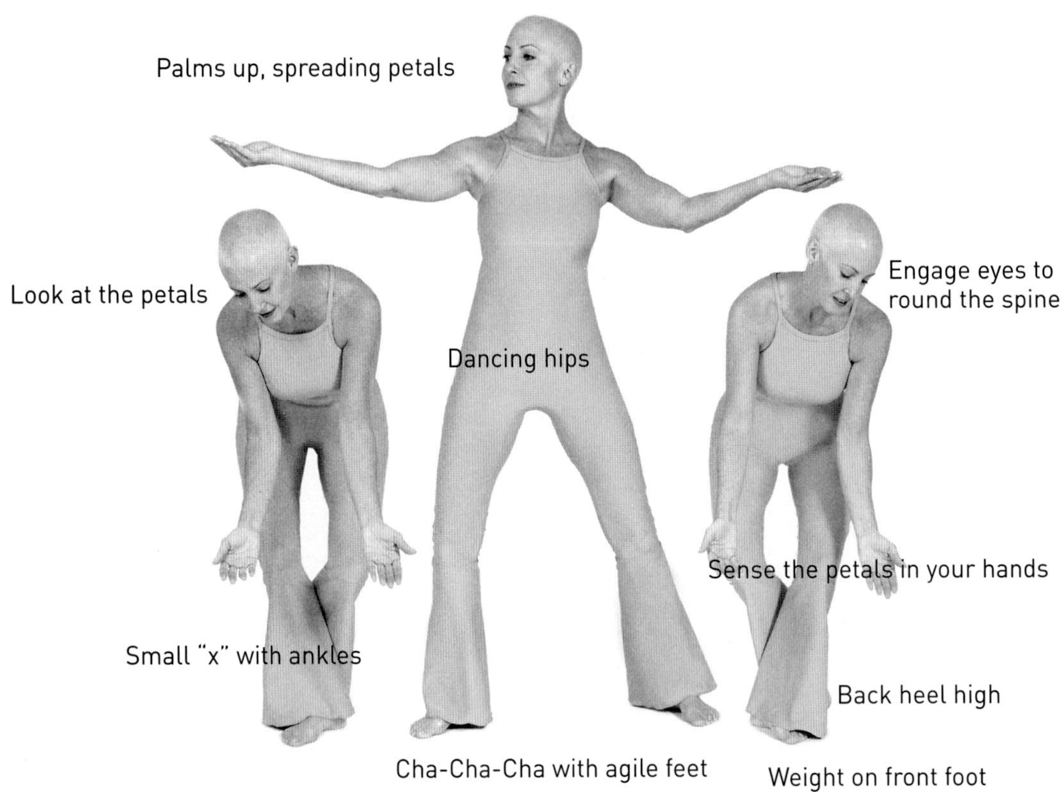

Standing in "A" Stance or Riding (Sumo) Stance, Cross Behind with your right foot, and sink, keeping your ankles close, gathering petals with your hands. Rise up, sounding *here* as you spread the petals, moving your arms out to the sides, as you step out into a rhythmic Cha-Cha-Cha. Now Cross Behind with your left foot and sink. Sense relaxation in all thirteen major joints as you sink and rise. Alternate sides.

Repeat 32 times—count each Cross Behind as 1 repetition—alternating sides or until your breath and body say, "We feel elastic and energetically pumped up."

IMAGINE GATHERING AND SPREADING ROSE PETALS.

BENEFITS: Increases strength in feet, legs, and buttocks and agility in ankle, knee, and hip joints. Improves abdominal, back, and Core strength and enhances mobility in the hands, arms, shoulders, and neck.

CLASSIC: Practice fluidly folding and unfolding your body.

ATHLETIC: Sink more deeply, and with your arms energetically prepare to gather and lift more and heavier petals. Vertically rise up with more explosive precision.

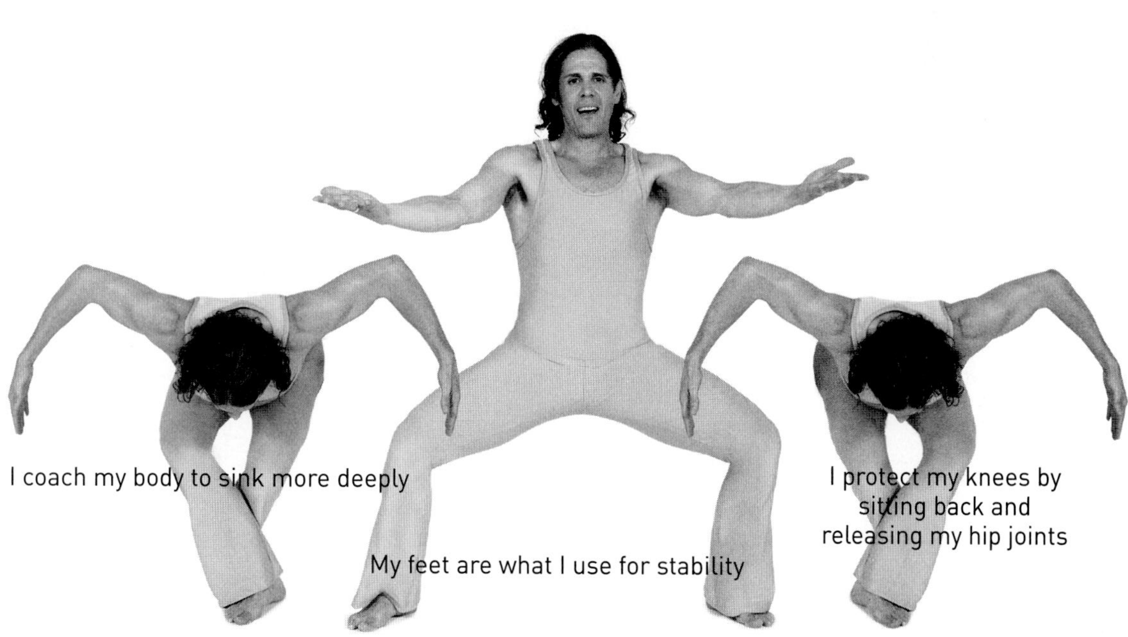

FREEDANCE

Be vocal
Play
Express
Emote
Fuel your dance with emotion
Self-expression
is the key
Let yourself go
Movement wise,
anything goes
Move in the whole space
with all parts of your body
No thinking—all feeling

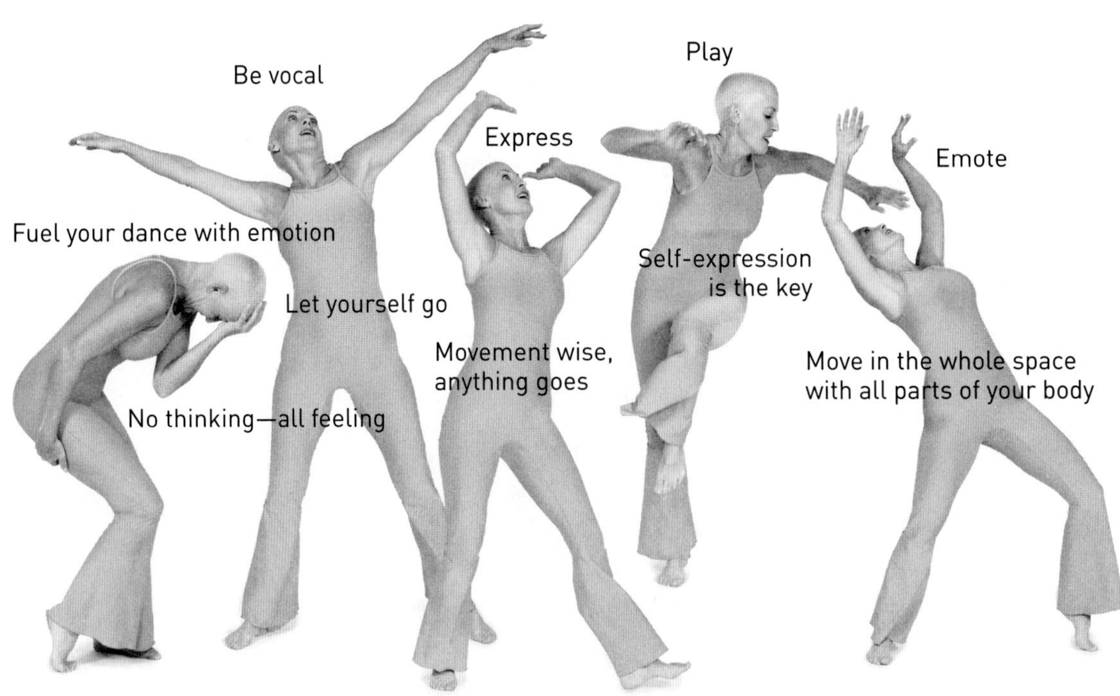

Dance your heart out. Be theatrical. Be spontaneous. Dance outside the lines. Create new ways of moving.

Repetitions: Dance until your body says, "Wow, I've peaked, and I'm ready to cool down."

IMAGINE YOURSELF DANCING IN A DREAM.

> BENEFITS: Encourages self-expression. Improves whole-body strength, flexibility, agility, mobility, and stability.

CLASSIC: Practice breaking your movement habits, and move in ways that deliver blasts of new sensations.

ATHLETIC: Challenge your dancing self and dance height, weight, depth, speed, and stillness. Make small, big, linear, and circular shapes. Change. Change. Change.

Lifting higher challenges my skill
I know crossing limbs strengthens and stretches
Jumping higher pushes my cardiovascular edge

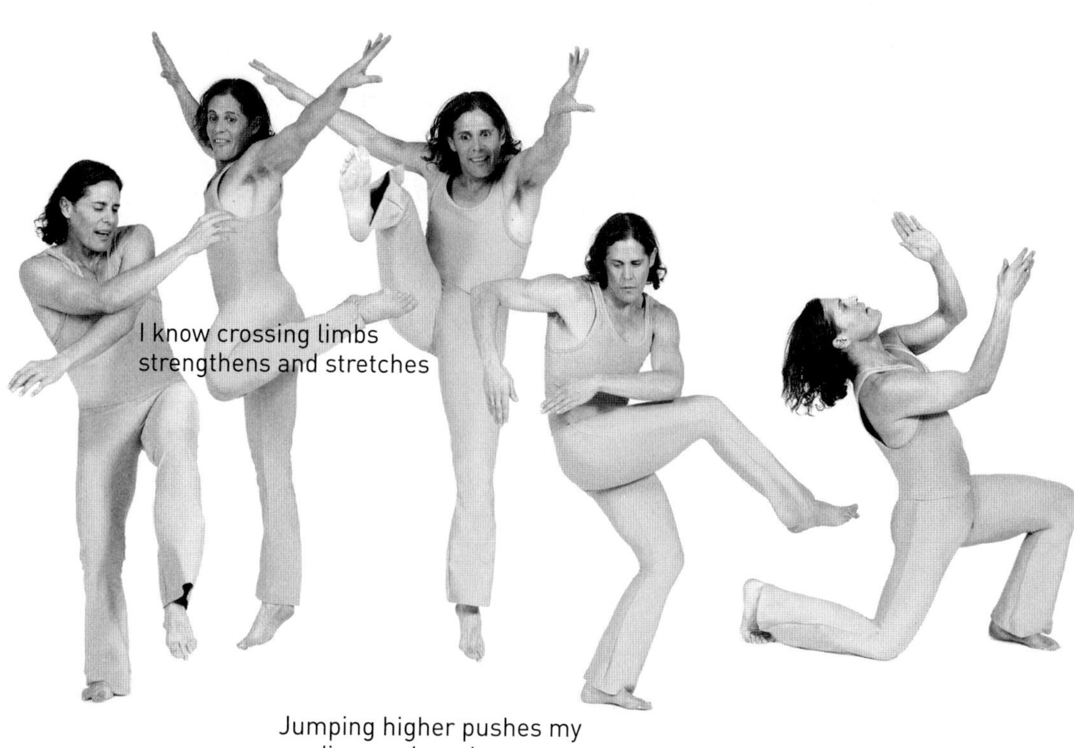

body check

Take a moment to perceive your exertion. Notice how you feel. Notice your breathing and your heart rate, and compare their activity with the intensity of the workout you have just experienced. You should feel energized, sweaty, and warm. You should be breathing fully, yet able to catch your breath, and speak. Now you are ready to cool down. If you feel you did too much, lighten the intensity next time you work out. If you feel you need more, load the intensity.

COOL DOWN

In Cycle 5 you take advantage of the heat and pliability generated from the previous movements, which will allow you to stretch more easily and open up your joints more fully. In this cycle, you begin to slow down, recenter, balance, and harmonize your body, mind, emotions, and spirit. Listen to the voices of your body. They will guide your physical actions, including the need to stretch specific areas of your body. Pay attention to breath and energy flow as you address any particular muscle or joint. Your heart rate should gradually lower, and you should sense your body getting ready for the next cycle. Depending on your body, you may need to take more time to cool down before you begin FloorPlay.

RELEVÉ HULA HOOP

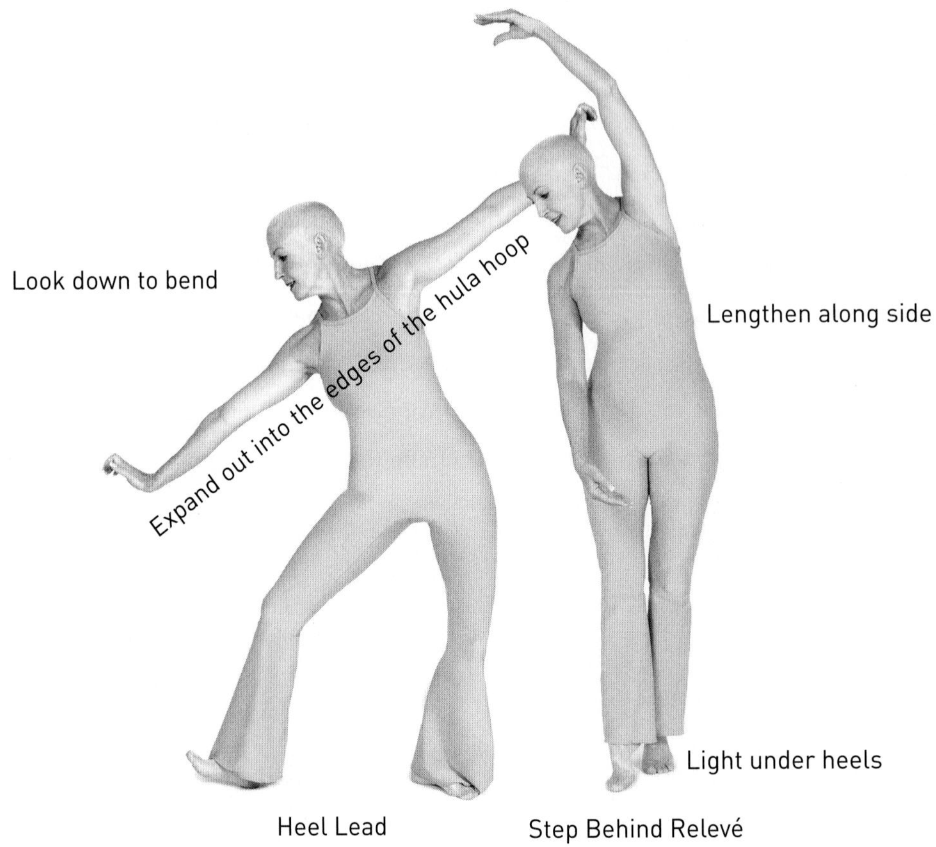

Starting in Riding (Sumo) Stance, hold on to the edges of an imaginary hula hoop. Lead with your left heel, sinking and rising up into Cross Behind Relevé, slowly bending to the left, opening and stretching the sides of your body. Smoothly move to the other side leading with your right heel. Breathe fully and deeply to slow down and decrease your respiration and heart rate. Sense your body calming down, regaining natural, steady breathing. Alternate sides.

Repeat 16 times—counting each Relevé, left and right, as 1 repetition—or until your body says, "My sides feel stretched out, my heart is calmer, and my breathing is slowing down."

IMAGINE YOURSELF HOLDING A HULA HOOP.

BENEFITS: Calms the heart and harmonizes body and breathing. Improves spine, arm, shoulder, and waist flexibility.

CLASSIC: Listen to the voices of your body and move in ways that address your body's need to slow down, calm down, stretch out, and lengthen.

ATHLETIC: Sink deeper and rise higher to achieve more flexibility in your muscles and joints.

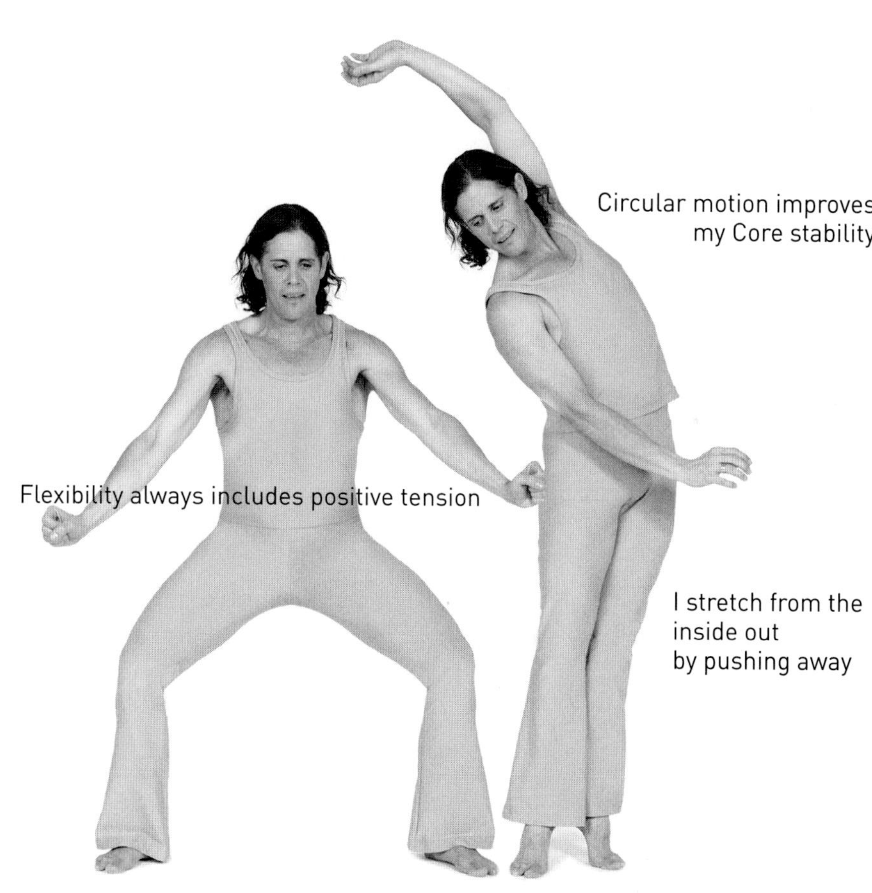

BODY PULSE

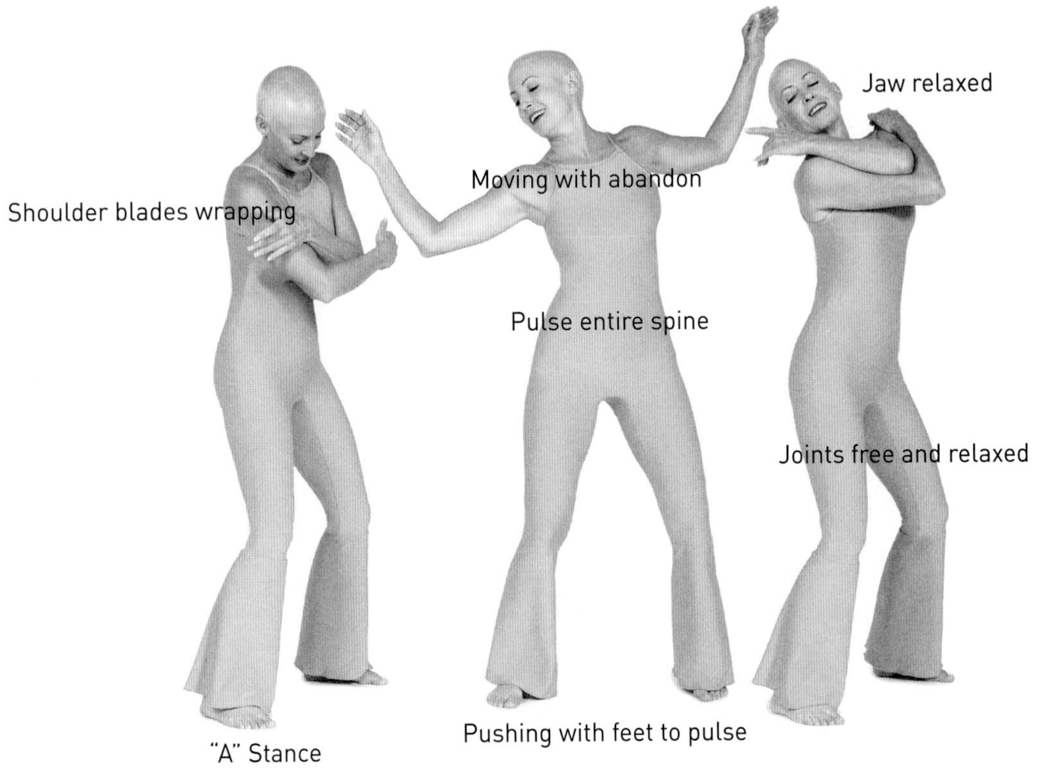

Standing in "A" Stance, rhythmically move your three body weights (pelvis, chest, and head) to create a whole-body pulse. Push with your feet as you cross and uncross your arms and sense energy moving through your entire Core, from your tailbone to the crown of your head. Let go of the muscular tension and free your bones, with loose abandon, like that of a rag doll. Exhale as you cross your arms and inhale as you open your arms.

Repeat 32 times—counting each cross and uncross as 1 repetition—or until your body says, "I feel harmony in my body, mind, emotions, and spirit; I'm more relaxed."

IMAGINE YOUR BONES AND MUSCLES FALLING INTO A DEEP STATE OF RELAXATION.

> BENEFITS: Lowers the heart rate and respiration, integrates upper and lower body, recenters you, and gives you time to listen to the voices of your body, so that you can make movement choices that will help you cool down and be prepared to move to the floor.

CLASSIC: Practice moving your three body weights and integrating your whole body to unify your body and breath. Move and seek deeper levels of relaxation.

ATHLETIC: Move more fully, freely, and with abandon to relax.

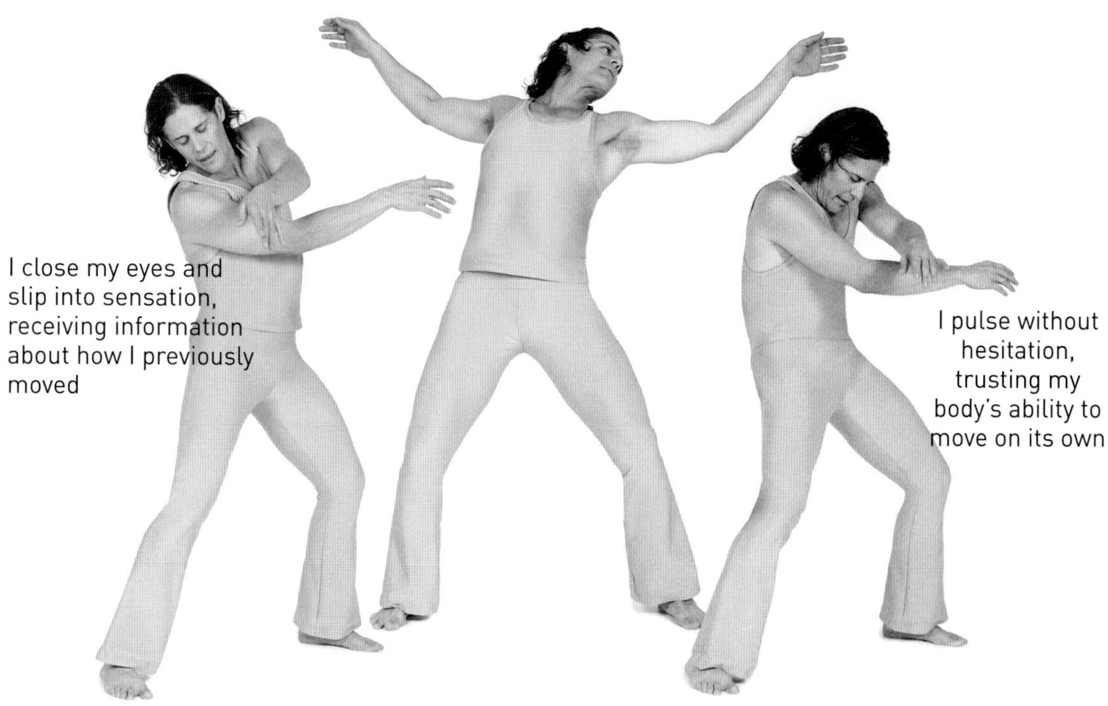

FLOAT UP RELAX DOWN

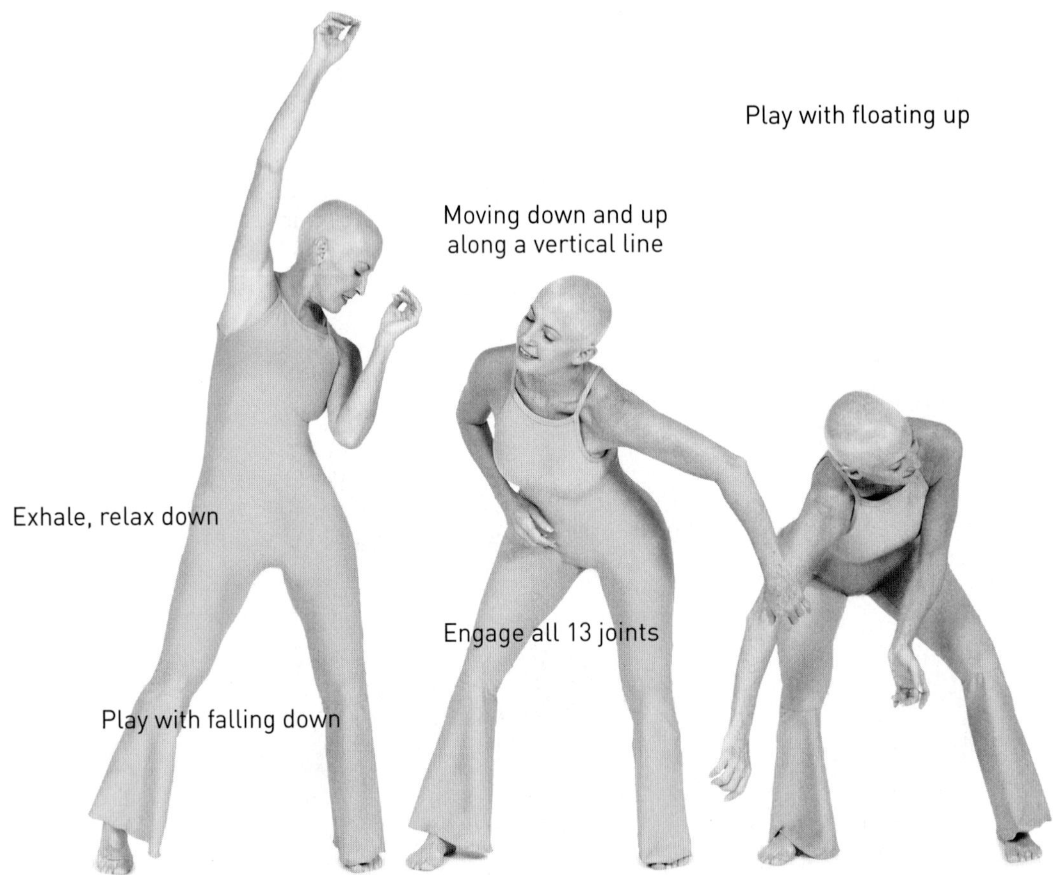

Standing in "A" Stance, inhale, floating up, and elongating and sensing your spine lengthen and your body open. Exhale, and release all of the thirteen joints, as you sink and slowly fall to the earth. Let go, and sense whole-body relaxation.

Repeat 8 times—counting each floating up and drifting down as 1 repetition—or until your body says, "I'm ready to move into FloorPlay."

IMAGINE YOU'RE A LEAF SLOWLY FALLING TO EARTH AND FLOATING BACK UP.

BENEFITS: Improves leg and back flexibility, mobility, and enhances spine agility. Promotes whole-body relaxation.

CLASSIC: Practice smooth transitions between the actions of floating up and drifting down in preparation for moving on the floor.

ATHLETIC: Look up and reach higher, shift weight, sink deeper. Round and hang your body into sensations of greater strength and flexibility.

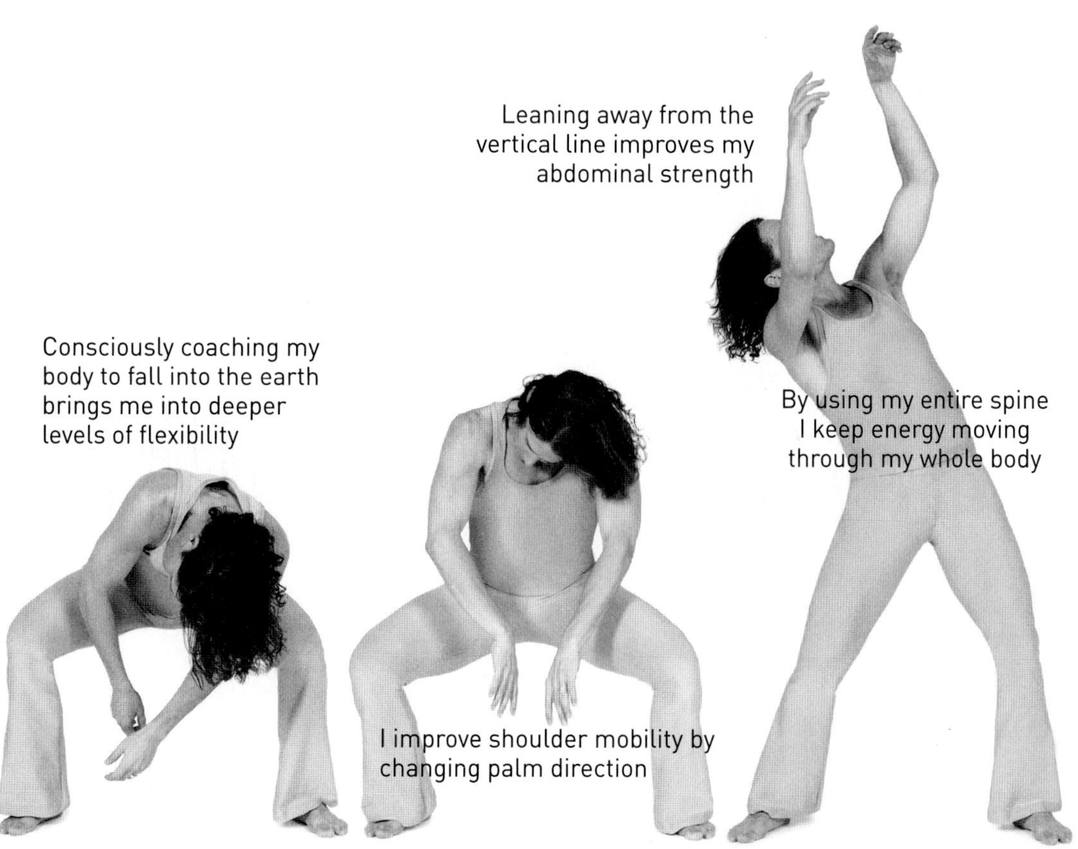

I use my Base to flood my upper body with energy

cycle 6 FLOORPLAY

In Cycle 6 you use the floor to stimulate your body. Using gravity, space, time, and sound, you use the art of play and the art of moving on the floor to become strong, stretched, defined, balanced, and fit. While the moves are described mechanically, the science behind FloorPlay relies on the internal wisdom of your body to seek places of comfort.

Throughout this cycle, you'll use the floor as a space to surrender into, move onto, and push away from. You'll use time and space to explore your own personal levels of strength, flexibility, mobility, agility, and stability. You'll play with gravity, falling into it and resisting it. You'll use your body parts as free weights, lightening and loading the muscle demand. You'll play with the dynamics of push and pull, open and close, in and out, up and down, under and through. In the end, it is the balance between stillness and movement that gives FloorPlay its power and offers you results, without the usual strain and boredom associated with conventional floor work.

These FloorPlay motions are designed to help work and relax your muscles from the inside out. To protect your bones and joints always practice FloorPlay on carpet or a mat. For additional knee protection use knee pads; they help you relax even more to get the most out of each stretch.

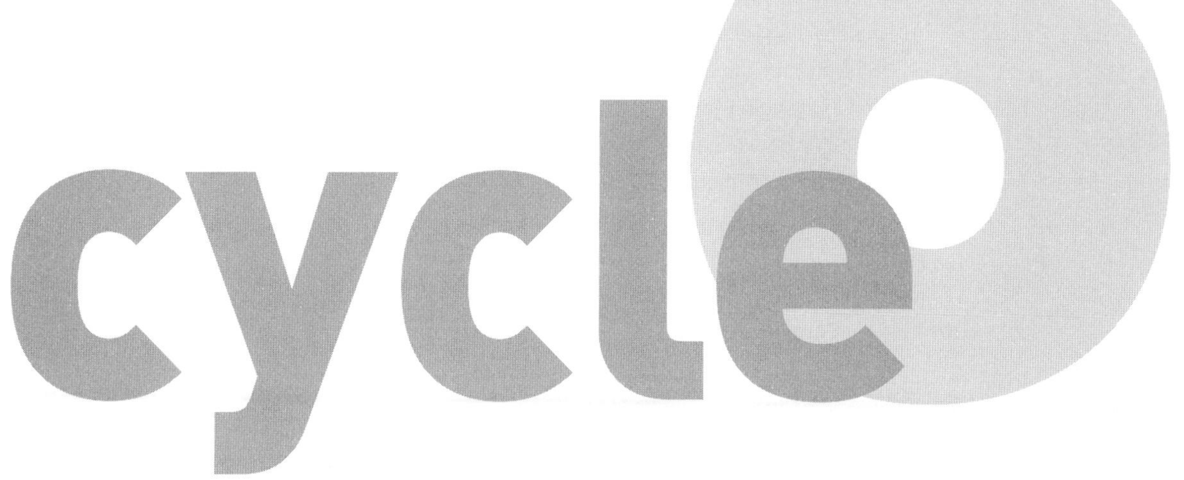

ROCKING ABS

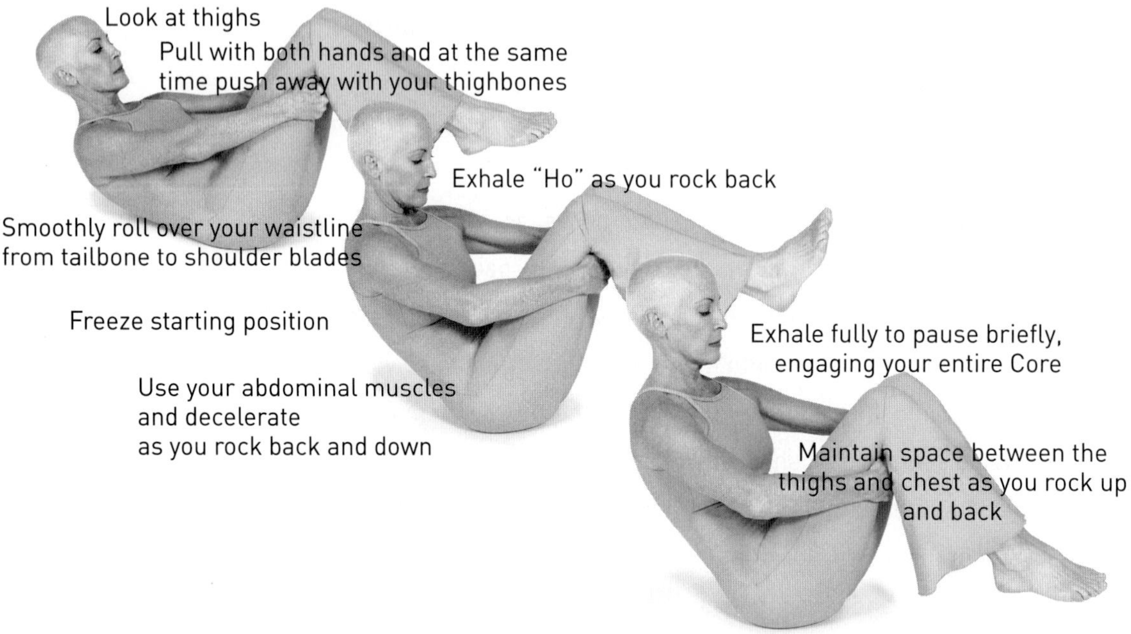

Look at thighs

Pull with both hands and at the same time push away with your thighbones

Exhale "Ho" as you rock back

Smoothly roll over your waistline from tailbone to shoulder blades

Freeze starting position

Use your abdominal muscles and decelerate as you rock back and down

Exhale fully to pause briefly, engaging your entire Core

Maintain space between the thighs and chest as you rock up and back

Starting by lying on your back; round up and grab the back of your thighs. With your knees bent, create a pull–push action between your hands and thighs and freeze into this Starting Position. Keep your thighs vertical by pulling with your hands and pushing with your thighs. Next, begin rocking back and forth in a very small range of motion, massaging your waistline while keeping your abdominal muscles engaged and your chin down. Exhale and sound *ho,* each time you rock back, keeping your eyes focused on your thighs. Eventually, increase the motion to rock from the tailbone to the shoulder blades. Never rock onto the neck! Keep your lower jaw relaxed.

Repeat 16 times—counting each rock back as 1 repetition—or until your body says, "My Core is stronger, and I'm ready for the next move."

IMAGINE YOUR WAIST AS A ROLLING PIN.

BENEFITS: Improves abdominal strength and spine flexibility.

CLASSIC: Practice pulling with your hands and pushing with your thighs as you rock in small and larger ranges of motion using your abdominal muscles, not leg action.

ATHLETIC: Rock up and down more fully and faster though never onto your neck.

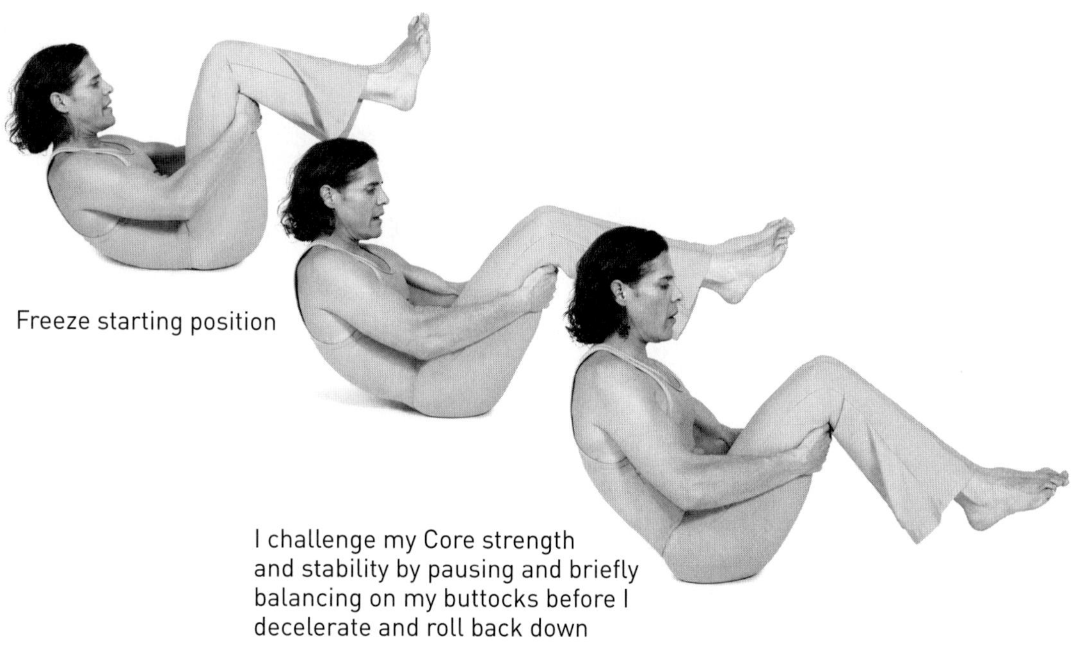

ARM AND LEG SHAKES

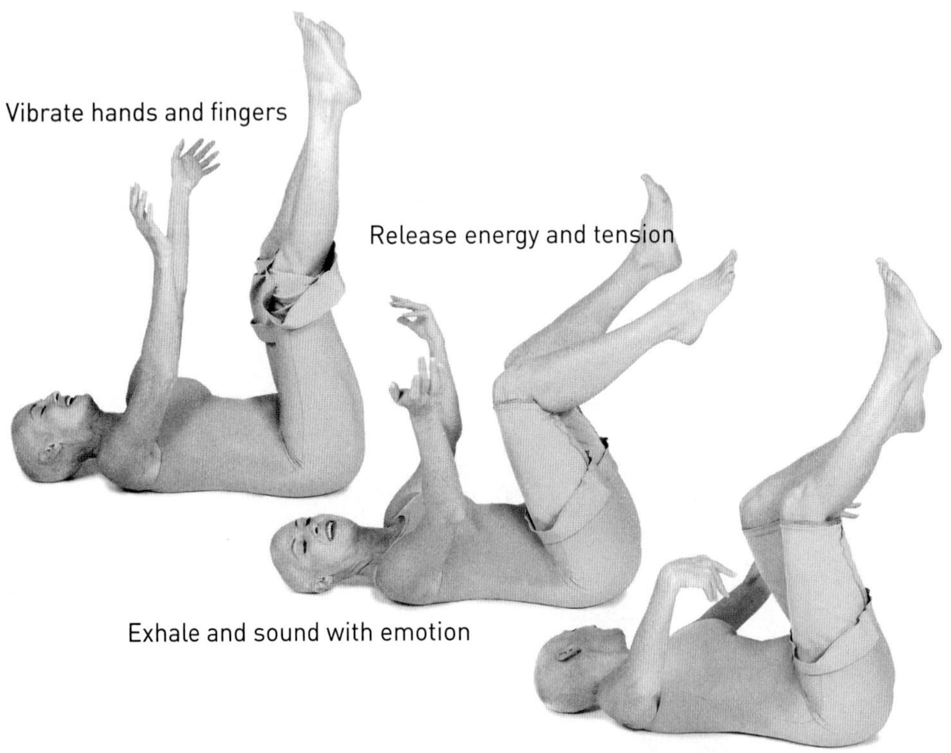

Starting on your back, keep your three body weights on the floor and vigorously shake your hands, arms, feet, and legs in the air. Say one vowel—*a, e, i, o, u*—at a time, shaking and vocalizing until you run out of air. Rest in between each vowel, then repeat shaking.

Continue, shaking and vocalizing, until your body says, "I am free of tension."

PLAY WITH SHAKING WATER OFF YOUR BONES AND JOINTS.

BENEFITS: Improves abdominal and Core strength and flexibility of the feet, legs, hands, and arms. Increases agility and releases tension.

CLASSIC: Use sound to naturally engage the Core and support your shaking limbs. Shake dynamically, infusing your movement with relaxation.

ATHLETIC: Reach higher, lift your head off the floor, and shake more vigorously.

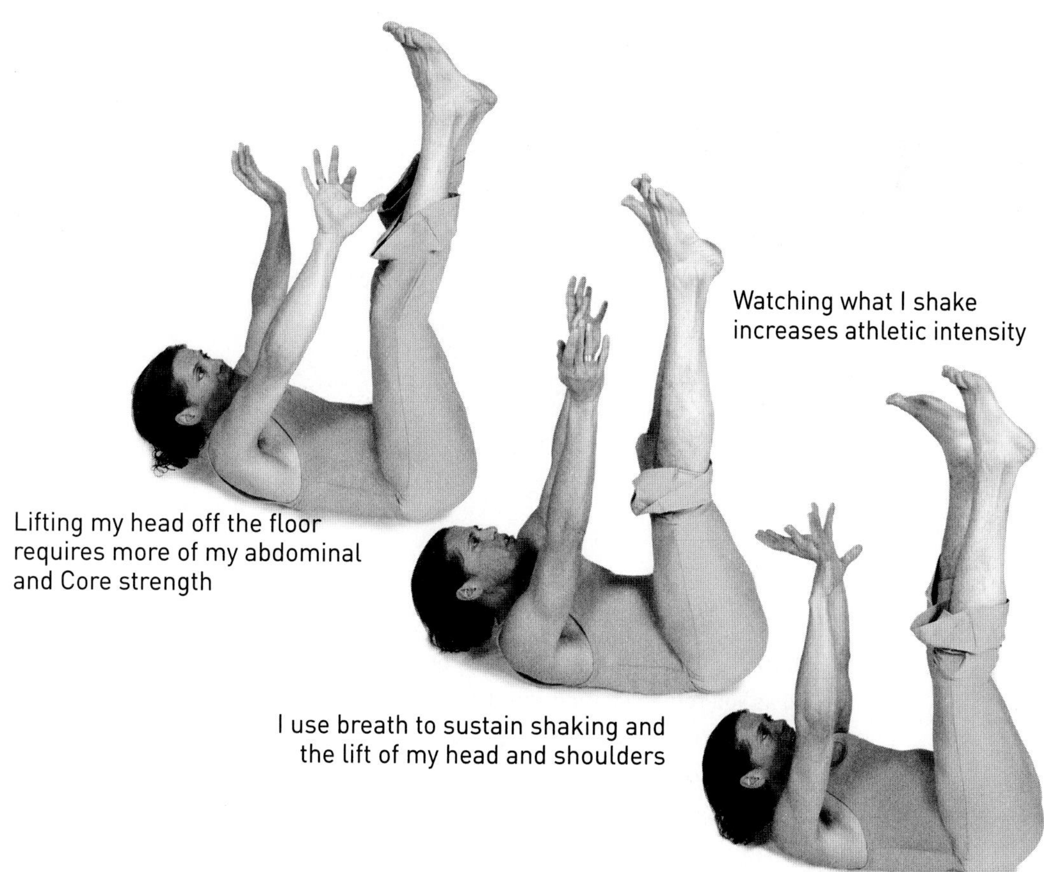

TOOTSIE ROLL

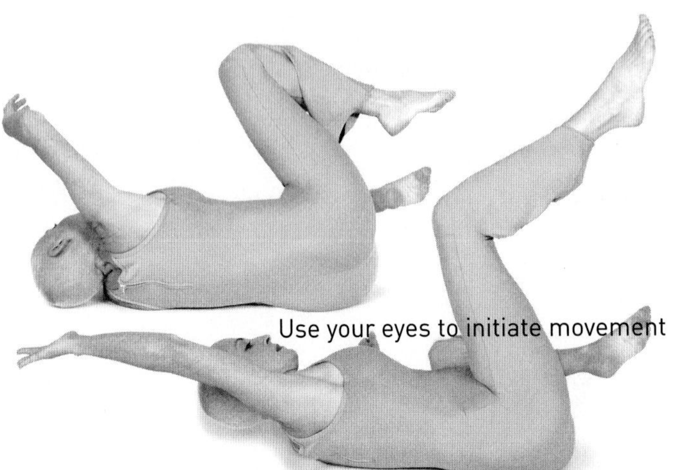

Use your eyes to initiate movement

Open and close your arms and legs like pages of a book as you roll from side to side

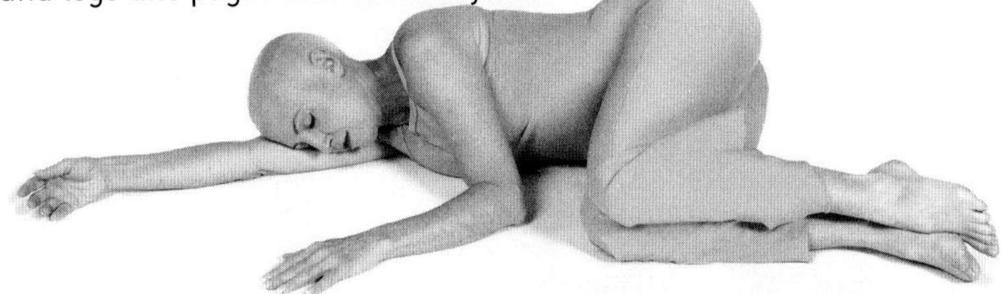

Rest fully into the earth until you are ready to roll again

Starting on your left side, roll freely onto your back and onto your right side, exhaling as you roll and letting your bones and muscles fall into relaxation. Stay loose, and as you roll from side to side, say *oh.* Rest into each side fully and play with the rolling motion. Sense ease and fluidity, and play with your arms and legs as you roll from side to side.

Repeat 16 times—counting each roll from left to right as 1 repetition—or until your body says, "I am so relaxed and loose."

IMAGINE YOU ARE A TOOTSIE ROLL, ROLLING IN SPACE.

> BENEFITS: Improves abdominal strength and provides a kidney and back massage. Stimulates the entire spine.

CLASSIC: Practice moving and relaxing.

ATHLETIC: Use more of your whole body and extend your range of motion.

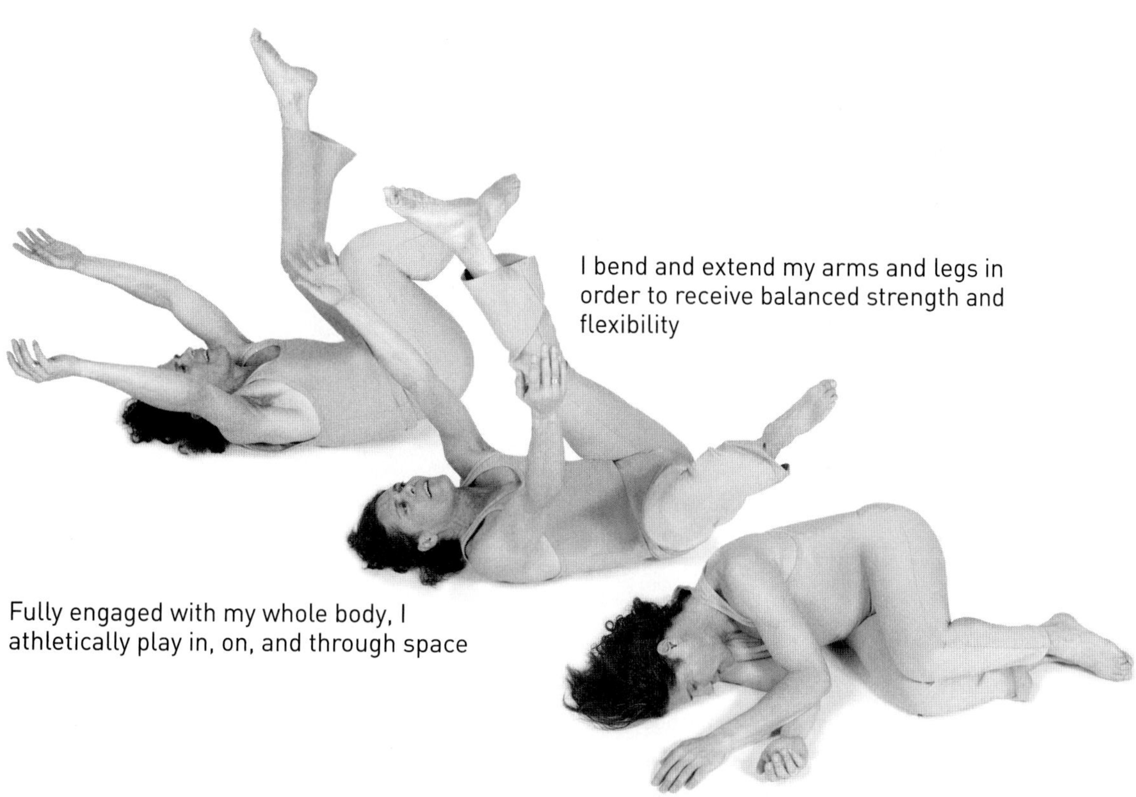

I bend and extend my arms and legs in order to receive balanced strength and flexibility

Fully engaged with my whole body, I athletically play in, on, and through space

I give in to gravity and move away from it to generate strength and flexibility

TWIST AND REST

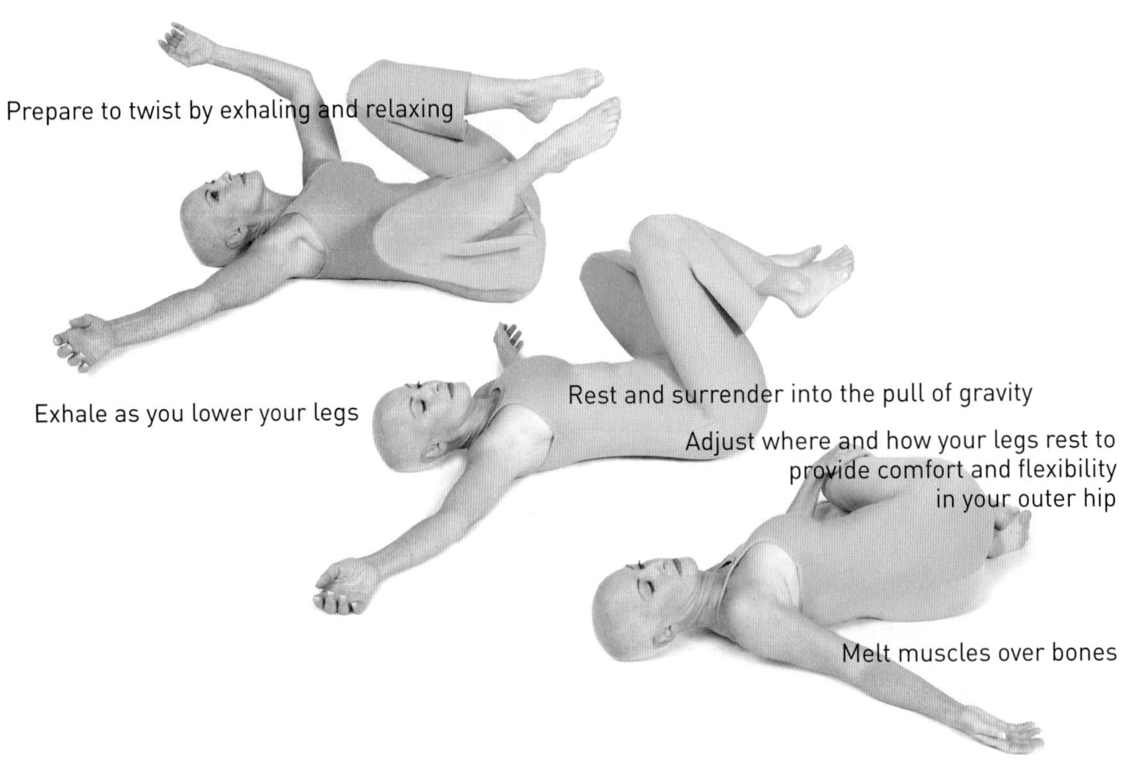

Starting on your back, draw both knees into your chest. Let both knees naturally fall across your body to one side, keeping your shoulders on the floor to achieve a relaxing twist and stretch along your spine and outer hip. Pause, and sound *ah* and rest until your body says, "I want to stretch the other side." Then inhale and exhale slowly as you twist to the other side. Alternate sides.

Repeat 4 times—counting each left and right twist as 1 repetition—or until your body says, "I am deeply relaxed, my hips and low back feel open, and I feel peaceful inside and out."

IMAGINE YOU'RE A PIECE OF TAFFY.

BENEFITS: Encourages deep relaxation, and improves spine and outer hip flexibility.

CLASSIC: On days when your outer hips feel tight, place a pillow between your knees, creating support for your muscles to let go.

ATHLETIC: Practice using the sensation of relaxation to reenergize your body, mind, emotions, and spirit. Breathe deeply and fully, to nourish your cells and harmonize your body and mind.

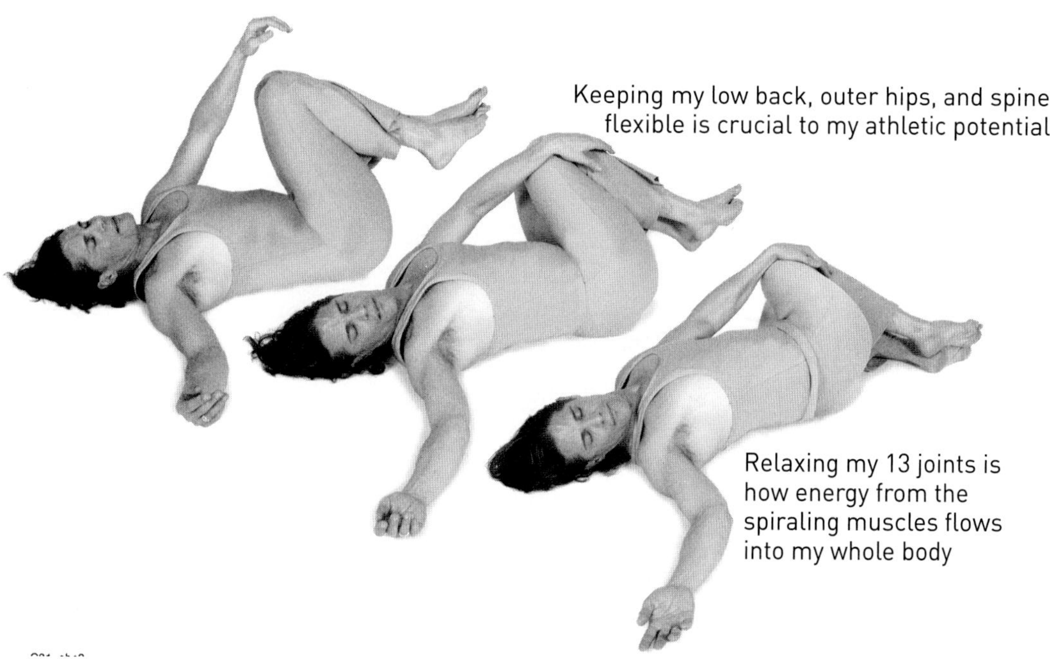

PSOAS YAWN

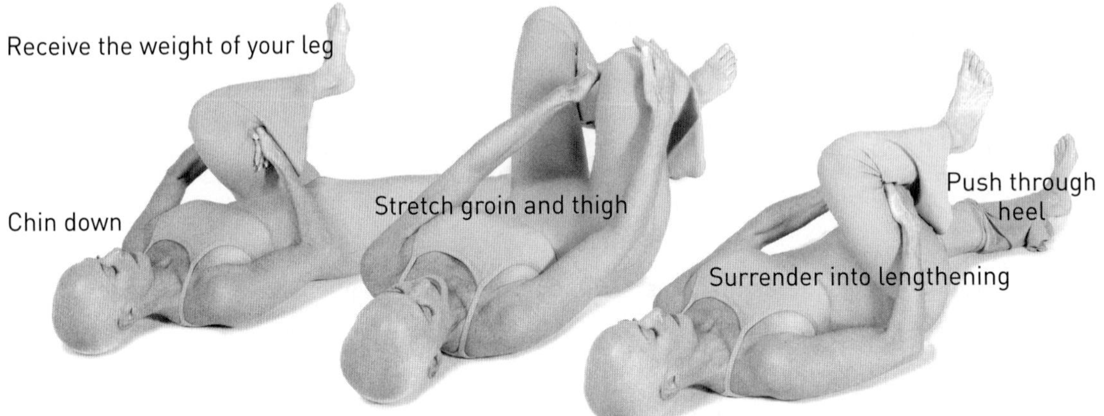

Lying on your back, both legs extended, bring your left thigh in close to your chest. Hug your left thigh as you extend your right leg through your right heel. Sense lengthening along the right side of your body and hum as you exhale. Keep the entire back of your body and the extended leg on the floor, and your chin down to help lengthen the back of your neck. Alternate sides.

Repeat 4 times—counting each left and right hug as 1 repetition—or until your body says, "I feel like I'm ironing out any kinks that may be hanging around."

IMAGINE YOU'RE TEN TIMES TALLER THAN YOU ARE.

BENEFITS: Lengthens the spine in a restorative fashion, stretches and relaxes the psoas and leg muscles, and integrates the upper body with the lower body, which allows you to move with greater power and grace.

CLASSIC: Practice lengthening and increasing the flexibility of your psoas muscle by pressing through the foot of your extended leg.

ATHLETIC: Hug your shin and fold your thighbone closer into your chest.

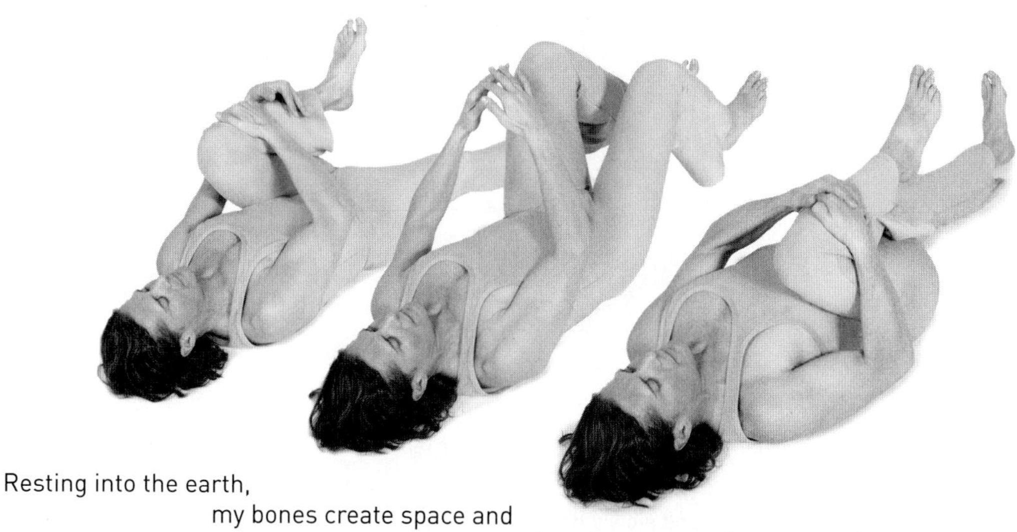

Resting into the earth,
my bones create space and
a place for my muscles to stretch

THIGH YAWN

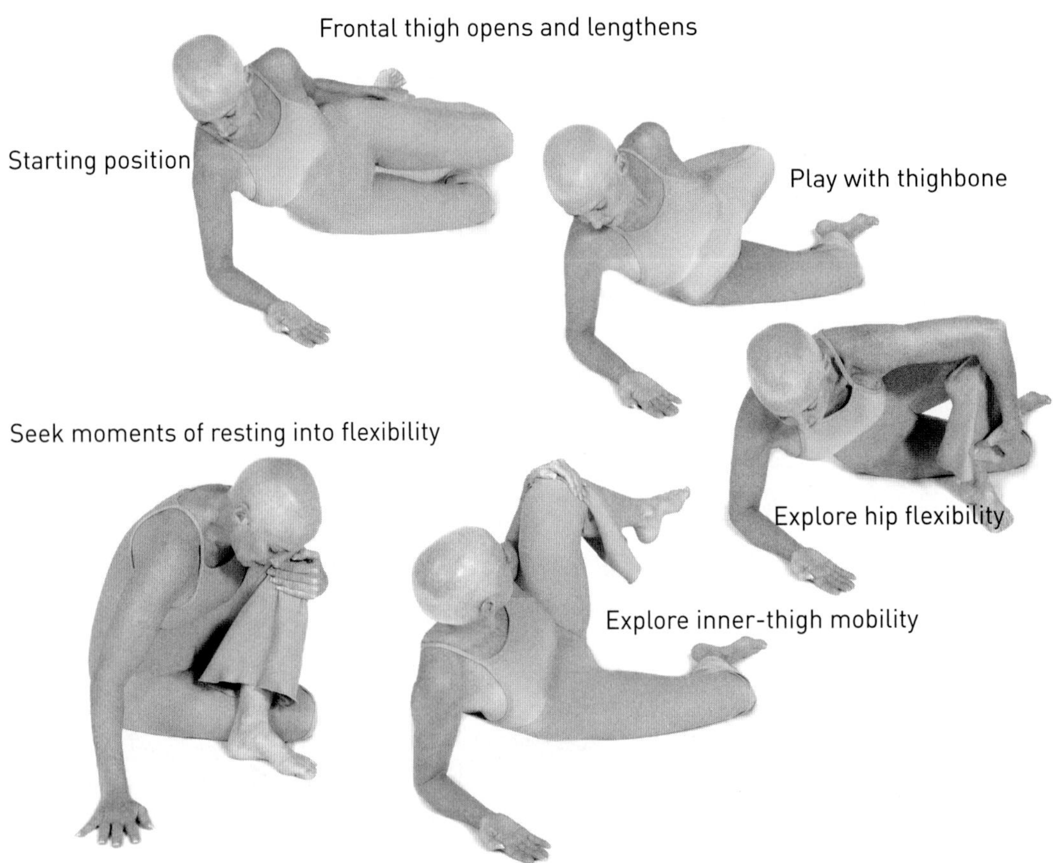

Starting on your left side, press your left elbow and forearm down with your palm up (place palm down if you need added stability). Hold your right ankle with your right hand and slowly draw your right thigh back toward your buttocks to a comfortable and pleasurable stretch, while sounding *ah.* Before you change to the other side, add mobility and flexibility by playing with your right leg. For example, bring your right foot to the front, lift your right thigh in the air, or extend your foot toward the ceiling. Play with changing shapes.

Repeat 4 times—counting each side as 1 repetition—or until your body says, "I love how I'm feeling."

IMAGINE YOU ARE A FLEXIBLE PRETZEL.

BENEFITS: Stretches and relaxes the frontal thigh, opens and relaxes the outer hip, and improves spinal agility and flexibility.

CLASSIC: Practice moving your thighs and changing shapes to achieve flexibility.

ATHLETIC: Energetically play in space with your whole body, rolling onto your belly and folding and unfolding your leg.

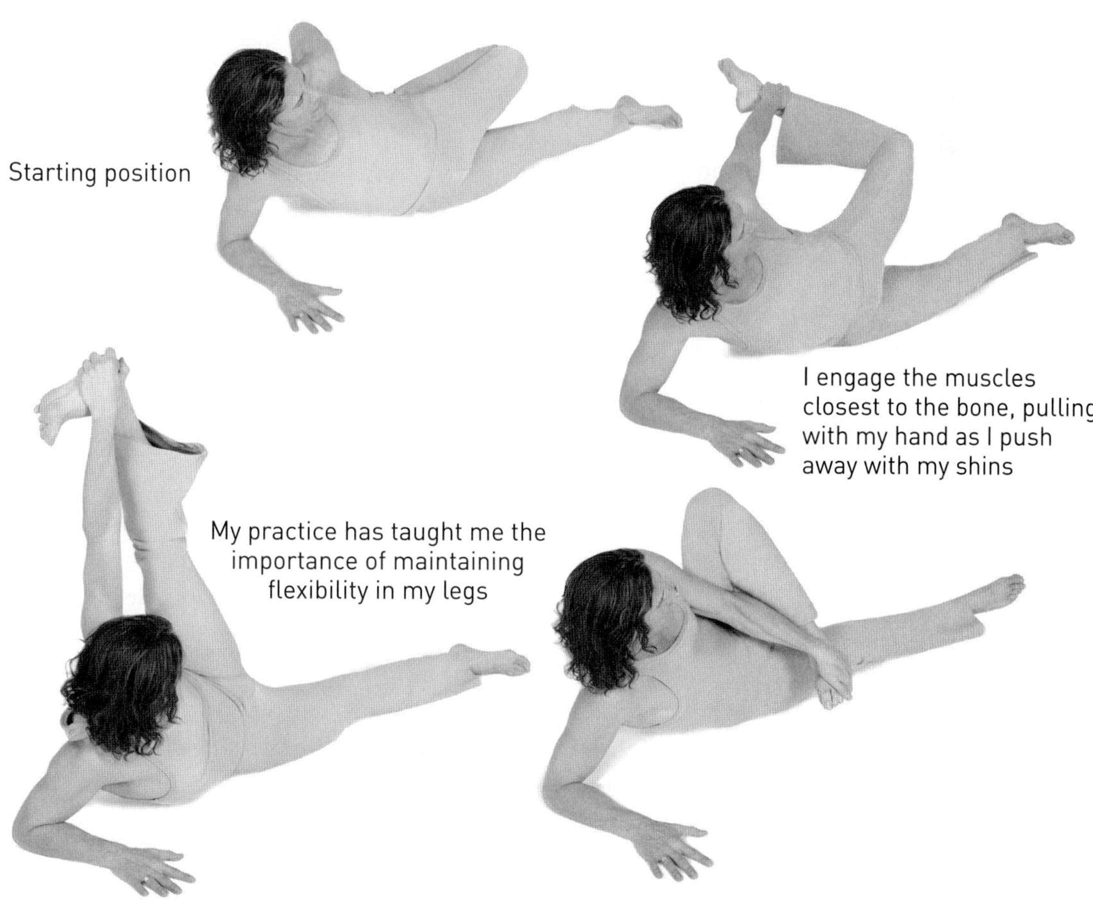

Starting position

I engage the muscles closest to the bone, pulling with my hand as I push away with my shins

My practice has taught me the importance of maintaining flexibility in my legs

SIDE YAWN

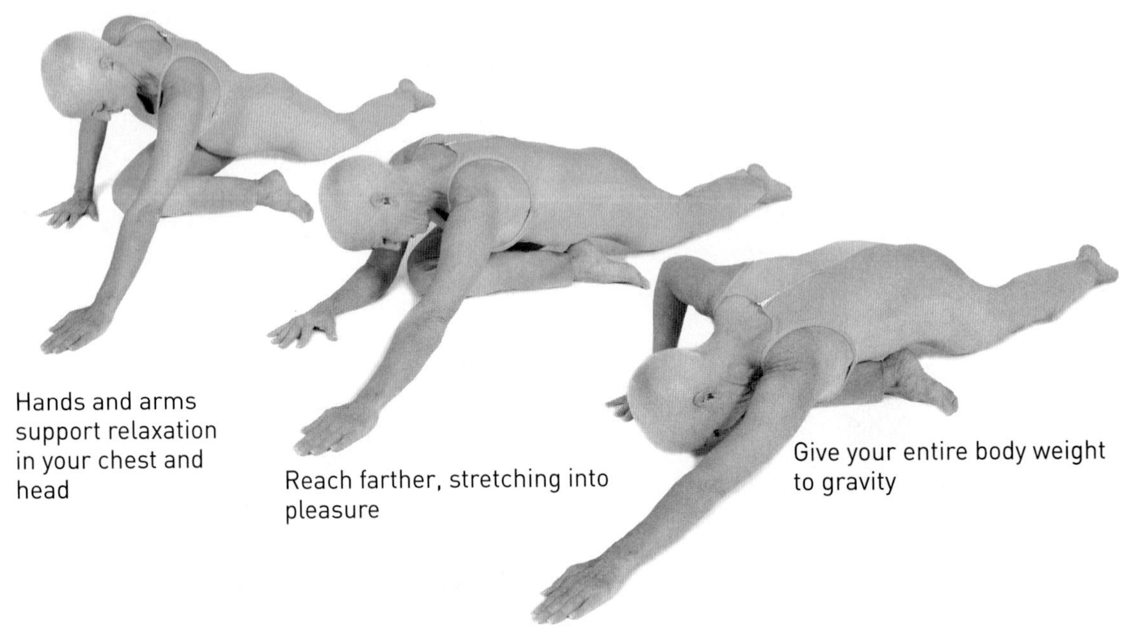

Hands and arms support relaxation in your chest and head

Reach farther, stretching into pleasure

Give your entire body weight to gravity

Sense the side of your body opening like a yawn

Kneeling over on all fours, slide your left leg back behind you, taking your whole body with you and lowering yourself as close to the floor as possible. Slowly roll over your bent knee and onto your outer right hip, using your hands and forearms for support. Wobble your hips back and forth, and sound *whoa,* sensing a comfortable spine and outer thigh stretch. Now, keeping your palm on the floor, extend the left arm beyond your head and stretch from fingers to toes. If need be, rest on your hands to lighten the body weight over your hip and knee joints. Draw both hands back under your chest and push away and back onto all fours. Alternate sides.

Repeat 4 times—counting each side as 1 repetition—or until your outer thigh says, "I feel open and relaxed, and I'm ready to move on."

IMAGINE MELTING INTO THE EARTH.

BENEFITS: Stretches your outer hip and thigh and helps lengthen your spine.

CLASSIC: Practice relaxing into gravity to gain flexibility. Micro-move to seek comfort in your hip joint, and wobble left and right to relax from the inside out.

ATHLETIC: Rest more body weight over your bent knee and add push-ups.

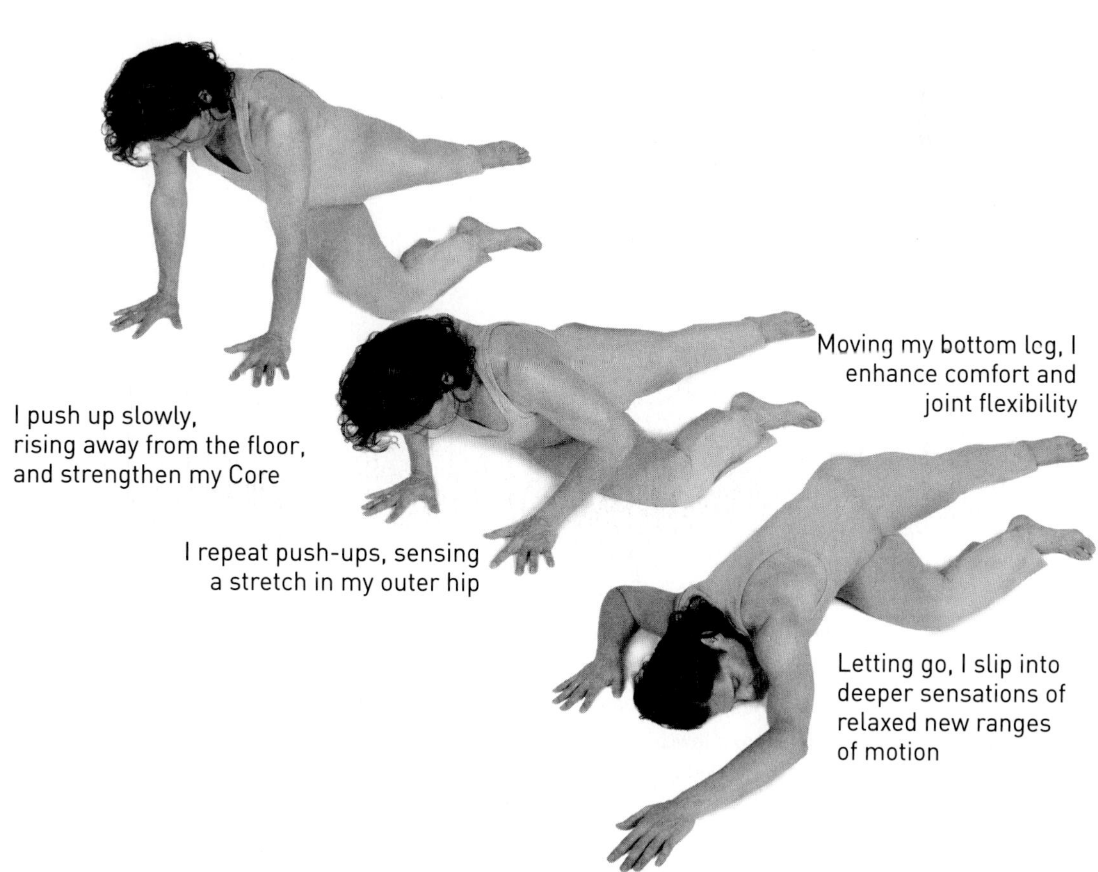

TAILOR YAWN

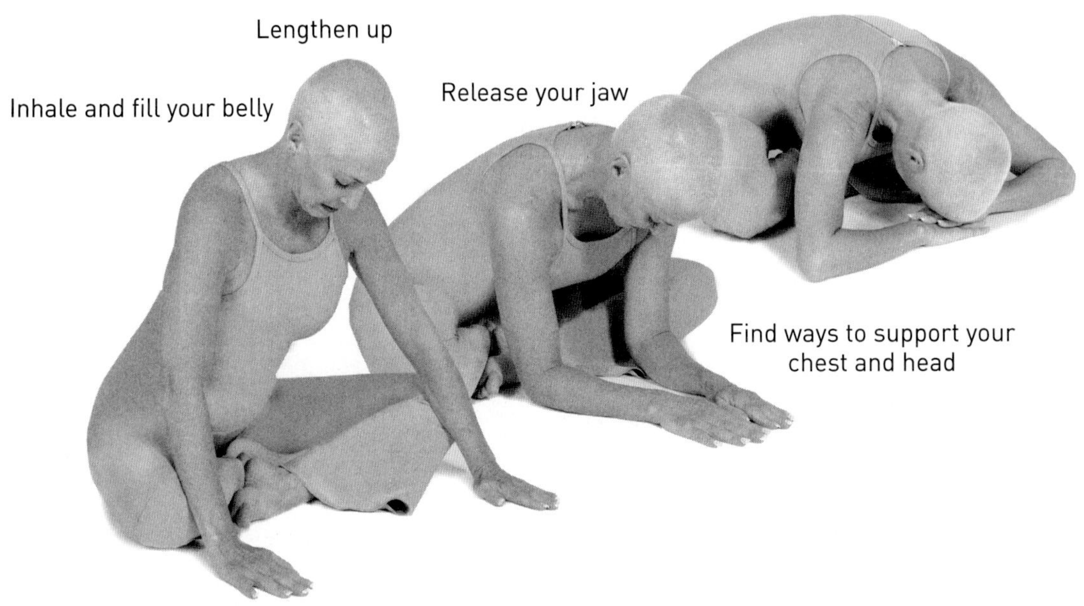

Starting in the tailor position, your legs comfortably crossed with your right leg in front, wobble your hips back and forth to find comfort. Inhale deeply and exhale the sound *ha* as you lengthen your spine and comfortably round your Core over your legs, resting into the earth using your hands and forearms for support. Sense flexibility in your low back, outer thighs, and spine. Inhale and lengthen through the crown of your head. Now cross with the left leg in front and repeat rounding over and resting.

Repeat 4 times—counting each leg in front as 1 repetition—or until your body says, "I feel relaxed and stretched out."

IMAGINE YOU ARE A CLAM, CLOSING ITS SHELL.

BENEFITS: Stretches the buttocks, outer hips, thighs, back, neck, and spine.

CLASSIC: Practice rounding and relaxing over your Base and become aware of the new sensation of integration of your body, mind, emotions, and spirit.

ATHLETIC: Play with movement detail, lengthen and round more.

With one last stretch, I push and pull my palms to get that extra inch of stretch that helps me lengthen intrinsically
As I exhale, I release all unnecessary tension
I pause to consciously appreciate my new levels of fitness

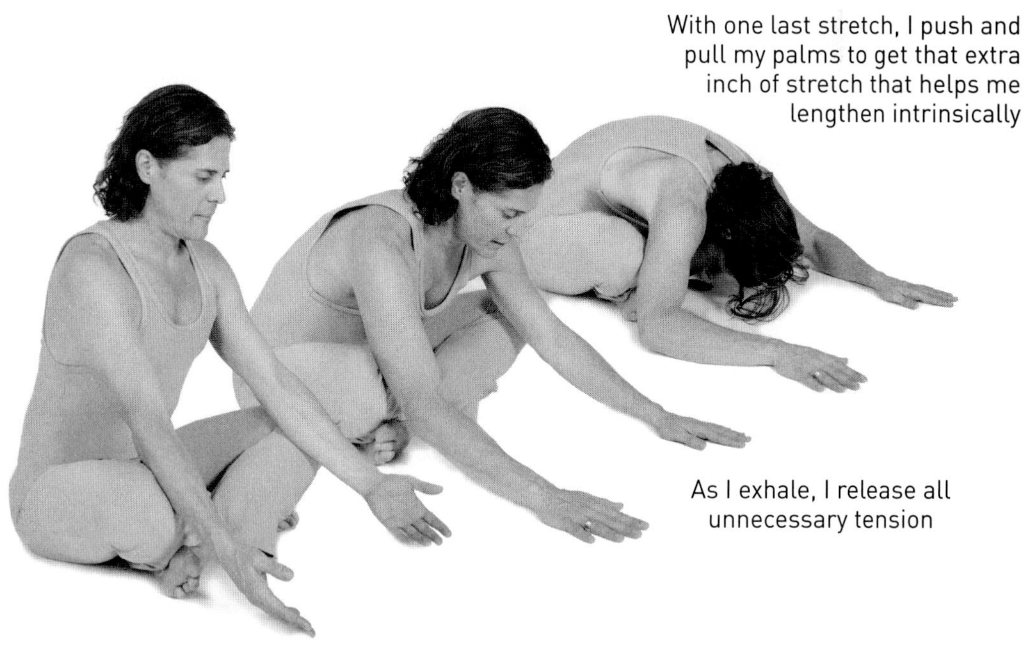

THIRTEEN JOINT RENEWAL

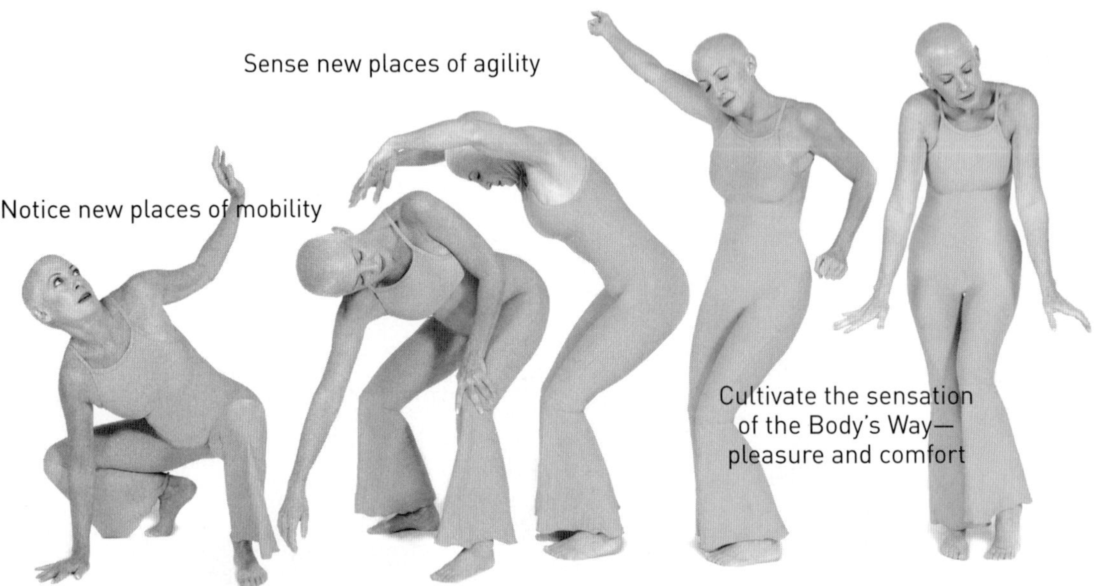

Starting from the ground up, playfully move all thirteen major joints and come into a standing position. In natural time, and in your own way, move and recognize the new levels of strength, flexibility, mobility, agility, and stability you have gained from the time and attention you have put into your workout.

Continue moving until your body says, "I feel aligned and connected."

IMAGINE ALL THIRTEEN JOINTS AWAKENING.

BENEFITS: Connects you to all of your thirteen main joints with a new awareness, greater sensitivity, and deeper appreciation of your healthier body, mind, emotions, and spirit.

CLASSIC: Regardless of what you perceive the intensity of your workout to have been, use this move to get to know your "now" body, the one you'll be Dancing Through Life with for the rest of your day!

ATHLETIC: Use this move to get to know how your joints and muscles have been affected by your athletic endeavor.

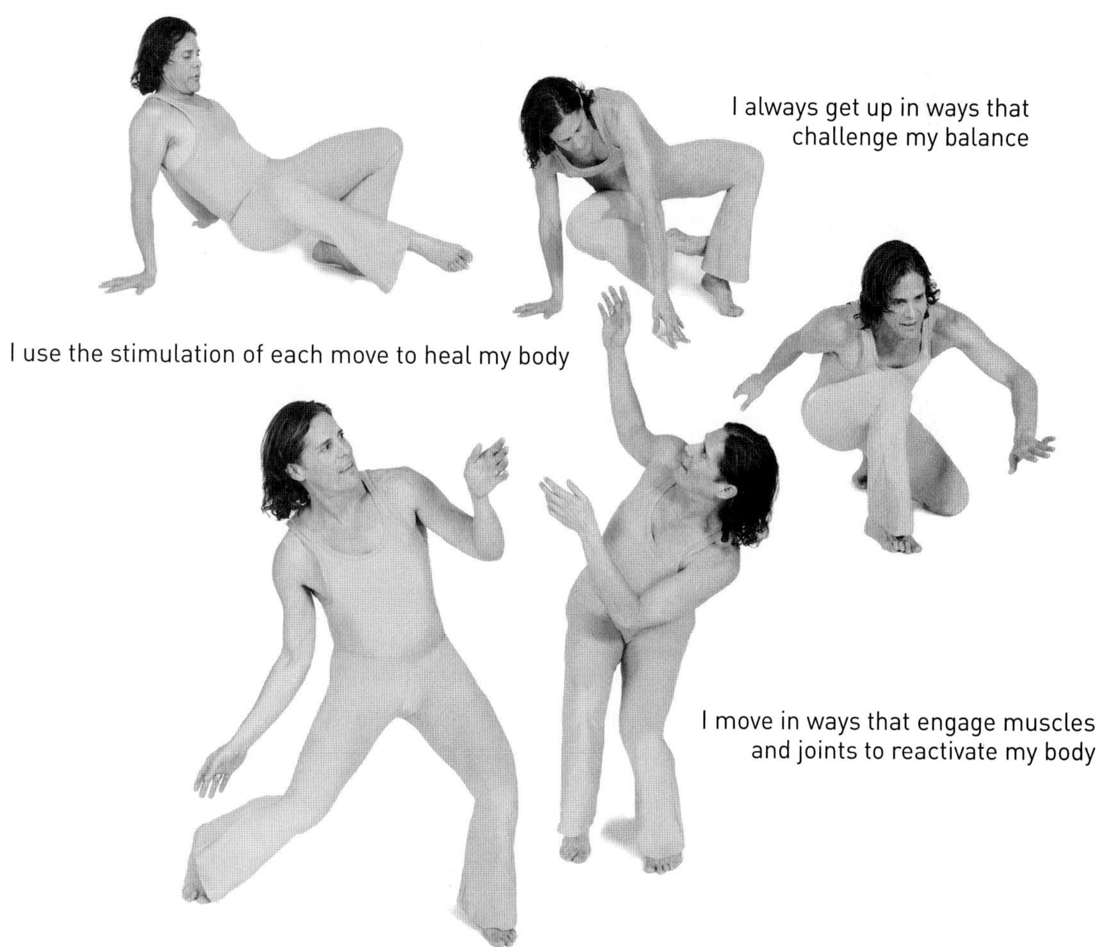

I always get up in ways that challenge my balance

I use the stimulation of each move to heal my body

I move in ways that engage muscles and joints to reactivate my body

LEG AIRBRUSHING

IMAGINE BRUSHING ENERGY ALONG YOUR LEG BONES.

BENEFITS: Tones arms and upper body, improves arm and leg circulation, increases lower body strength and hip joint agility, and invigorates the lungs.

CLASSIC: Practice using your hands to improve circulation.

ATHLETIC: Brush more briskly.

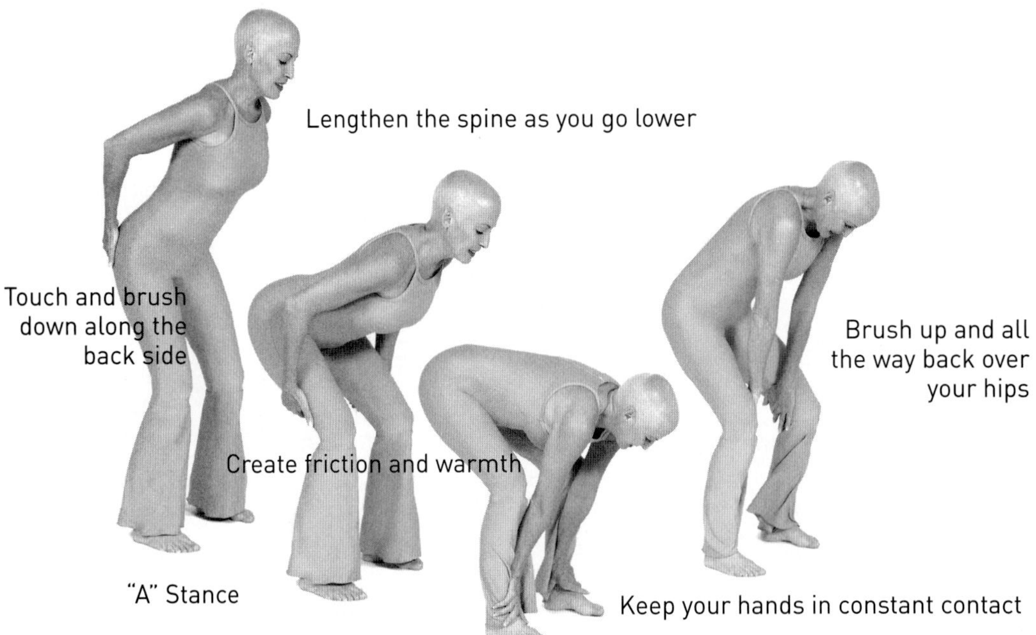

Starting in "A" Stance, with your hands at the top of your buttocks, with knees soft, use your hands to brush energy down the backsides of both legs, all the way down to your ankles as you sound *hey.* Now brush up the insides of both legs. Brush down and up quickly until you feel a warm heat generated in your leg muscles. Brush off any excess energy your muscles have accumulated during your workout, releasing any energy blocks.

Repeat 16 times brushing down and up, or until your legs say, "We feel energetically warm."

ARM AIRBRUSHING

IMAGINE BRUSHING ENERGY ALONG YOUR ARM BONES.

CLASSIC: Practice brushing all the way out and over your fingertips and rotate your palm before your brush up.

ATHLETIC: Brush more briskly, rotate your palms more.

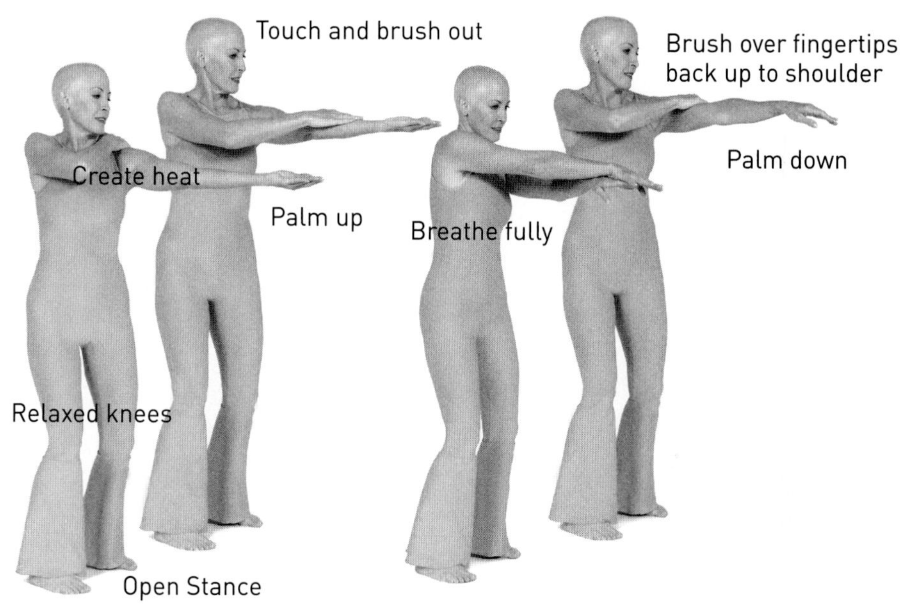

Starting in Open Stance, airbrush your arms. Extend one arm with the palm up, and use the other hand to swiftly brush from the shoulder all the way out to the ends of your fingertips as you sound *ho,* and then turn your palm over and softly brush back up toward your shoulder. Brush away any tension in your shoulder and arm and release any energy blocks. Alternate sides.

Repeat 16 times, each arm brushing out and in as one repetition or until your arm says, "I feel energetically warm and I'm ready to do the other side."

cycle 7 STEP OUT

In Cycle 7 you consciously recognize the self-healing and fitness benefits you have just received. In this cycle, you will establish your intent for the rest of your day and step out into your life with a sense of renewed health.

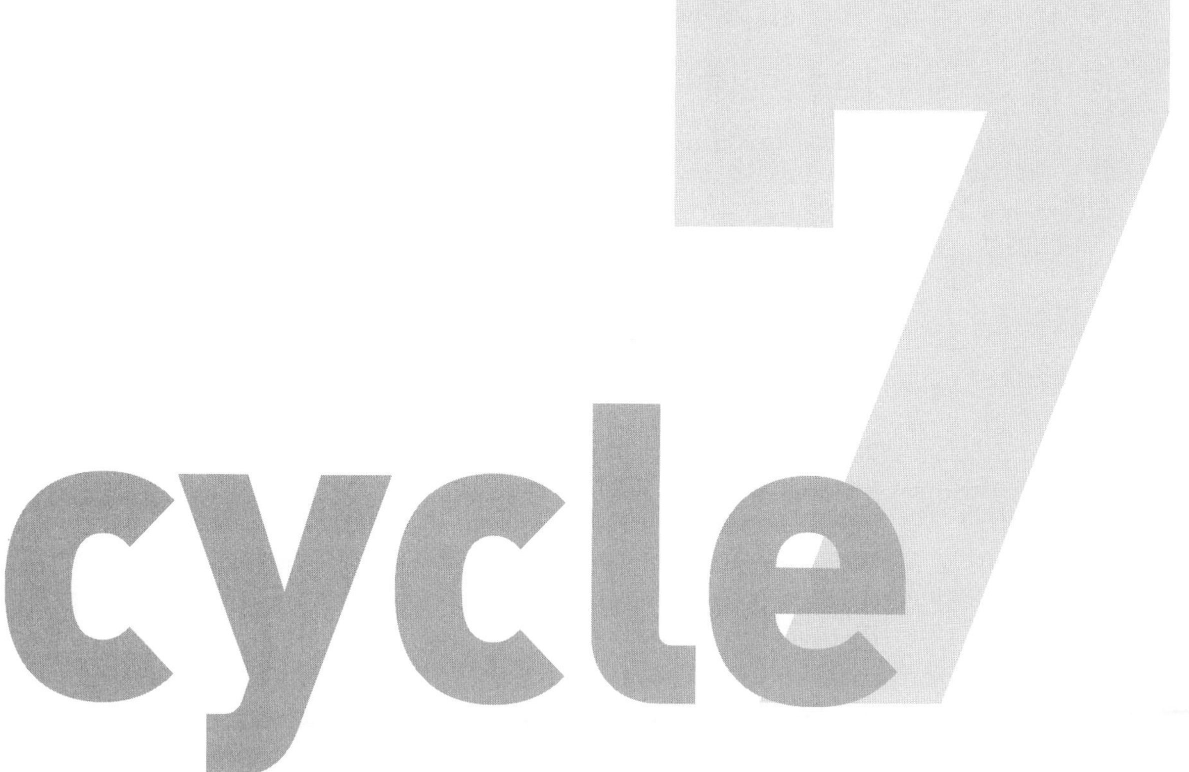

STEP OUT

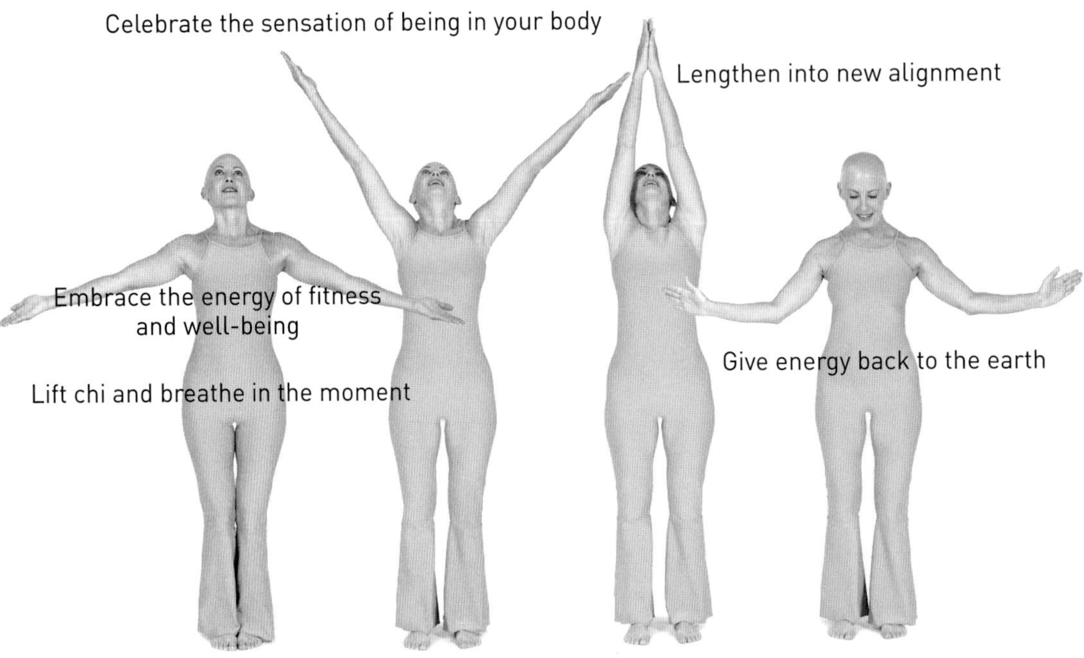

Starting in Closed Stance or Open Stance, inhale and with palms up, draw your arms up from the sides of your body ending above your head. Feel the sensation of renewed fitness and health. Now exhale and with palms down, lower your hands in preparation to rub your palms.

Briskly rub your palms together, building up a good heat and breathe in and out. Turn your palms up to feel the energy and heat you have created in your body during your workout or place your hands on your belly and heart and close your eyes to sense peace and harmony in your body, mind, emotions, and spirit. When your body says, "I'm ready to move on," open your eyes, and step out of your Nia experience and into the magic of your next moment.

IMAGINE PREPARING FOR A JOYOUS EVENT.

BENEFITS: Helps create mindful and conscious endings—and positive new beginnings.

CLASSIC: Practice connecting to the ending of your experience, because it is as important as the beginning. Enjoy the sensation of this end and the sensation of the new beginning.

ATHLETIC: Be fully present to the new you, the one who emerges from the end and into the new beginning.

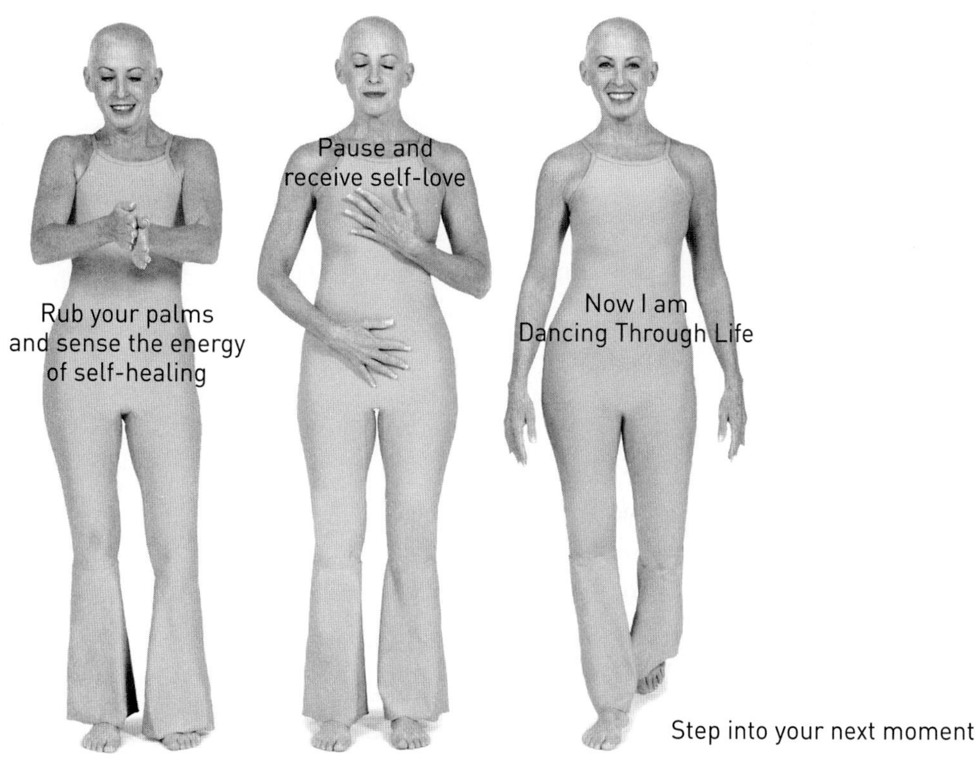

Sense your new body dynamically aligned, full of love, and awakened to deeper sensations of pleasure and joy

JOURNAL QUESTIONS FOR AFTER YOUR WORKOUT

As we mentioned earlier, there is nothing more powerful than writing about your experience. Oftentimes writing reveals details not noticed as you were moving. Use these questions to learn even more about you and your workout and use this information to improve the way you consciously train and guide your body.

1. How did I generally feel while doing my Nia workout today?
2. What new physical sensations did I discover, and in what part of my body did I discover them?
3. What new technique or movement skill did I develop?
4. How can I change what I do to feel even better after each workout?
5. How can I get more of what I want from moving my body the Nia way?
6. Where did I sense the most strength in my body today? The most flexibility? The most mobility? The most agility?
7. Where did I sense the most weakness in my body?
8. What gave me the most joy?
9. What movement form positively affected my nervous system, helping me to move with grace and ease?
10. What is my neck telling me about the way I used my jaw, eyes, and head?
11. What is my back telling me about the way I used my three body weights?
12. What are my knees telling about the way I used my Base?
13. What is my lower back telling me about the way I used my pelvis?
14. What are my shoulders telling me about the way I used my hands and arms?
15. What is my energy telling me about the way I listened to my body today?
16. What moves can I practice to get the most out of my next workout?
17. What focus will make my movements more dynamic and efficient?
18. What was the most important discovery for me today?
19. What can I consciously do in my real life that will positively add to my physical, mental, emotional, and spiritual well-being?
20. What can I physically do to Dance Through Life today?

A **Nia** *Story*

TAKING CHARGE OF YOUR DREAMS

STUDENT: Nancy

CLASS LOCATION: Milford, Connecticut

OCCUPATION: Owner, Sound Mind and Body, LLC

When Nancy was first introduced to Nia, she already had an extensive background in dance. While she was young, she had studied ballet, tap, jazz dance, modern dance, Duncan dance, and folk dancing. She had also had extensive aerobics and gymnastics training, and had studied karate, yoga, and t'ai chi.

Unfortunately, while participating in these activities, she had suffered an injury—herniation of a spinal disc. This caused significant chronic pain, and made further participation in conventional aerobics quite difficult. She also developed chronic, debilitating headaches.

Nia, however, proved to be exactly the kind of exercise her body needed. It allowed her to be extremely active without any significant risk of pain or injury. Nia did much more, though, than just help Nancy physically. It also reignited her spirit.

"From the time I was five years old," Nancy relates, "my big dream in life was to dance, or to teach dance and own my own studio. But like many other people, I put my dream on hold, because I didn't think it was practical. I did dance professionally for a short time when I was just out of high school, but I gave it up. I did all the things I was supposed to do: I went to school, got married, put my husband through school, and raised a child. I listened to everyone but myself.

"I tried very hard to live up to the ideal of success. But my heart was never in it! I hated the corporate ladder. I was even fired from three jobs because I didn't 'fit the mold.' My marriage ended in divorce. And to top it off, I learned afterward that my ex-husband, the most vocal of my naysayers, had become a dance critic! I was angry, unfulfilled, and trapped in an empty life. I blamed everyone else for the choices I had made.

"I decided to move to Connecticut, and I when I arrived I joined the Southport Racquet Club. Southport had an excellent aerobics program; they offered traditional aerobics plus traditional dance classes. Then they invited Debbie and Carlos to visit, and Nia classes were instituted at the club.

"The first thing I noticed was that everyone in class began learning everyone else's name. It's amazing how you can go to conventional fitness classes for years with the same people and never speak to anyone. Nia brought such a wonderful noncompetitive energy to the group. It made us feel connected. It really stirred the energy. It was such a breath of fresh air after a day at the office!

"My back began to get better, and the chronic headaches from which I'd been suffering began to dissipate. I gathered strength—emotionally, physically, and spiritually. My friendships flourished, and my negative attitude turned positive. I got over the anger of the past and took responsibility for my life.

"Good things began to happen. I took up acting and became active in community theater. I even got a few professional roles. A few women from my Nia class formed a circle, and we began to celebrate holidays as I grew spiritually. I began to heal my relationship with my family, and settled into a supportive romantic relationship.

"The Nia connection is one of the best things that's ever happened to me. It has changed my life completely. It taught me to take charge of my dreams."

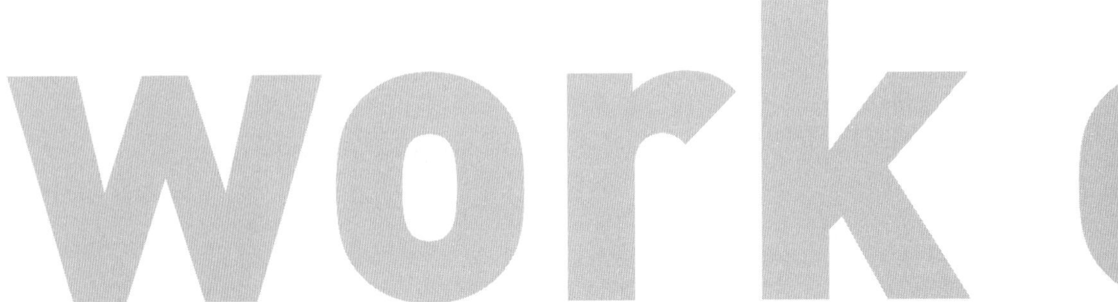

THE NIA WORKOUT MENU

As discussed at the beginning of the chapter, you should begin every Nia workout by choosing a focus from the Nia Workout Menu. This menu contains information that will help you grow and change over time, both mentally and physically. Based on the Thirteen Principles of Nia outlined in Chapter 1, each principle includes the following:

- ***Focus and intent:*** the target of your attention as you work out
- ***Pearls:*** words that help you connect to the unique energy and central ideas of each principle
- ***Workout tips:*** help you reap the benefits of each principle
- ***Visuals:*** help you connect to whole-body sensation
- ***Conscious personal training:*** statements that help you coach and guide your own practice

Each time you work out, refer to this menu to vary your experience and the benefits received.

PRINCIPLE 1. THE JOY OF MOVEMENT

Joy is the primary sensation you should seek from all movement. If you momentarily lose joy, tweak your movement until joy again arises. When joy is present, sustain it. When joy is not present, look for it.

Focus and Intent

Focus on the joy of movement with the intent to find ease, efficiency, and pleasure. Focus on joy as the energy and sensation you seek in every workout.

Pearls

Love, light, honesty, play, freedom, trust, listening, honoring, integrity, humility, grace, respect, passion, achievement, personal, pleasurable, ecstasy

Workout Tips

- Move and feel one with your physical truth—with what you can realistically do.
- Move and seek a relationship with joy.
- Move and return to joy when and if you lose it.
- Move and make joy something you cultivate and nurture, a part of every movement.

Visuals

- Seek the sensation of liquid joy running through your veins.
- Stay connected to joy by seeing it in your mind as a person you can dance with and talk to.
- Sustain joy by imagining that your body is becoming fuller and fuller with joy, light and airy like a helium balloon.
- When joy is not present, play hide-and-seek with it. Find joy by peeking under rocks, behind walls, and up in the clouds.
- Imagine that your whole body is a pair of dancing sunglasses that have eyes only for joy.
- Keep the physical sensation of joy alive by dancing and breathing in white energy light, which grows into a pasture of joy throughout your whole body.

Conscious Personal Training

- I am seeking joy and making it a personal choice as I move and work out.
- I am alive and joy is in me, fluid, soft, relaxed, and available so that everything I do heals me.

- I am choosing and sustaining joy so that my body is getting stronger, healthier, and more vital.
- I am filled with cells that vibrate joy in my body, mind, spirit, and emotions.
- I am running wild with images of joy that feed my body and invite me to choose pleasure.

PRINCIPLE 2. NATURAL TIME AND THE MOVEMENT FORMS

Natural Time

Nia movements are done in your own personal, natural sense of time. Move the main thirteen joints of the body and use your body sensations to measure movement. Move your body, respecting its natural timing and way of moving.

Focus and Intent

Focus on moving all thirteen joints to create systemic movement. Witness yourself and notice in every move the joints that are connected or disconnected. This is your tool for discovering the healing benefits from functioning as a whole person.

Pearls

Joints, bones, sensing, explore, timeless, connected, personal, authentic, movement, measure

Workout Tips

- Move in your own way, and in your own time, getting to know how you move and what you need to do to feel more pleasure and comfort.
- Move and consciously connect to sensation by listening to the voices, your body's messages that guide you to move in healthier and more functional ways.
- Move your joints, seeking the sensation of balance.
- Move your joints and sense the flow of energy through your whole body.

Visuals

- Imagine your body is mostly liquid and space.
- Visualize each joint as a mouth that can open and close.

- Visualize your joints as windows that move air in and out.
- Imagine creating more space in your joints.
- Visualize helium balloons in every joint.
- Imagine sounds coming out of each joint as they open and close.

Conscious Personal Training

- I am moving all thirteen joints to move healing energy into and through my body.
- I am using my bones, both long and short, to measure, sensing where to place my body as I seek comfort and pleasure.
- I am becoming more body aware by sensing my bones and joints dancing together to create harmonious movement.
- I am more of the real me by dancing in my own way and in my own time.
- I am learning more as I dance me, and adopting a new way of doing what I do using the Nia tools and techniques.

The Movement Forms

All of the Nia moves are derived from nine classic movement forms: three each from the martial arts, the dance arts, and the healing arts. Use the movement forms to add movement and energy variety into your workouts.

Focus and Intent

Each of the nine movement forms has its own special focus and intent. You could choose to focus on one movement form every time you experience Nia, or mix several forms into one workout. The forms are your best tool to become physically, mentally, emotionally, spiritually, and energetically intelligent about the healing benefits of movement and energy variety.

The Martial Arts

T'ai Chi

Focus and Intent

Focus on the slow dance.

Pearls

Soft, relaxed, like the wind, fluid, water, grounded, timing, internal, harmonized, equality, rooted, oneness, connected, sensory, liquid, patient, focused, balanced, meditative, graceful, integrated, breath, efficient, strong, agility, energy, compassionate, effortless, natural time, gentle, flowing, circular, supple, quiet, receptive power, open, chi, dynamic ease, wise, floating ribs, mystic column of the spine, systemic, fingers and hands, eye and hand coordination, weight shifting, inner calm, earth, sky, water, wind, nature, waves, God, clouds, a mountain

Workout Tips

- Move as a tender being.
- Move and keep every part of you flowing.
- Move and remain centered and connected to the world through your feet, eyes, breath, and hands.
- Move and create beauty through how you act in the world.

Visuals

- Like the wind, allow your spine to move freely.
- Be rooted like a tree, deeply connected through your roots into the depths of the earth.
- Sense fluid energy flowing through your limbs, like water running along a stream.
- Move like a balloon, your belly empowered, full of fertile chi.
- Move like a soft willow tree, feeling the moisture of rain melting into the surfaces of your "leaves" (your arms and hands).
- Like the ocean, adjust and be in relationship to all things.

Conscious Personal Training

- I maintain a soft vertical alignment, keeping my body perpendicular to the ground.
- I eliminate all unnecessary tension from my body by sensing the grace of this form of movement.
- I maintain a low center of gravity by keeping my joints soft and pliable, open to the sensation and flow of chi.
- I use my whole body as one connected unit, moving systemically.
- I gain balance and more power when I use my feet.

Tae Kwon Do

Focus and Intent

Focus on the dance of precision.

Pearls

Antagonist, attack, defend, react, sharp, solid, masculine, protective, thrust, aware, danger, survival, life and death, speed, start and stop, forceful, cutting, direct, quick, blast, intentional, conscious, precise, focused, directed, sudden, no hesitation, strong Base, slice, strike, kick, punch, block, fear, alert, contact, power, passion, male, warrior, pushing, aggressive, productive, adrenaline, instinct, discipline, timing, resistance, rage, anger, hand, fist, feet, knuckles, elbow, keen, now, present, calculated, creative force

Workout Tips

- Move as a powerful and focused being.
- Move and be aware of your body and the surroundings you move and live in.
- Move with the intent to be seen and felt.
- Move with confidence, without hesitation.

Visuals

- See the power of fire moving the sensation of speed and agility through you.
- Imagine your limbs as flexible cords, and then feel the sensation of your muscles squeezing and tightening around them.
- Visualize pushing out red liquid through your heel or fist as you kick or punch.
- Imagine lightning coming out of your fingertips as you thrust energy into space.
- Imagine your feet are magnets, grounded into the earth.
- As you exhale and deliver a punch, imagine a shield of armor lighting up, covering the entire front and Core of your body.

Conscious Personal Training

- I use every part of my body to effectively ground and deliver energy.
- I am maximizing my power, concentrating on all of my body parts working together.

- I am practicing dynamic ease, working on the timing of my technique, the correct use of my power, and the swiftness and slowness of my craft.
- I am aware of the explosive release of my power, which comes at the point when I finish the kick or punch.
- I am delivering a punch, kick, block, strike, or power move using my hips and Core.
- I am cultivating my ability to work with chi as the source of my energy.

Aikido

Focus and Intent

Focus on the dance of harmonious spherical motion.

Pearls

Win–win, entering, continuous, flowing, spirals, circles and lines, recycling energy, centering, perpetual motion, seamless, turning, belly, intent, focus, earth, sky, in and out, infinity, figure eight, cooperative, harmonizing, energy, peaceful and powerful, rotating around an axis, yielding, bending, swirling, adapting, going with, grounding, relaxation, awareness, connected

Workout Tips

- Move by connecting and blending with everything outside of you.
- Move and be aware of your physical body and the energy that moves you.
- Move with intent and focus.
- Move by turning lines into circular and spiral motions.

Visuals

- Visualize swirling yellow light moving around you as you walk and dance.
- Blend and imagine yourself melting into everything you touch and connect with.
- Imagine your arms and hands as long powerful swords, supporting them with grace as you dance and move through life.
- Imagine that you have a body double, who steps into you as you move forward—another you filling your physical body with added power.

- Visualize two headlights streaming their light out in front of your hip bones, shining the way into all spaces.
- Imagine every cell of your body as an eye that can see out in front of you, behind you, and all around you.

Conscious Personal Training

- When I turn, I remain balanced, feeling myself in the center of a spiral, grounded along my vertical axis.
- I allow my movement to come from my center, from the inside to the outside.
- I move as if my feet had eyes that can see deeply into the earth.
- I am extending my energy out into space without force, using less muscle effort and more focused energy.
- I direct my energy so that it follows where I place my attention.

The Dance Arts

Jazz Dance

Focus and Intent

Focus on the dance of fun, showmanship, and expression.

Pearls

Snap-crackle-pop, interpretive, playful, angular, attitude, jazzy, soulful, vital, happy, hands, impulsive, lusty, sassy, demonstrative, showy, exploration, alive, fun, electrifying, shimmy, uninhibited, teeth and smiles, sudden, up and down, short and fast, choppy and linear, fluid and percussive, pulsating, variety, rhythmic, asymmetrical, upbeat, sensual, release, contract, isolated, burst, energetic, spontaneous, expressive, surprising, wild, skillful, quick, diagonal, projection, free, magic, motions, spontaneous, total attention, hips, hands, fingers, shoulders, entertaining, outward, to the audience, sexy

Workout Tips

- Move and express yourself with pizzazz.
- Move and be aware of isolated body parts.
- Move and use your face and hands to speak to the world.
- Move and play with small gestures that speak with passionate emotion.

Visuals

- Become popcorn, popping out one motion after another, using all of your body parts.
- Project hot, red fiery beams of light from your expressive arms and hands.
- Imagine the color orange flowing into any body part you want to turn on and electrify.
- Vibrate and shake energy off, imagining you are a dog shaking off water.
- Become the sexy entertainer, visualizing yourself as a seductive cat on a hot tin roof.
- Flashdance and imagine the lights are on you.

Conscious Personal Training

- I use my joints to support easy and free movement, regardless of the speed.
- I am firmly connected to the floor through my feet and moving at a speed that allows me to isolate.
- I am using dynamic tension to increase my speed.
- I bump my hips, moving energy up my vertical axis.
- I embrace fun and feel free to express myself.

Modern Dance

Focus and Intent

Focus on the dance of creating shapes in space.

Pearls

Moody, serious, free, bound and unbound, introspective, cubic, cylindrical, long and short, up and down, percussive, somber, lively, languid, space and time, on and off balance, above and below, tight and loose, full and empty, form and formless, momentary, recovery, sharp, slippery, silk and metal, wildly emotional, balance, shapes, space, fluid, connections, heavy, light, round, square, angles, circles, lines, corners, retrospective, playful, contrasts, gravity, surprise, aloof, collapsed, rocking, expressive, endless, start, stop, continuity, mechanical, natural, stride, linger, stop, freeze, hot, cold, staccato, explosion

Workout Tips

- Move and consciously create a different shape with your body.
- Move and play with being off balance.

- Move and become different textures.
- Move and play with temperature, weight, sound, and emotion.

Visuals

- Imagine you are surrendering into blue illuminated liquid.
- Visualize moving your legs as if they were taffy, softening and growing longer.
- Imagine squeezing yourself into and out of spaces, as if your limbs were toothpaste coming out of the tube.
- Fall off balance, imagining you are splashing your energy onto the ground like green raindrops.
- Visualize your rib cage as an accordion, allowing the sun's energy to slip into the spaces, penetrating your internal organs with warmth and healing light.
- Imagine yourself as a ball, rolling from one spot to the other.

Conscious Personal Training

- I am improving my sensory awareness.
- I am moving through thick and thin spaces, feeling everything.
- I am contracting and releasing, becoming physically and emotionally connected.
- I am giving life to my movements, creating a sensation that can be felt and perceived by others.
- I am using my eyes to energetically connect my outside world to my physical body.

Duncan Dance

Focus and Intent

Focus on the dance of free-spirited, honest movement.

Pearls

Movement from the soul, child, spirit, angelic, freedom, flow, spontaneity, natural, nature, walking, running, playing, skipping, harmony, line, form, communicating, social, interactive, hope, positive, assertion, joy, response, rediscovery, awakening, remembering, joy of play, coordinated, effortless, ease, unbound, listening, a spark, fresh, the pulse of the legs and feet, rhythm, steps, spring like, thrusting up, descending down, fairy-like magic, slow, moderate, primal body, inner-core energy, sequencing, smoothly sliding waltz, bouncing polka, melodic phrases, gestures, imaginary scenes, creative, within, connected to, elements, discovery, fascination, exploring, unfolding, center, emoting, emotional, radiating up and out, becoming a part of the surrounding space, immediate, limitless

Workout Tips

- Move with the freedom of spontaneity in your heart.
- Move and play with your body and the worldly delights around you.
- Move to feel the child within who is mesmerized by life.
- Move and turn the world on with your angelic presence.

Visuals

- Imagine your arms are golden wings of light—and fly, feeling the wind ruffle through your feathers.
- Visualize your arms and hands offering love-filled droplets of rain.
- Visualize sunlight streaming down on your chest, with light particles glistening on your skin as sunlight glistens on a clear blue lake.
- Undulate your body up into the sky, and imagine silvery smoke rising from the heat of your internal passion.
- See yourself dancing freely and spontaneously, being one with your animal self.
- Imagine being seduced by the talking trees, animals, and plants; dance to their messages.

Conscious Personal Training

- I let the music seduce my movement from the ground up.
- I am looking up, reaching into the sky, into possibility and hope.
- I am unleashing all parts of me to fly, as if I were a bird.
- I am letting my child dance and play in the sea of movement.
- I am rising high onto the balls of my feet, making space for light to fill the dark undersides of my feet, dancing on the light of love.

Teachings of Moshe Feldenkrais

Focus and Intent

Focus on the dance of conscious awareness of sensation.

Pearls

Somatic, individualized experience, energetically coherent, living, biological, genetic, functioning, animalistic, simple, felt, perceived, psyche, self-conscious, layered, ancient, reflective, threaded, patterns in time, optimal, behavioral, healthy, healing, body, mind, spirit, emotions, transparent, adapting, proprioception, undulation, useful, life line, unified, systemic, human, body education, self-adjusting, body centered, individualized, therapy, internalized, assimilating, applicable, species, creature, responsible, holographic, connected, oneness, biofeedback, completion, body conscious, newness, creative, meditative, mindful, supersensitive, internally directed, reflection of the nervous system, accessible to awareness, sensation, feeling, thought, senses, states of existence

Workout Tips

- Move with sensory awareness and feel life as it happens.
- Move along a path of least resistance to increase sensation.
- Move to turn all experiences into sensations that deepen and improve your experience of living in a body.
- Move fast and slow, with mindful awareness of how to move so that you are efficient and remain energy-full.

Visuals

- Visualize your movement evolving like a white string, unwinding away from your center.
- Imagine resting into the internal softness of billowy clouds, supported by breath.
- See you and your body moving with the efficiency and attitude of a black sultry cat.
- Imagine you and your body as a tiger, and allow your primal animal self to organize your movement.
- Visualize your nerves as golden threads that pulse calm energy.

- See you and your body resting into the glowing amniotic fluid of life and swim your motions.

Conscious Personal Training

- I am intentionally relaxing, decreasing the rate of nerve impulses sent to my muscles.
- I am learning how to vary my speed from as fast as possible to as slow as possible.
- I use my mind's energy to control and direct my physical actions.
- I am accumulating intelligence and knowledge by feeling and sensing my body in space.
- I feel my body as it moves.

Alexander Technique

Focus and Intent

Focus on the dance of movement from the top.

Pearls

Internal, subtle, not doing, consciousness, exploration, three-dimensional, ease, flexibility, health, physical freedom, sensing, perceiving, transforming, operative, physical, emotional, imaginative, natural, resourceful, beneficial, carriage, body weight, organism, attitude, relationships, unbound, free, method, available, accessible, healthy joints, new approach, conscious mind, aware, whole, neuromuscular, discovery of patterns, effortless, equalized, balanced, continuous, simple, useful, authentic, organic, don't try, easy breathing, automatic, grace, naturalness, easy involvement, no overdoing or underdoing, breaking habit, thinking and moving, total conditioning, head up and out—body follows, lightness, upward direction, visualize instead of doing

Workout Tips

- Move and fall up.
- Move with the sensation of your head moving up and out, away from your torso.
- Move as a whole person, with all of your body parts connected and relating to each other.
- Move and direct your body and self mindfully.

Visuals

- Imagine your head magnetized by the sun's golden rays.
- Visualize you and your body moving like an amoeba, whole and fluid.
- Imagine breathing and seeing white smoke flowing through your spine, elongating your neck.
- Imagine you have feet under your torso that can push down into your hips as your head moves up and away from your torso.
- Visualize large white wings expanding over your back, to lighten your body weight.
- See your head floating like a blue cloud over the center of your spine.

Conscious Personal Training

- I am connected to every part of my body.
- I find balance in the way I approach myself.
- I think consciously about how I wish to direct myself.
- I allow my back to lengthen and widen.
- I am using my potential.

Yoga

Focus and Intent

Focus on the dance of conscious alignment of bones and joints.

Pearls

Bones, alignment, counterforce, postures, muscles, ligaments, extensions, strengthening, flexibility, stretch, agility, gentle, powerful, focused, conscious, long, receptive, unity, oneness, balance, presence, harmony, internal, effortless, endurance, guided, light, unending, length, lying, sitting, prone, inverted, backbends, infinity, spiritual, expansive, long bones, short bones, liquid, supportive, restful, restorative, distance, projected, energy, line, easy, peace, stillness, active, elongate, committed, opening, closing, soft, supple, breath, belly, tangible, sensed, perceived, somatic, body centered, fingers, toes, systemic, aware, triangles, angles, sympathetic and parasympathetic nervous system, external and internal, attentive, timeless, ageless, letting go, surrender, soft eyes, open mind, multidirectional

Workout Tips

- Move and sense the loving relationship between your bones and joints.
- Move and create healthy posture in motion and in stillness.
- Move and be connected to your body, mind, and spirit.
- Move to self-heal.

Visuals

- Imagine you're being held in the arms of Mother Earth, and rest into your bones.
- Become a tree and imagine the roots of your trunk going deep into the earth.
- Visualize your breath as wings, allowing breathing to give flight to places where you need extra strength and support.
- Visualize your legs as pillars supporting you.
- Imagine that your spine is a vine, growing up into the clouds.
- Visualize extending energy through your arms and beyond your fingertips, like rays of sunlight.

Conscious Personal Training

- I practice regularly to create change.
- I take time to sense alignment.
- I am continuing to stretch and breathe evenly, correcting my moves by seeking pleasure and comfort.
- I give as much attention and care to moving out of a position as when I moved into it.
- I feel my spine move as I stretch.

PRINCIPLE 3. MUSIC AND THE 8BC SYSTEM

Nia is almost always practiced to the sounds and silences of music, using an eight-beat counting system to organize the movements. Master the art of listening and connect to sound and silence.

Focus and Intent

Focus on listening to music with the intent to develop an intimate relationship with all kinds of sounds, including silence.

Pearls

Sound, silence, rhythm, harmony, melody, beat, resonance, vibration, tone, frequency, note, syncopation, rest, styles, listen, ears, skin, silence, patterns of sound, track, mapping sound and silence, seduction, calming, agitating, healing, creative, expressive, stimulating, speeds, excitation, instruments, sections, code, voice, appreciation, mood, inspiration, violins, horns, bells, bass, drum, waves, reverberation, filters, variety, harmonizing, tangible, discordant, creative force, primordial, feminine, masculine, accent, measure, meter, tempo changes, off-beat, double-time, slow, fast, cadence, phrase, pause, jazz, Celtic, reggae, hip-hop, classical, salsa, ethnic, notation system

Workout Tips

- Move and become a metronome, using your body to find the beat.
- Move and listen to your favorite music, and mark the beat—stepping with your right foot on, "one," and your left foot on "and," until you get to "eight-and." At that point, begin again to count from one.
- Move and dance to a piece of music and listen to the drummer, using what you hear to guide your Base.
- Move to silence and recognize the internal music of your emotions, which inspire you to dance.

Visuals

- Imagine each sound as a raindrop that touches a part of your body, seducing it to move.
- When you hear bells, tambourines, or triangles, dance your belly with the sound.
- When you hear stringed instruments, imagine playing a violin.
- Each time you hear a different instrument, see yourself conducting an orchestra with different body parts.
- Imagine you are nothing but ears; apply filters and listen to the subtler sounds in the background.

- Imagine communicating with the sounds you hear, listening for their voices and responding with the voice of your body parts.

Conscious Personal Training

- I listen to the beat and connect to the flow of masculine energy.
- I feel the seduction that sound and vibration have on my whole body.
- I use the music to alter the way I move.
- I allow the wind of sound and silence to move the sails of my body.
- I allow music to touch and awaken my spirit.

PRINCIPLE 4. FREEDANCE

Anything goes, movement wise. Let go of structure. Break out and move in spontaneous, free ways.

Focus and Intent

Focus on cultivating and expressing your authentic self with the intent to break movement habits. FreeDance provides you with a foundation to be free and creative each time you dance.

Pearls

Empty mind, anything goes, seduced by the music, feelings and emotions, creative source, authentic movement, Witnessing, the right fit, body expression, body gesture, radical, change, act, pretend, no judgment, creativity, evolve, no thinking, go shopping for new motions, more like a mime or a puppet or like someone else.

Workout Tips

- Move and freely express yourself.
- Move and use emotions to fuel your dance.
- Move and make radical movement changes.
- Move and be spontaneous and theatrical.

Visuals

- Imagine you are a panther stalking prey quietly.
- Imagine dancing in a room filled with helium balloons.
- Imagine you are holding a lemon under your chin, opening up the back of your neck.
- Imagine rubbing your ear on a fuzzy shoulder.
- See your head as a windshield wiper, long and moving from side to side.
- Imagine yourself wiping off a bench with your fanny, your pelvis free.

Conscious Personal Training

- I am experiencing body-centered choreography.
- I am exploring new ways to move.
- I am shifting my attention from my dance to the music.
- I am acting to become emotionally flexible.
- I dance subtle and demonstrative gestures.

PRINCIPLE 5. AWARENESS AND DANCING THROUGH LIFE

In Nia, you become aware that every movement in life is a dance and that every movement can be used to self-heal. Pay attention to body sensations and heal your body by doing little repair work all throughout the day, choosing pleasure over pain. Sense, perceive, and use every movement as a dance to support self-healing.

Focus and Intent

Focus on the sensation of pain and pleasure with the intent to observe what you do to increase ease, comfort, and pleasure and to self-heal.

Pearls

Healthy choices, conscious decisions, Sensory IQ, messages, voices of the body, observe, reference, recognize, feeling, sensation, stimulation, pain, pleasure

Workout Tips

- Move and make a conscious, sensory connection between your body and your movement experience.

- Move and particularly notice one part of your body, and pay attention to what you are doing, how you are doing it.
- Move and make one tiny, small adjustment to enhance the quality of the experience.
- Move and repeat what feels good, what brings you peace and harmony, what releases old habits and ways.

Visuals

- Imagine your entire body as one sensory nerve.
- See your feet and hands as ears that receive subtle feedback.
- Imagine your tailbone as a long tail that picks up and transmits information along your entire spine.
- Imagine your joints breathing in and out.
- Imagine your abdominal muscles chewing and activating sensation in your Core.
- Imagine another set of arms and hands at the back of your body, connecting you to the space behind.

Conscious Personal Training

- I am slowing down and paying attention to what I sense, connecting to the sensory impulses I receive.
- I use my physical body to become aware of what I do that creates comfort.
- I am becoming aware of my touch, how I stand, how I feel, what I think, what I smell, what I hear, what I see, and what I perceive as art.
- I am connected to everything going on inside and outside of me, energetically connected to my body and my world.
- I make choices based on what I feel and I choose pleasure over pain.

PRINCIPLE 6. THE BASE—FEET AND LEGS

Your feet are the hands that touch the earth and through your legs they carry the energy of the earth to your whole body. Connect to your foundation, your feet, the hands that touch the earth.

Focus and Intent

Focus on your feet and legs with intent to move in a grounded, functional, and safe way.

Pearls

Steps, stances, kicks, Relevé, Duck Walk, Squish Walk, Rock Around the Clock, Whole Foot, heel, ball, strong, agile, foundation, flexible, support, balance, connected, platform, hands that touch the earth

Workout Tips

- Move and use your feet like hands.
- Move and use different parts of the feet, your heel, ball, inner and outer arch, and five toes.
- Move and change the direction of your feet.
- Move and let knee and hip comfort dictate how you place your feet.

Visuals

- Imagine your shins as straws, drinking energy from the earth.
- Imagine your feet like suction cups, firmly planted.
- Imagine the ball of your foot as an ink stamper and avoid smearing the ink.
- Imagine your shins as fence posts, vertically aligned.
- Imagine the ball of your hip as a baseball that rests and moves in a mitt.
- Imagine the end of your thigh as a pendulum that freely swings.

Conscious Personal Training

- I change the direction of my feet to improve hip mobility.
- I use my whole foot to sink into and push away from.
- I use my foot and ankle together for agility and stability.
- I am picking up and placing my feet to protect my knees.
- I lead with my heel to support my movement from behind and underneath.

PRINCIPLE 7. THE THREE PLANES AND THREE LEVELS

Every movement can be done within three planes—low, middle, and high—and can be done with three different levels of intensity. Mixing the three levels and three planes creates a wide repertoire of movement choices. Transfer body weight along a Smile Line, moving from low to middle to high. Use three levels of intensity to vary your rate of exertion.

Focus and Intent

Focus on three planes and three intensity levels with the intent to vary the range of motion and intensity of your workout.

Pearls

Low, middle, high, slow, moderate, fast, small, big, bigger, subtle, acute, sinking deeper, rising higher, contracting inward, expanding outward, Smile Line, open and closed joints, movement variety, levels one-two-three, low, moderate, high intensity.

Workout Tips

- Move through the three planes, opening and closing your joints.
- Move and shift your body weight along the Smile Line as you sink and rise from one side to the other.
- Move and vary the range of motion and muscle intensity.
- Move and sink and rise vertically.

Visuals

- Imagine your torso slipping below the waterline as you sink.
- See yourself rising high into the clouds as you rise.
- Imagine water in your joints, splashing as you vary your movement, speed, and intensity.
- Imagine your feet as batteries that vary the electrical charge that moves through your body.
- Imagine your body as a helium balloon that fills and empties as you move through three planes.
- Imagine your bones five times their length, reaching out into space, lower, higher, wider to increase intensity.

Conscious Personal Training

- I move gracefully and powerfully through low, middle, and high planes.
- I am exploring my own safe ranges of motions and intensity.
- I am discovering my comfort level in a deep plane.
- I play with movement forms to vary the energy intensity.
- I use my three body weights to load and lighten the intensity.

PRINCIPLE 8. THE CORE—PELVIS, CHEST, AND HEAD

The three body weights are the home of your emotions, and your energy centers. The pelvis is a container of energy, the chest transmits and receives energy, and the head processes energy. Integrate the three body weights—your head, chest, and pelvis.

Focus and Intent

Focus on the three body weights—pelvis, chest, and head—with the intent to integrate your entire spine and Core.

Pearls

Pelvis, chest, head, container, spine, organs, breathing, balance, eyes, ears, nose, mouth, receive, direct, transmit, chakras, emotions, posture, unit, alignment, sound, rib cage, sternum, sacrum, coccyx

Workout Tips

- Move and establish equality among your pelvis, chest, and head.
- Move and use breath to integrate your Core.
- Move and consciously talk to your pelvis, giving it freedom to move as you walk and dance.
- Move and change the volume of your movement if you feel the desire to emotionally shut down.

Visuals

- Imagine your coccyx as a long tail that adds grace and power to your movement.
- Imagine your pelvis as a bowl filled with healing water.
- Imagine your chest as a birdcage that protects and nourishes your heart and lungs.
- Imagine your head as a vase, a container for beautiful thoughts and dreams.

Conscious Personal Training

- I am vertically aligned, while respecting the natural curves in my spine.
- I use my voice, sending the resonance of tone through my chest.
- I say yes and think yes to move my head.
- I move my pelvis, chest, and head from the inside out.
- I am adding emotion and feeling organic movement in my three body weights.

PRINCIPLE 9. THE UPPER EXTREMITIES—ARMS, HANDS, AND FINGERS

The Upper Extremities are tools for healing, touching, directing energy, and creating connections. They are extensions of your feelings and thoughts and allow you to express yourself in personal and purposeful ways. Use your hands and arms as tools for healing and expressing yourself.

Focus and Intent

Focus on the natural use of your hands and arms with the intent to generate powerful, graceful, and expressive gestures.

Pearls

Messengers, five fingers, voices of emotions, give and receive, hold, pull, push, move, build, direct, definition, shoulder girdle, shoulder blades, touch, efficient, imaginative, creative, hands, wrists, fingers, forearms, upper arms, elbow, punch, strike, block, blade side, Webbed Spaces, inner and outer arch of hand, chop, fluff, open doors, chop wood

Workout Tips

- Move with emotion to organically initiate arm movement that includes the hand.
- Move and extend energy into and out of your hands.
- Move and touch the space outside of you, integrating upper and lower body.
- Move and change the direction of your palms.

Visuals

- Visualize the joints of your arms as flexible springs.
- See colors of paint flowing out the ends of your fingers into space.
- Imagine your arms and hands as beautiful wings that include your shoulder blades.
- Imagine your hands as paintbrushes, playing with different strokes and textures.
- See your hands and arms as powerful long swords that cut through space.
- Imagine your arms fifty times longer, touching the walls of the space around you.

Conscious Personal Training

- I bring my hands back to my heart, relaxing my shoulders, before I reach out.
- I combine linear and circular energy flow, giving my muscles exactly what they need.
- I play with emotion and visuals to move systemically and more powerfully.
- I remain energetically relaxed until the very end, when I release power in my movement.
- I use contrast to stimulate intrinsic and extrinsic muscle action, moving slow and fast, up and down, big and small, and in and out.

PRINCIPLE 10. X-RAY ANATOMY

X-Ray Anatomy is the practice of using your eyes, your other sensory organs, and your intuition to see inside you. You can penetrate the veil of your flesh to reveal the proper placement of your bones, tendons, ligaments, and muscles. Use your eyes and intuition to see inside.

Focus and Intent

Focus on the position of your bones and joints with the intent to use your real eyes and Sensory IQ to perceive alignment.

Pearls

Bones, joints, vertical, horizontal, skin, sensation, pain, pleasure, realign, heal, physical, emotional, balance, integration, support, precision, online, offline, individual, energy flow, potential, power, relationship, comfort, ease, efficiency, grace, leverage, levers, structure

Workout Tips

- Move and sense the relationship between your feet, ankles, and shins.
- Move and redirect the position of your feet to establish energy flow along the bones from the ground up.
- Move and adjust the height of your chin to establish a dynamic vertical line from head to toe.
- Move and adjust the position of your knees to free your hip joints and spine.

Visuals

- Imagine your bones are lightbulbs, shining from the inside out.
- Imagine your bones as the frame of a house, and vertically align your structure.
- Imagine your bones as a light, porous, alive substance that feels and thinks.
- Imagine your bones as fence posts that your muscles hang on.
- See your joints as well-oiled machines.
- Imagine your self as a marionette whose appendages respond to the energy strings of life.

Conscious Personal Training

- I use my bones to spiral and stretch my muscles.
- I use my joints to balance the sensation of strength and flexibility.
- I use my bones and joints to move and measure, seeking dynamic ease, pleasure, and comfort.

- I adjust the placement of my feet to support dynamic alignment.
- I place my sensory attention on my bones, rather than muscles, to efficiently generate relaxed power.

PRINCIPLE 11. FITNESS IS THE BUSINESS OF THE BODY

Fitness can be achieved by listening to the voices of the body, setting goals, creating plans, reaching decisions, and attaining results. Like all businesses, fitness is a process of making changes. Listen to your body; set goals and achieve results.

Focus and Intent

Focus on the Body's Way with the intent to achieve your personal fitness and health goals.

Pearls

Honoring, developmental, voices of the body, voices of your body, process, ongoing changes, realistic goals, plans, choices and decisions, results, benefits, personal desires, adaptability, lifestyle, personalization, body–mind–spirit–emotions, holistic, attention, details, cause and effect, love, pleasure, consistency, joy, expressive, path of least resistance, internally guided, self-regulated, conscious personal trainer

Workout Tips

- Move and recognize your small, subtle fitness accomplishments, as well as the big ones.
- Move and set realistic goals that help you continue to develop.
- Move to address the specific needs of your body, mind, emotions, and spirit.
- Move and consider your lifestyle, so that what you do adds to your fitness and health.

Visuals

- Imagine you are the CEO of your body's corporation and act with wisdom and integrity.
- Imagine your body parts as team members that collectively contribute to your success.

- See the business of your fitness and health like a body with a heart that has compassion for your successes and failures; with a mind that visions and dreams the future; with feet and legs that take action and move in the right direction; with a pelvis, chest, and head that remain emotionally connected and expressively interactive.
- Imagine being on the cover of *Forbes.* What would they say about how you run the business of your body?

Conscious Personal Training

- I make choices that integrate movement into my lifestyle.
- I make decisions that enhance the quality of my life.
- I choose pleasure over pain.
- I am trusting that the Body's Way is the way to heal.
- I am consciously coaching my self.

PRINCIPLE 12. CONTINUING YOUR BODY–MIND–SPIRIT EDUCATION

Healing the body is a practice that never ends. Every new workout is an opportunity to reeducate your body, mind, and spirit. Reeducate, explore, transform, and learn.

Focus and Intent

Focus on lifelong learning with the intent to keep yourself fascinated and motivated to seek higher levels of fitness and health for the rest of your life.

Pearls

Review, observe, seek, explore, learn, question, isolate, integrate, read, practice, books, videos, lectures, workshops, classes, the Internet, discussion groups, the library, life, notice, grow, change, improve, transform, new out of the old, evolve

Workout Tips

- Move and seek a new-to-you skill every time you dance.
- Move and desire the ability to improve your craft and skill through practice and education.

- Move and integrate a new focus or a new piece of information that changes what you did yesterday into something new and fascinating for your body and mind today.
- Move and discover how you learn, what motivates you, and what you can do that will ensure your on-going growth and transformation.

Visuals

- Imagine receiving a Ph.D. in mastering the voice of your Body's Way.
- See your body and mind transforming into higher levels of Sensory IQ.
- Imagine every cell of your body as a brain, hungry for more and more information food.
- Imagine your body as a plant whose nourishment comes from the cognitive and experiential information you give to it.
- Imagine a lightbulb lighting up to transform what is old into something new every time you think, "Ah, ha! Now I understand and embody the information."
- Imagine training for the Fitness Business Olympics and settle for nothing less than your best.

Conscious Personal Training

- I accept responsibility for the business of my fitness and health.
- I am taking charge of my destiny, finding answers that lead me to greater fitness and health.
- I am creating goals and personal plans that support me in developing and growing without sabotaging my efforts.
- I am self-empowered and my own best personal trainer.
- I am making movement a part of my life forever.

PRINCIPLE 13. DANCE WHAT YOU SENSE

When you experience the primary lesson of Nia—that life should be lived through sensation—you become connected. Connect to the sensations of your body before you fully express your dance.

Focus and Intent

Focus on sensation with the intent to communicate and express what you sense.

Pearls

Sensation, Sensory IQ, relaxed, alert, waiting, receiving, transmitting, choosing, dancing, expression, personal, interactive, body centered, stimulating, healing, dynamic, connected, in the now, one with, inside to outside, listening, communicating

Workout Tips

- Move and seek the voice of any body part encouraging you to dance with it more freely.
- Move and wait until you feel connected to a body part before you let go more fully.
- Move and dance to stimulate the awareness of sensation, and express the sensation through your dance.
- Move and seek the sensations of pleasure, joy, and comfort throughout your whole body.

Visuals

- Imagine every cell in your body smiling and expressing joy as you dance.
- Imagine that your entire body is a foot whose nerve endings connect you to the earth.
- Imagine yourself as an animal who relies on sensation and intuition to guide choices and decisions.
- Imagine the voices of your body as loudspeakers conveying sensory truth.
- Imagine speaking without speaking, using the preverbal communication of sensation as your language.
- Imagine teaching the entire world a primary lesson of Nia, that life is a sensation, felt and experienced through the body.

Conscious Personal Training

- I sense every part of my body, from the inside out.
- I am relaxed in my body, alert in my mind, and waiting for a sensation to arrive before I really let go.
- I am dancing the sensation of bones and joints.
- I am dancing the sensation of liquid light through my bones.
- I am dancing and expressing my unique spirit.

. . .

And there's more! The Nia Web site (nia-nia.com) offers additional menu choices and tips. Variety is a major part of staying connected and committed to any fitness regimen—and our Web site offers a plethora of inspirational ideas for keeping your workouts fresh and making sure that the physical, emotional, and mental growth you have now started to experience never stops.

six *Dancing Through Life*

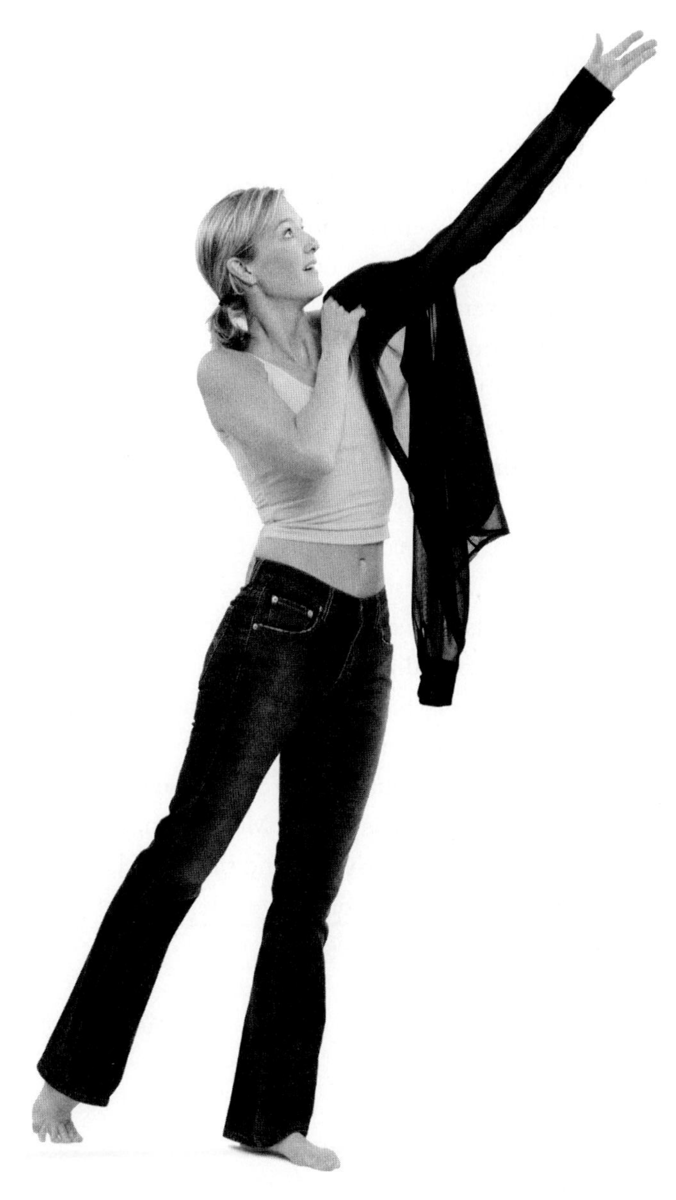

By now, you know a great deal about Nia. Good for you! Learning a new way to stay healthy and strong is always exciting, and now it's time to learn one final concept that can change your life forever.

That concept is *Dancing Through Life.*

Other exercise programs end when you leave the gym. But that's when Nia really *begins.*

Let's face facts: We live almost all of our lives *outside* the gym. Therefore, what we do outside the gym is far more important than what we do in it. Because of this, one of the most important concepts we teach Nia students is that of Dancing Through Life. This means integrating all fifty-two moves into your daily life and carrying over to *real life* all the healthy movement choices that we practice during Nia classes. It means turning everyday movement into a dance of fitness and life.

In Nia, dancing is not just what we do when the music comes on. It is any movement our bodies make. Ultimately, dancing is not even something we *do:* It is what we *are.* This ubiquitous dance of life cannot be confined to any specific place. It requires the largest possible stage: life itself.

Dancing Through Life is movement as pleasure. It is Nia's prescription for enjoying life in a human body. It actively integrates healthy movements into *every* aspect of living, from the mundane activities to the sublime. It can consist of washing the dishes, mowing the lawn, or making love: It doesn't matter what you do, but how you feel when you do it. It is also a waltz of movement and stillness, silence and sound. It's a method for finding meaning, beauty, and connection—magic!—in a world that may once have seemed dross and pointless.

Turning the movements of life into a dance is one part of Dancing Through Life, but there are also two other important elements that contribute to it. One is Living Meditation, a system for bringing the meditative state to ordinary life, and the other is Life as Art, a system of finding beauty and inspiration in every part of the world around us.

THE DANCING THROUGH LIFE TRIAD

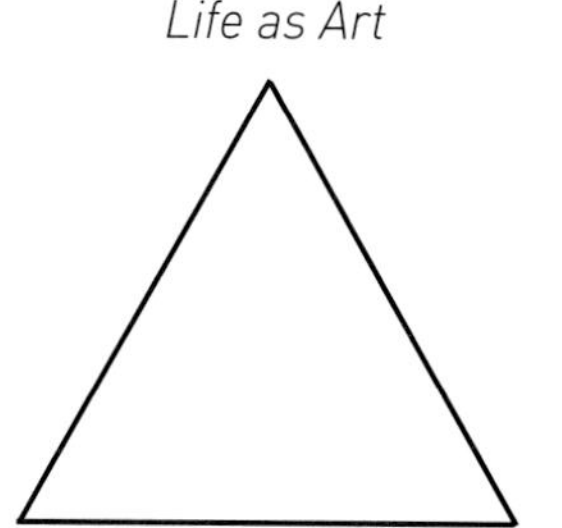

These three elements work synergistically to create a dance. When you incorporate all three into your life, you will find new meaning and a new sense of peace. Now we'll explore each of the elements in the triad.

A **Nia** *Story*

FEMININE AGAIN

STUDENT: Julie

CLASS LOCATION: Dallas, Texas

OCCUPATION: Teacher

Julie was very physically active before she began to do Nia, but her workouts weren't really working. One major problem was that they weren't stopping her stress.

She was overwhelmed by the ongoing tension associated with being the program director for a hospice organization, and this stress was physically manifested by extreme tension in her jaw, neck, and shoulders. She tried to release some of this physical stress through conventional aerobics, but the results were unsatisfying. The pain remained, and her body was not thriving. Her exercises only made her feel more tense and gave her body, as she now puts it, "a hard, masculine" look.

All that changed with her very first Nia class. "I immediately felt the tension melting from my body," she says. "I felt myself moving with grace and creativity—things I'd never felt before in aerobics classes. For the first time, I felt like a dancer!"

Nia reawakened Julie's sense of femininity. "Nia has made me a 'softer' person," she notes. "When I was director of the hospice program, I had a great deal of energy tied up in my success and career. It was very masculine energy. I felt imbalanced and desperately needed to find my feminine self again. I needed to find that part of myself that was creative, nurturing, surrendering (in a good way), soft, and curvy. I felt rigid and full of linear angles.

"After several weeks of Nia, though, my teacher said that she saw me as softer. I could have cried! It was a revelation! In the past, exercise had made me only very hard and angular. Nia has given curves to my shape and has given me a more feminine look."

Nia's softening effect carried over to Julie's mental and emotional outlook. "Mentally," she says, "I manage stress much better. Also, the creativity I developed from Nia has carried over to all the other parts of my life. Now my life has more flow. Spiritually, I praise God with my movement. I feel myself giving and receiving energy. I feel connected to all living things, including the earth. Emotionally, I feel more. Before Nia, I always kept my emotions at bay, to avoid appearing weak. Now, I am happy to cry tears of joy or sadness and to be authentic about who I am."

the dancing through life system

Dancing Through Life is a system we use to integrate the sensations of healthy movements into every aspect of living. It is a dance that weaves together sound and silence, action and inaction, and perception and reality. Its movements are based on the Body's Way, but its forms of expression are limitless.

Arising from any stillness—as naturally as air bubbles rise through water—are the sounds of the earth. To the attuned ear, the sounds of the earth are like music. This music invites us to dance.

In Nia, we teach people to think of dancing as anything the body does.

For example, when you swing your arms while walking to catch the bus, the movement may be identical to one you perform in a Nia class. Nia is not separate from life. It is not separate from the body. It *is* the body: the body in action.

As you learn to Dance Through Life, your awareness will grow. You will become cognizant of your breath surging in and out, and you'll even become aware of that moment of stillness between breaths. This awareness is a gift. It is your natural reward for living in a body. It is, however, also a tool. It is the tool that empowers you to improve the way you move. It enables you to choose pleasure over pain, and thus arrive at the Body's Way.

The conscious awareness that comes from Dancing Through Life teaches you to let go of the unconscious impulses that may so often rule your life. You stop sleepwalking through your short stay on this earth and start to *wake up.* Instead of being driven by longstanding habits, you begin to change these conditioned responses into conscious, intentional actions.

So how do you begin to Dance Through Life? You begin simply by choosing to be *alive in your own body,* instead of divorced from it. When you do this, you will become connected not just to your body but to the entirety of your existence and to the earth on which your life is unfolding.

As you become more in touch with the sensations of your body, mind, emotions, and spirit, you will experience the sensation of holistic union that exists among these four most basic elements of selfhood. We refer to this union as the *nexus of cooperation.* Cooperation is more than just an abstract reference; it is an actual, physical *sensation,* difficult to describe but unmistakable once you've experienced it. It is, to some extent, similar to the feeling of comfort and confidence that people experience when they are in the zone, or in a state of flow.

When you begin to employ the techniques of Nia and to experience the sensation of full-being cooperation, your body will guide you, by itself, toward balance, awareness, stillness, movement, and inspiration. Your body will show you the most comfortable postures and the most efficient ways of moving. Thus your body itself will show you how to Dance Through Life. You will reclaim the perfection that has always been within you and is still there now, waiting.

We all know that our attitudes affect our bodies, but the converse is also true: Our bodies influence our attitudes. When your body becomes fully alive and abundantly aware, your general attitude toward life will become more serene, and you will discover mental and emotional strengths that you've never before experienced.

This ascension to a higher physical and mental plane will require practice. Each day you will need to practice the techniques of Nia and integrate them into your everyday movements. The rewards for this work, however, can be astonishing. With dedication, you will be able to achieve a condition of physical grace that we call *body wisdom,* which leads inexorably to peak mental and emotional function. If you work at Nia consistently and efficiently, this achievement will not only be possible but will be virtually inevitable.

When you begin to Dance Through Life, you will see many remarkable changes:

- You will experience more physical pleasure in almost every aspect of your life.
- You will begin to experience *Joy* with a capital *J*—the universal Joy that transcends personal joy.
- Your life will have greater meaning. You'll stop asking yourself, "What's it all about?"
- You will experience a wealth of sensations each day.
- Your body will feel lighter and stronger, and fear and pain will slowly become a part of the past.
- Your mind will be calmer and more clear.
- You will be able to find truth and reality through somatic awareness.
- You will be able to experience the union of your body, mind, emotions, and spirit as a physical sensation.
- Your Sensory IQ will skyrocket.

living meditation

Perceiving each of your movements as a dance, though, is just the first element of Dancing Through Life. The heightened awareness created by seeing life as a dance will enable you to participate in another vitally important aspect: Living Meditation. Just as dance should be broadened to include almost every movement you make, meditation should be integrated into the fabric of each day. Every moment of every day is the appropriate time to meditate.

The fundamental goal of Living Meditation is simply to *stop.*

- Stop the inner dialogue in your mind.
- Stop being attached to external illusions that are created by false assumptions.
- Stop indulging in emotions that cause unhappiness and stress.

With practice, stopping these actions isn't much more difficult than stopping physical movement after a period of activity. Your body loves being active, but it also loves to stop, in order to rest and repair itself. Thus activity is natural, but inactivity is also natural. Your body knows when to stop, and your mind should learn this skill, too.

Stopping movement and stopping your internal mental activities are both analogous to the Dancing Through Life technique of experiencing silence. Silence, as we've noted, is a part of music. Without spaces of silence, the sounds of music would be chaotic and meaningless. Silence confers order and harmony to sound. Similarly, Living Meditation brings order and harmony to the cacophony of life.

We can begin to experience Living Meditation only when we choose to open ourselves to the pause of silence that can be found in each moment. In this pause is stillness, which is a portal to the inner world. When we open ourselves to stillness, we are better able to see life as it really is—devoid of our preconceptions, subjectivity, and fears. The stillness that you will find within yourself is just as much a part of Dancing Through Life as the movements you make. The body and mind crave stillness as much as movement. There is as much to be gained from one as the other. They are each part of the Body's Way and are part of the dance of life.

Imagine, for example, that you have come to a stoplight in your car and for a moment *everything* stops—no inner dialogue, no negative thoughts, no attachment to external actions. Your body remains at an alert, resting state, and you are free from desires, goals, and fears. You are in a place of absolute neutrality. This moment becomes one of Living Meditation. In this moment of stillness, you become actively engaged in the process of nondoing. This may sound oxymoronic, but it's not—there is truly a state of active inactivity.

You can learn to identify this state as a *physical sensation.* Experiencing this sensation of stillness will bring great pleasure to your body and mind. It will also bring you a special kind of energy. This energy is not overtly stimulating but is very empowering. It is the energy of healing.

Capturing these moments of inner silence can be difficult, especially at first. There is no shortcut to stillness, although many people try to reach the meditative state quickly by repeating various mantras. Mantras can help, but reaching stillness is mostly just a matter of exercising discipline. You have to simply *tell yourself* to stop the movements of your mind and emotions—and then you have to *do it.*

Doing it doesn't mean leaving your body for some other plane of existence, and it doesn't mean repressing your emotions. Instead, it means learning to find the stillness within you that already exists, stopping within this stillness, and opening yourself to the feeling of neutrality. With practice, you will be able to focus on these moments of nondoing just as effectively as you can now focus on moments of extreme mental and physical exertion.

For example, you will learn to focus on the sensations of your feet when you stop walking just as intently as you may now be able to focus on them while you are walking. This moment of nonwalking, or stillness, will provide you with sensations that are just as real as those of walking.

When you do capture a moment of stillness, you should fully commit your energy to it, just as wholeheartedly as you now commit your energy to moments of great effort. When thoughts arise, allow them to pass, as you return to silence and neutrality. *Listen* to the silence.

Some people, though, find it rather difficult to reach a meditative state. They have a lot on their minds and tend to be preoccupied. Carlos, however, has devised a system for helping these people integrate meditation into their lives. He named this system *RAW.* RAW is an acronym for relaxed (body), alert (mind), and waiting (spirit). Carlos found that when people focused on achieving these three simple states, they became much more adept at meditating.

The big difference between RAW and other approaches to meditation is that RAW teaches us to get into and stay in our bodies. It is consistent with Nia's body-centered philosophy. We don't trip out or travel out of our bodies but instead seek to go deeper and deeper into our bodies. RAW doesn't even require us to set aside time for meditation, because when RAW is mastered, the meditative state becomes accessible in each moment.

Once you develop your skills at achieving the condition of RAW—simply by relaxing, staying alert, and waiting—RAW will become an organic element of your personality. It will become as natural to you as breathing.

When you practice RAW, you will begin to feel many changes. You will feel energized, alert, confident, calm, patient, and grounded. Living Meditation can become an oasis in every hour of your life—and RAW will help get you there.

Living Meditation will enable you to:

- Sense stillness without taking time out, or withdrawing from life.
- Gain wisdom from stillness and neutrality.
- Actively engage in nondoing, just as you now engage in doing.
- Feel a palpable sensation of oneness, as your body, mind, emotions, and spirit unite.
- Gain physical strength from stillness—more power, flexibility and agility.
- Be better able to vanquish stress.
- Experience relaxation in the muscles and connective tissues surrounding your joints, particularly those of the jaw.
- Have a stronger sensation of universal Joy and enjoy all activities even more.

life as art

The dance of life would be incomplete, however, without the third element of the Dancing Through Life triad: Life as Art. Most of us have been trained to believe that art consists of objects such as paintings, drawings, sculptures—and little else. We're taught to appreciate these objects and to hold them in higher aesthetic esteem than the ordinary things that surround us. But what would happen if we instead viewed *everything* with the wonder and admiration we generally reserve for art?

If this were to happen—and it *does* happen among Nia students—we would perceive Life as Art.

Perceiving Life as Art is similar to bringing meditation to every moment, and dance to every movement. It is a way of vastly enriching the human experience and fully achieving the state of Dancing Through Life.

The most fundamental benefit of seeing Life as Art is that it can make ordinary life as *inspiring* as viewing a great painting. This inspiration is not just figurative. It is literal. When we are inspired by art and beauty, we inhale the ethereal energy, or chi, that surrounds all great art and all physical beauty. In fact, the Latin root word for *inspire* means "to inhale." When you learn how to perceive the whole world as art, you will feel inspiration from this art flow into you. You'll feel it as a physical sensation. You will actually inhale the beauty, with its chi, that is all around you. The world becomes your masterpiece!

Like the other elements of Dancing Through Life, this inhalation of chi is not figurative or symbolic but can be felt as a real, physical sensation. If you give enough attention to perceiving Life as Art, you will almost certainly begin to feel abiding blasts of energetic inspiration, as chi infiltrates your body, mind, emotions, and spirit.

Let's try an exercise. Right now, as you're reading this book, allow your eyes to unfocus, to broaden your peripheral vision. Look at the image of your hand holding the book, and notice your hand's color, texture, and shape. See the veins on your hand, as they move life through your body. Experience the background behind the book, with its vast variety of shapes and shades. Look at light and shadow, and white and black on the page. Notice all of this, at once . . . and wait . . . and wait . . . and wait—until, suddenly, your body inhales the chi that surrounds you. Remember that RAW cannot be achieved without waiting and that in the stillness of this waiting lies Living Meditation. When you arrive at this state of being, you will see that everything around you is art.

The benefits you will experience from perceiving Life as Art are remarkable:

- You will have a constant source of inspiration: the world around you.
- You will be able to change your body, mind, and emotions by changing your perceptions.
- Your senses of sight, hearing, taste, and smell will become more acute.
- You will lose the blind spots that keep you from seeing the world as it really is.
- Your ability to appreciate beauty will have a healing effect on your body and mind.
- You will appreciate your body's beauty without indulging in negative judgments.
- You will spend more time in awe of life.
- You will become more artistically creative.

Every single day, without exception, make at least *one* attempt to open yourself to neutrality, using Living Meditation, and then open to seeing life as it really is—a work of magnificence! When you do this, you will begin to Dance Through Life as if it were the only possible way of living.

Soon, with practice, every moment, every movement, and every pause of stillness will lead ineluctably to Dancing Through Life. And when you have mastered the practice of Dancing Through Life, you will be well on your way to the most precious gift that Nia has to offer: awareness.

awareness

Awareness—the ability to fully comprehend life—might seem to you to be a mystical ideal that can be achieved only through years of meditation. But there is really nothing mystical about it. At its core, awareness is simply *knowing what's going on around you at any given moment.*

Many people think that awareness is a primarily mental function, but its not. The mind, in fact, is notoriously unreliable at achieving complete awareness, because so much of the mind is cut off from the present moment. The mind tends to be preoccupied with the past and the future. Many people spend most of their time thinking about things that have already happened, or things that might happen. Only sporadically do they focus their full attention on what is happening in the moment. For some reason, the past and future seem important to us and the current moment often seems trivial—it's just another day at work or another evening at home.

Furthermore, the thoughts that rocket through the mind are often at odds with actual reality. Unfortunately, they're frequently colored by our preconceptions, our fears, and our regrets. These thoughts may seem utterly real, but they're often illusory. Moreover, even when our thoughts do reflect reality, they're still just *reflections*—not the real thing. They are *interpretations* of the moment, not the moment itself.

Therefore, there is only one extremely effective way to enter the realm of awareness, and that way is the same as most other Nia pathways: through the body.

Awareness begins as a somatic process. Unlike mental and emotional activities, physical activities can take place *only* during the present moment; the only sensations the body knows are those of the present. The brain and nervous system process the body's information and then relay this information to the mind, emotions, and spirit. To be fully aware, your body, mind, emotions, and spirit must all be on the same page, focusing on the same thing.

Many people, unfortunately, cannot get this process started, because they have buried their abilities of somatic awareness. This burial often starts early in life. As children, we are commonly urged to repress and ignore the physical sensations that teem within us. We're often told to sit still, to be quiet, to wait until later to eat or drink, and to put our energies into our minds instead of our bodies. As a consequence, we tend to end up living in our heads instead of our bodies. Divorced from physical reality, we cram our brains with facts and mistakenly believe that these facts constitute awareness of the world around us.

But this *isn't* awareness. It's alienation wearing a thinking cap.

To help people overcome this alienation from real life, we generally recommend that they begin by focusing on their skin. The skin is the largest organ in the body and is an exquisitely sensitive sensory organ. No matter where you are or what you're doing, there are always sensations available to you through your skin. The skin is especially valuable for showing us the Body's Way, through the language of pleasure and pain.

The skin and the body's other sensory organs—the eyes, ears, nose, and mouth—can awaken the mind to awareness. In fact, they *must* awaken the mind—and the emotions and spirit, too—for complete awareness to occur.

As awareness increases, people become more attuned to what their bodies need in order to achieve self-healing. To self-heal in accord with the Body's Way, extra stimulation through movement may be required. Stimulation is, in fact, a major component of self-healing. It not only feels good but also helps improve physical function. It also, in turn, further increases awareness, and spurs a cycle of regenerative healing.

self-healing

When people learn the concept of Dancing Through Life, they don't need to take time away from their normal lifestyles to generate stimulation. Because life gives us the opportunity to move almost all the time, we have the opportunity for stimulation whenever we want. For example, if you're sitting at work and your back hurts, all you have to do is find the stretches and postures that will make the pain go away. By doing this simple act, you create a biofeedback loop that connects you to your body's needs. You have, in fact, healed yourself.

Stimulation creates self-healing, which is the *ultimate expression* of self-awareness. When you Dance Through Life, self-healing occurs every day, all day long. You become your own healer, guided by awareness of your own body.

Self-healing usually does not consist of a single, dramatic act, but instead is generally composed of a long series of small acts of self-kindness, guided by pleasure. Over time, as these individual acts accumulate, people become eminently skillful at exercising their self-healing powers.

One major advantage of performing self-healing acts in small increments is that it allows healing to become a part of each day. In this regard, self-healing is similar to adding dance to every movement of life, adding meditation to every moment of life, and seeing art in every vision of life. That is why performing small acts of self-healing is an integral aspect of Dancing Through Life.

Learning to perform acts of self-healing does not, however, eliminate the need for occasional assistance from professional health-care practitioners. On the contrary, it makes these visits significantly more effective, because people who practice self-healing are invariably better able to partner with health-care professionals than are people who are essentially divorced from their own bodies. People who feel responsible for their own healing generally have more information to share with their doctors and are more adept at remaining compliant with treatment.

Furthermore, when you learn to sponsor your own healing, it changes the way you perceive your physical problems. You naturally tend to become more positive and proactive, and feel more in control. You replace the attitude of "My shoulder is hurting" with one of "I am healing my shoulder."

EXERCISE: A SELF-HEALING RITUAL

The Self-Healing Ritual is our all-time favorite exercise because it is the Body's Way. Once a day, move through these five stages and Dancing Through Life will become a totally new experience in a new body.

These five stages are the same stages you used in Chapter 3 to support your incremental successes on the path to self-healing. Now you will physically experience these stages. These five stages are the preverbal stages we

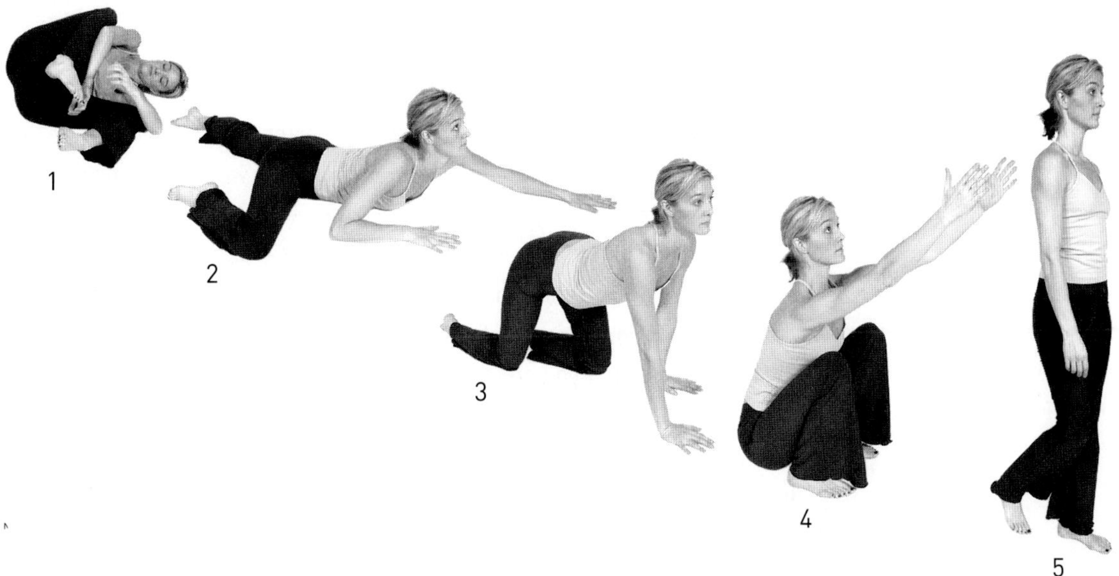

all went through to develop physically as a child. Not only did they prepare you physically to stand up, each stage strengthened your body's bones, joints, muscles, ligaments, tendons, organs, emotions, senses, and thinking and intuiting parts at the right time. Each of these stages is a foundation for the next. They organically realign your body by helping you reclaim physical mobility, flexibility, and agility in parts of your body that exercise alone cannot affect.

Every morning, or in the evening, move through these five stages, spending as much time in each stage as your body wishes. They are an excellent FloorPlay sequence to include in any workout. Make sure the surface you will be moving on is clean and clear of any obstruction. Wear clothing that allows you to move freely. Begin on the floor and move through the five stages, transitioning slowly from one to the another. Because these stages are organic and take you back in time, they may awaken in you emotions. Do not be surprised if feelings of vulnerability arise. Trust your body and listen to its signals that say, "I'm ready to move from this stage into the next." Because these five stages are preverbal, your instinct and intuitive sense guide you.

1. **Embryonic fish.** You are moving in the womb. In water. Nurtured. Fed. Supported. All your basic needs are met. Think of no edges, no separa-

tion, no sense of linear line, and no up or down. You are coiling and uncoiling in a movement that is fluid and soft.

2. **Creeping lizard.** This stage strengthens the entire body, mobilizes all of the joints—particularly the hip joint, cervical vertebrae, and Core—and coordinates the upper body with the lower body. Now you are moving on the earth, physically dragging your pelvis on the ground. Pull yourself with your hands and forearms. Your eyes look ahead, not down. Push with your feet as you pull with your arms. You look up and out to perceive life, creep with your inner thighs, forearms, and hands.
3. **Crawling bear.** Now you are on all fours. Your ability to move forward, back, to the left and right strengthens your bones, joints, and muscles. You can look and see more of the world around you, and your energy centers, the chakras, trigger your nervous system so you begin to interact with the world inside you and outside more energetically. Look out into the world. Hang your belly and spine. Soften your wrists, elbows, and shoulder blades as you move. Drag the knee, or lift it slightly, like a baby.
4. **Standing ape.** Standing is actually like squatting. It moves the spine into vertical alignment, and exposes your body's energy centers in the front and in the back, making your physical body more interactive with the energy fields. Your body is now supported on two feet, rather than two feet and two hands. Squat with your legs folded and your spine lengthened up, with your arms and hand free. Look up, reach out into life.
5. **Walking human.** Now your body is fully extended, upright, moving freely around a vertical axis. Your arms hang, your feet move you. This stage is all about integration. You are walking, looking out at a three-dimensional world, and you can exercise free will, desire, and conscious choice.

This is Nia.

We hope it has touched you—physically, mentally, emotionally, and spiritually.

What began as merely a way to lose weight or to tone your muscles has, we hope, become much more than that for you.

Nia, after all, is more than just a way of moving.

It is a way of living.

Welcome to your new life.

> *The* STUDENT FORUM *available on the Nia Web site, (nia-nia.com) offers you a place to talk and get advice. There you'll receive support and feedback from Nia teachers and trainers. You'll also find information on products, workshops, classes, special events, and prizes.*

appendix a The Nia Glossary

aikido. One of the three martial arts, in the nine movement forms of Nia; known as the dance of harmonious spherical motion.

Alexander Technique. One of the three healing arts, in the nine movement forms of Nia; known as the dance of movement from the top.

awareness. Part one of the fifth of Nia's Thirteen Principles, which teaches you to constantly pay attention to your physical sensations to promote self-healing. The conscious starting point of all action.

Base, the. The sixth of Nia's Thirteen Principles, which guides you to use your feet, knees, and legs as the foundation for all movements.

body awareness. The ability to be conscious of your body, moment to moment.

body centered. The ability to remain focused on your physical sensations, not your thoughts.

body euphoric phenomenon. Self-acceptance of one's own body.

body image. The image one has of one's own body, composed of reality and perception.

body–mind–spirit. The triad of being that Nia affects.

Body's Way, the. The specific design and structure of the body, which dictates its proper use.

Business of Fitness. The eleventh of Nia's Thirteen Principles, which directs you to nurture your body in an organized, structured way.

center. The physical center of the body, from which support comes. In Nia, moving through center keeps the body balanced and supported.

chakras. Ethereal energy centers located at seven points along the front and back of the body that, when balanced, help maintain health and homeostasis in the body.

chi. Ethereal energy that provides life force.

conscious personal training. Using specific information to guide yourself, as if you were the personal trainer of your consciousness.

Continuing the Body–Mind–Spirit Education. The twelfth of Nia's Thirteen Principles, which directs you to continue focusing on your craft and technique perpetually.

cooperation. The actual, physical sensation of feeling the linkage of body, mind, emotions, and spirit in holistic union, sometimes referred to as being in the zone, or in a state of flow.

Core, the. The eighth of Nia's Thirteen Principles, which directs you to integrate your pelvis, chest, head, and spine with all of your movements.

Crawling. The third stage of the five stages of self-healing, in which you venture into new movement territories, taking calculated risks to discover new skills that improve the way you move.

Creeping. The second stage of the five stages of self-healing, in which you begin to consciously guide your body to move in new ways that include healthier patterns, recognizing and acknowledging subtle improvements.

Dance What You Sense. The thirteenth of Nia's Principles, which guides you to dance and live through sensation.

Dancing Through Life. Part two of the fifth of Nia's Thirteen Principles, which empowers you to enjoy the dance of your every movement and to carry over to real life all the healthy movement choices of a Nia workout.

Duncan dance. One of the three dance arts, in the nine movement forms of Nia; known as the dance of free-spirited, honest movement.

dynamic ease. A distinct physical sensation of effortless power, consummate balance, the perfect mix of mobility and stability, and an unparalleled blend of yin and yang energies.

earth. The magnetically charged ground and the lowest plane of movement (as in moving to and connecting with the earth).

Embryonic. The first stage of the five stages of self-healing, in which you explore your present condition and become aware of what needs healing.

extrinsic muscles. Large, superficial muscles responsible for gross movement.

feedback. The information you receive from your body, from noting the sensations of pain and pleasure.

Feldenkrais Teachings of Moshe Feldenkrais. One of the three healing arts, in the nine movement forms of Nia, known as the conscious awareness of sensation.

five stages of self-healing. The five developmental stages of optimal movement: embryonic, creeping, crawling, standing, and walking.

FreeDance. The fourth of Nia's Thirteen Principles, which encourages the use of unfettered, unrehearsed movement to stimulate somatic creativity.

fusion fitness. The combining of classic movement forms.

heightened awareness. Awareness that includes the body, mind, and spirit, which is stimulated by moving with purpose and focusing on physical sensations.

imagery. Consciously creating visual images to trigger whole-body movement in a personal way.

intrinsic muscles. Small muscles, closer to the bones and joints, responsible for detailed movements and internal support.

Jazz dance. One of the three dance arts, in the nine movement forms of Nia; known as the dance of fun, showmanship, and expression.

Joy of Movement. The first of Nia's Thirteen Principles, which directs you to seek and experience joy in every movement.

Life as Art. Receiving inspiration—as a physical sensation—from everyday life.

Living Meditation. The process of including stillness in every moment, in order to bring balance and harmony to life.

meridians. Ethereal energy pathways that run throughout the body.

mindfulness. The ability to focus all your attention on one area while staying alert, calm, and relaxed, as you witness your own body, mind, emotions, and spirit.

mobility. The freedom to move, provided by flexibility in the joints.

Modern dance. One of the three dance arts in the nine movement forms of Nia, known as the dance of creating shapes in space.

Movement Forms. Part two of the second of Nia's Thirteen Principles; what you use to change the chemistry and energy of a movement.

muscle memory. Neural networks in the body that retain memories of physical movement.

Music and the 8BC System. The third of Nia's Thirteen Principles, which directs you to master the art of listening.

Natural Time. Part one of the second of Nia's Thirteen Principles, which encourages you to move your body in its own way, in its own time, with individualized and personalized movements that allow you to build proper neural connections.

Neuromuscular Integrative Action (Nia). A program using physical activity to integrate one's neurology with one's body or musculature.

neutral. The resting phase in movement, in which you gain power from relaxation. Also known as coming back to neutral.

Nia moves. The set of fifty-two moves of the Base, Core, and Upper Extremities, which, along with the Thirteen Principles, make up the Nia Technique.

Nia Technique. A cardiovascular program that uses whole-body, expressive, grounded movement to achieve fitness and wellness.

path of least resistance. The effortless way to move; it's always the right way.

pleasure principle. The act of creating pleasure in your body, which connects you to your body and to its own way of moving.

positive tension. A state of healthy physical stress that supports healing and builds strength.

Prepare Position. A Base starting position that powers martial art kicks.

psoas muscle. One of the most important muscles in the body, which originates in the lumbar vertebrae and is attached to the thighbone, and plays a major role in coordinating your upper and lower body movements.

RAW. The quality of being relaxed, alert, and waiting, which teaches you to get into and stay in your body, as a way to reach the meditative state.

Ready Position. The Upper Extremities starting position that powers martial art arm and hand motions.

self-healing. The conscious act of addressing personal needs, which results in greater pleasure and improved function.

Sensory IQ. The measurement of somatic intelligence, or awareness of the body.

somatic memory. See *muscle memory.*

stability. The ability to support, provided by strong and flexible joints, muscles, and connective tissues.

Standing. The fourth stage of the five stages of self-healing, in which you can enjoy the benefits of your heightened attention and actions.

tae kwon do. One of the three martial arts, in the nine movement forms of Nia; known as the dance of precision.

t'ai chi. One of the three martial arts, in the nine movement forms of Nia; known as the slow dance.

thirteen joints. The main joints in the body, including both ankles, knees, hips, wrists, elbows, and shoulders, plus the whole spine. The joints are designed to provide optimum mobility and stability throughout the whole body.

Thirteen Principles. The set of tenets that, along with the Nia moves, make up the Nia Technique.

three body weights. The pelvis, chest, and head, which are used as free weights to load and lighten action, and improve alignment.

three levels of intensity. Part two of the seventh of Nia's Thirteen Principles, which distinguishes the three rates of exertion: low, medium, and high.

three planes of movement. Part one of the seventh of Nia's Thirteen Principles, which distinguishes the low, middle, and high postural positions that support the flow of energy through the whole body.

Three Stages of Practice. The practice of learning the move, moving the move, and energizing the move.

Upper Extremities. The ninth of Nia's Thirteen Principles, which reminds you to use your arms, hands, and fingers as tools for self-expression.

vertical axis. Any center line that distributes energy vertically or horizontally, such as the spine.

voices of the body. The somatic feedback that teaches you how best to move.

Walking. The fifth stage of the five stages of self-healing, in which you have reached your ideal goal and are ready to set another self-healing goal, beginning from the embryonic stage.

well-being. A reflection of optimal health.

Witnessing. Observing yourself, without judgment, while focusing on what you sense and what you feel.

X-Ray Anatomy. The tenth of Nia's Thirteen Principles, which teaches you to sense and observe your skeletal structure and alignment.

yang. Outward-directed, or "male" energy, such as that used when exhaling. It is the opposite of yin energy.

yin. Inward-directed, or "female" energy, such as that used when inhaling. It is the opposite of yang energy.

yoga. One of the three healing arts in the nine movement forms of Nia; known as the dance of conscious alignment of bones and joints.

your Body's Way. The current design and function of your own body.

appendix b Sources

Applegate, Edith. *The Anatomy and Physiology Learning System,* 2nd ed. Philadelphia: Saunders, 2000.

Baptiste, Baron. *Journey into Power.* New York: Simon & Schuster, 2002.

Bartenieff, Irmgard, with Lewis, Dori. *Body Movement: Coping with the Environment.* Langhorne, PA: Gordon & Breach, 1980.

Bisacre, M.; Carlisle, R., Robertson, D.; and Ruck, J., eds. *The Illustrated Encyclopedia of the Human Body and How It Works.* New York: Exeter Books, 1979.

Bolles, Edmund Blair, ed. *Galileo's Commandment.* New York: Freeman, 1997.

Brennan, Richard. *The Alexander Technique Workbook.* Longmead, UK: Element Books, 1992.

Bridgman, George B. *The Human Machine: The Anatomical Structure and Mechanism of the Human Body.* New York: Dover, 1939.

Cailliet, Rene. *Low Back Pain Syndrome,* 2nd ed., Philadelphia: Davis, 1968.

Calais-Germain, Blandine. *Anatomy of Movement.* Seattle: Eastland Press, 1993.

Calais-Germain, Blandine, and Lamotte, Andree. *Anatomy of Movement Exercises.* Seattle: Eastland Press, 1996.

Cerver, Francisco Asensio, ed. *The Human Body.* Cologne: Könemann, Italy, 2000.

Coulter, H. David. *Anatomy of Hatha Yoga.* Honesdale, PA: Body & Breath, 2001.

Cumbaa, Stephen. *The Bones and Skeleton Book.* New York: Workman, 1991.

De Beauport, Elaine, with Diaz, Aura Sofia. *The Three Faces of Mind: Developing Your Mental, Emotional, and Behavioral Intelligences.* Wheaton, IL: Quest Books, 1996.

Delavier, Frédéric. *Strength Training Anatomy.* Paris: Éditions Vigot, 2001.

Desikachar, T.K.V. *The Heart of Yoga: Developing a Personal Practice.* Rochester, VT: Inner Traditions, 1995.

Edelman, Gerald M., and Tononi, Giulio. *A Universe of Consciousness: How Matter Becomes Imagination.* New York: Basic Books, 2000.

Feldenkrais, Moshe. *Awareness Through Movement.* New York: Harper & Row, 1977.

Grindel, C. G.; Crowley, L. V.; and Johnston, C. A., eds. *Anatomy and Physiology.* Springhouse, PA: Springhouse, 1997.

Hafen, Brent Q.; Frandsen; Kathryn J.; Karren, Keith J.; and Hooker, Keith R. *The Health Effects of Attitudes, Emotions, Relationships.* Ashland, OH: BookMasters, 1992.

Halpren, Steven, with Savary, Louis. *Sound Health: The Music and Sounds That Make Us Whole.* San Francisco: Harper & Row, 1985.

Hanna, Thomas. *Somatics: Reawakening the Mind's Control of Movement, Flexibility, and Health.* Cambridge: Perseus Books, 1988.

Howley, E. T., and Franks, B. D. *Health/Fitness Instructor's Handout.* Champaign, IL: Human Kinetics, 1986.

Hunt, Valerie V. *Infinite Mind: Science of the Human Vibrations of Consciousness.* Malibu, CA: Malibu Publishing, 1996.

Johnston, Victor S. *Why We Feel: The Science of Human Emotions.* Cambridge: Perseus Books, 1999.

Keleman, Stanley. *Embodying Experience.* Berkeley, CA: Center Press, 1987.

——. *Emotional Anatomy,* Berkeley, CA: Center Press, 1985.

Krucoff, Carol, and Krucoff, Mitchell. *Healing Moves.* New York: Three Rivers, 2000.

Licht, Sidney, ed. *Therapeutic Exercise,* 2nd rev. ed., Baltimore, MD: Waverly, 1965.

Lowen, Alexander. *Pleasure: A Creative Approach to Life.* New York: Penguin, 1970.

Marieb, Elaine N. *Anatomy and Physiology Coloring Workbook,* 5th ed. Menlo Park, CA: Benjamin/Cumming, 1997.

McCall, Lisa Ann. *The McCall Body Balance Method: Simple Concepts for Ageless Movement.* Dallas: Brown, 2001.

Moore, K., and Dalley, A. *Clinically Oriented Anatomy,* 4th ed., Baltimore, MD: Lippincott Williams & Wilkins, 1999.

Olsen, Andrea. *BodyStories: A Guide to Experiential Anatomy,* Barrytown, NY: Station Hill, 1991.

Preventative and Rehabilitative Exercise Committee of the American College of Sports Medicine. *Guidelines for Exercise Testing and Prescription,* 3rd ed. Philadelphia: Lea & Febiger, 1986.

Rolf, Ida P. *Rolfing—The Integration of Human Structures.* New York: Harper & Row, 1977.

Rosas, Debbie, and Rosas, Carlos, with Martin, Katherine. *Non-Impact Aerobics: The Nia Technique.* New York: Random House, 1987.

Rossi, Ernest Lawrence. *The Psychobiology of Mind-Body Healing: New Concepts of Therapeutic Hypnosis.* New York: Norton, 1986.

Rywerant, Yochanan. *The Feldenkrais Method: Teaching by Handling.* New Canaan, CT: Keats, 1983.

Samuels, Mike, and Samuels, Nancy. *Seeing with the Mind's Eye.* New York: Random House, 1975.

Scaravelli, Vanda. *Awakening the Spine.* San Francisco: HarperCollins, 1991.

Schultz, R. Louis, and Feitis, Rosemary. *The Endless Web: Fascial Anatomy and Physical Reality.* Berkeley, CA: North Atlantic, 1996.

Shioda, Gozo. *Dynamic Aikido.* New York: Harper & Row, 1968.

Siler, Brooke. *The Pilates Body.* New York: Broadway, 2000.

Sugawara, Tetsutaka; Xing, Lujian; and Jones, Mark B. *Aikido and Chinese Martial Arts,* vol. 2. Tokyo: Sugawara Martial Arts Institute, 1998.

Thibodeau, Gary A. *Structure and Function of the Body,* 9th ed., St. Louis: Mosby-Year Book, 1992.

Thompson, Clem W. *Manual of Structural Kinesiology,* 10th ed. St. Louis: Times Mirror/Mosby College, 1985.

Walker, Richard. *Encyclopedia of the Human Body.* New York: DK, 2002.

Wildish, Paul. *The Book of Ch'i: Harnessing the Healing Force of Energy,* Boston: Tuttle, 2000.

Winsor, Mari, with Laska, Mark. *The Pilates Powerhouse.* Cambridge, MA: Perseus Books, 1999.

acknowledgments

We are forever thankful to the many thinkers and movers who knowingly and unknowingly have inspired us and taught us to keep asking questions, persevere, and dream big. First, to our agent, Matthew Guma, for following his inner voice and for calling and asking us if we wanted to write a book! To Cameron Stauth, for personally delving into Nia and helping to give this work an elegant, user-friendly voice that was first brought to life by our friend and author, Katherine Martin. To Dr. James Garrick from the Center for Sports Medicine, St. Francis Hospital, San Francisco, who was the first to give a stamp of approval to the healing benefits of Nia. To Deborah Szekely, who first gave us an opportunity to share Nia with the public when she invited us to teach at her spa, Rancho La Puerta. To Debbie's parents, Jeanne and Arthur Bender, for instilling in her the belief and understanding that wisdom comes from within and for teaching her how to love and give unconditionally; to her children, Jennifer and Jessica, for allowing her to be the unconventional mother she was and still is; to her stepchildren, Colin and Monica, for their embracing love and respect; and to Debbie's sister, Jennifer Fox, and her husband, Paul Gould, for their endless support. To Carlos's family, Martha Eugenia, Luz Maria, Beto, and Antonio, for the love they continue to share; and to his partner, Jasmine, for the freedom to be and experience life so magically. To the visionaries of movement and thought, particularly Isadora Duncan, Martha Graham, Jose Limon, Ruth St. Denis, Doris Humphrey and Charles Weidman, Al Huang, Thomas Crum, B.K.S. Iyengar, Dan Millman, Ken Wilber, Gary Zukav, and Stanley Keleman, for reminding us of the power in breaking old paradigms. To Ann Campbell, our editor at Broadway Books, and her assistant, Ursula Cary, as well as her entire design team, for helping to make Nia beautiful to experience. To our very first group of Nia students from Marin County, who believed in and fully supported our vision of the future. To the Nia teachers and trainers, who believe in us and continue to share our voice and vision, and to the Nia students, who provide us with the opportunity to learn and explore. To the amazing Nia staff, who meticulously tend to the day-to-day business of keeping Nia alive and healthy. To Lenore Ooyevaar, for creating the book's beautiful illustrations. To Kim Dawson, who keeps us on track and focused, and who steps in whenever needed, always delivering the very best, no matter what it takes. To Carol Gonzalez, for her impeccable proofreading. To all our models, and to Jeff Hinds, our photographer, who so brilliantly captured Nia in motion, and our mechanical support team, Jodi Turner and Earth Oliver, who made our life easy. To Sandra LeBel, for holding space and keeping Kali happy and healthy. To all of you, we offer from the heart our deep appreciation, gratitude, and love, love, love. To Jeff Stewart, Debbie's husband, our business partner and the CEO of Nia, we offer respect, and personal and professional gratitude, love, and friendship for his creative energy, support, and belief in the work and in us. To Patricia Leigh Brown, for her courage in sharing her Dancing Through Life experience so eloquently. Finally, to Kali Rose, our assistant, whose personal vision was to be part of writing this book, who gave selflessly, sharing her insights, time, attention, and love, working far and above the call of duty.

about *the authors*

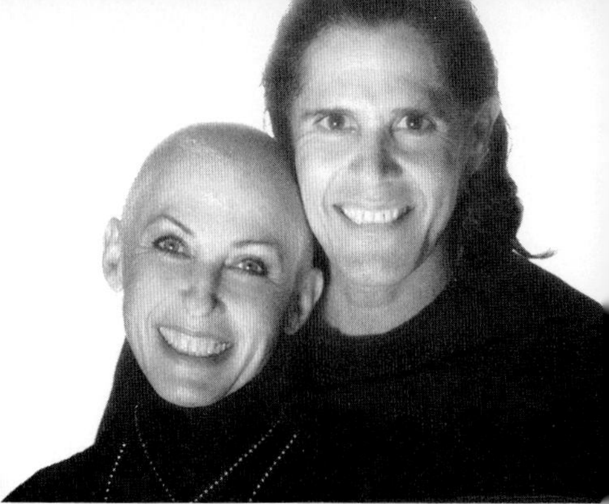

DEBBIE ROSAS and **CARLOS ROSAS** met in 1981, when Carlos—a tennis teaching professional—began taking classes at the aerobics studio owned and operated by Debbie. In 1983, they developed Neuromuscular Integrative Action (Nia), the first fusion fitness technique ever created. Since that time, Nia has become one of the most prominent fitness programs in the world, and Debbie and Carlos are widely regarded as the innovaters of fusion fitness—the combining of two or more classic exercise approaches.

Growing up near St. Louis, Missouri, Debbie experienced dyslexia, which led her to discover the power of kinesthetic learning. Her appreciation for the kinesthetic approach was enhanced in college, when she mastered human anatomy while studying to be a medical illustrator. Later she worked as an illustrator for the Missouri Institute of Psychiatry.

Debbie's early interest in physiology, anatomy, and health care propelled her to a career in the fitness industry; and in the early 1980s she became the founder and director of one of California's largest aerobics companies, The Bod Squad. Her company had more than fifty teachers, who together taught more than a hundred classes per week.

Carlos Rosas grew up in Mexico City, where his father was a sales representative for an international pharmaceuticals firm. A natural athlete, he played baseball and soccer; he also studied music. In the 1970s, he moved to San Francisco, where he was a college Spanish instructor and a tennis teaching professional.

Married during the 1980s, Carlos and Debbie went on to author *Non-Impact Aerobics* in 1987. Their non-impact approach was considered revolutionary in the 1980s, but is now an integral part of mainstream aerobic exercise. Today, though they are no longer married, they continue to build the Nia network worldwide.

Their work has been chronicled in more than 600 newspaper and magazine articles, they have appeared on numerous radio and television programs, and they speak regularly at the health and fitness industry's major conventions and symposia. They are also the authors of the chapter "Holistic Fitness," in the training manual of the American Fitness Aerobic Association, and have produced innovative videotapes for the general public. Together with their staff of trainers, they educate and license fitness and health professionals to teach Nia in traditional and nontraditional settings. They live in Portland, Oregon.